Pi

The Parent to Parent Handbook

"Our culture has hidden disability so well, a child with a disability seems to come as a complete shock to each new family. And yet, childhood disability is not as rare as we are brought up to believe. Many parents know the challenges and joys of raising a child with a disability, but we often can't find each other. Or we assume that everybody else knows what they're doing, and we are the only ones who are confused and hurt and lonely. *The Parent to Parent Handbook* will help us connect to each other in new ways. Watch out! Sharing our experience makes us strong. Together we will bring our children and our families out of the shadows."

—Sue Swenson, Commissioner, Administration on Developmental Disabilities, U.S. Department of Health & Human Services

"*The Parent to Parent Handbook* is a superb guide to developing not only Parent to Parent programs but also other grassroots initiatives. . . . Every pediatrician and other health professional who works in the community will find this book to be a valuable asset to pull off the shelf, to help answer some difficult questions."

—Thomas Tonniges, M.D., Director, Department of Community Pediatrics, American Academy of Pediatrics

"This book is both reflective and visionary—it is testimony to the strengths of families as pathfinders and the spirit and generosity within the Parent to Parent movement. We are tremendously grateful to the authors for this gift to the field of family support."

—Nancy DiVenere, Executive Director, Parent to Parent of Vermont

"Santelli, Poyadue, and Young have produced an invaluable resource. . . . I only wish I could have had this handbook in my desk drawer during my early years as founder and director of the Federation for Children with Special Needs!"

—Martha Ziegler, Former Director, Technical Assistance to Parent Projects

"In *The Parent to Parent Handbook*, our author friends map out a clear and direct path to . . . parent to parent power and hope for the future."

— Ursula Markey, Grassroots Consortium on Disabilities

"An easy-to-read resource, offering concrete examples to guide the process of program development, operation, promotion and evaluation. The Arc enthusiastically recommends this handbook to parents and organizations seeking to create supports for families raising a child with a disability."

—*Steven M. Eidelman, Executive Director, The Arc of the United States*

"As families who have the privilege and responsibility of raising our sons and daughters with disabilities or special needs, we understand the importance of finding other families who share our circumstances. We know that this basic connection with another parent helps to break down our sense of isolation and confusion, especially as we first embark on this remarkable journey. . . . Thank you to the authors for taking their experiences and giving us a book that will help all families whose children have special needs."

—*Polly Arango, Executive Director, Family Voices*

"Beautifully organized and presented . . . this handbook offers family leaders wise and practical guidance for creating parent to parent programs in a community, at the state level, and finally extending these efforts nationally. Thank you, thank you for writing this book."

—*Beverley H. Johnson, President, Institute for Family-Centered Care*

"A long awaited national and international resource for parents and professionals. . . . The authors are to be congratulated."

—*Pam Winton, Ph.D., Frank Porter Graham Child Development Center, University of North Carolina at Chapel Hill*

"This book offers eloquent evidence of the power of parent to parent support. Health care providers can join with families in looking to this book for innovation and insight."

—*William Schwab, M.D., Professor, Department of Family Medicine, University of Wisconsin*

"What a treasure! A wealth of valuable 'pearls of wisdom,' based on years of experiences by many families and programs, all in one place."

—*Merle G. McPherson, M.D., Director, Division of Services for Children with Special Health Needs, Maternal and Child Health Bureau*

The Parent to Parent Handbook

The Parent to Parent Handbook

Connecting Families of Children with Special Needs

by

Betsy Santelli

Florene Stewart Poyadue

and

Jane Leora Young

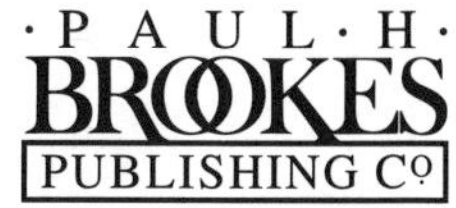

Baltimore • London • Toronto • Sydney

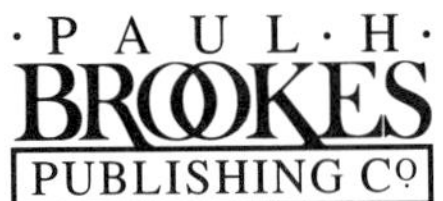

Paul H. Brookes Publishing Co.
Post Office Box 10624
Baltimore, Maryland 21285-0624

www.brookespublishing.com

Typeset by Integrated Publishing Solutions, Grand Rapids, Michigan.
Manufactured in the United States of America by
The Maple Press Company, York, Pennsylvania.

The individuals featured in the vignettes in this book have kindly granted permission for their actual names and stories to be used.

Purchasers of this book may download free of charge from the Brookes Publishing web site the usable forms. These forms are available at the following address: www.brookespublishing.com/ptop/. The duplication and distribution of these forms for commercial use is prohibited.

Library of Congress Cataloging-in-Publication Data

Santelli, Betsy.
The parent to parent handbook: connecting families of children with special needs / by Betsy Santelli, Florene Stewart Poyadue, and Jane Leora Young.
p. cm.
Includes bibliographical references and index.
ISBN 1-55766-497-8
1. Parents of handicapped children—Social networks—Handbooks, manuals, etc. 2. Parents of handicapped children—Services for—Handbooks, manuals, etc. 3. Self-help group—Handbooks, manuals, etc. I. Poyadue, Florene Stewart. II. Young, Jane Leora. III. Title.

HQ759.913.S35 2001
649′.15—dc21 00-069671

British Library Cataloguing in Publication data are available from the British Library.

Contents

About the Authors

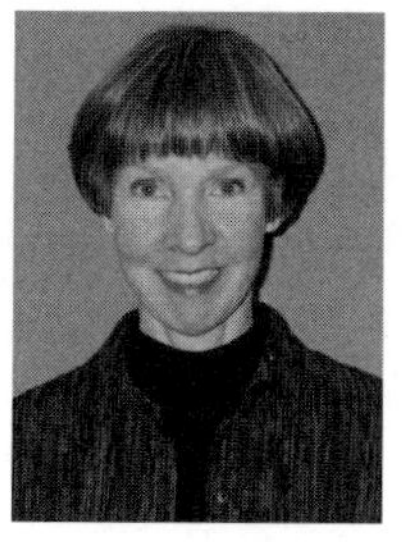

Betsy Santelli, M.Ed., received her master's degree in special education from the University of North Carolina at Chapel Hill and certification in parent and family education from the University of Minnesota–Twin Cities campus. Her professional experiences include teaching in special education, facilitating parent support and education classes, and training early childhood special education teachers. Since 1988, she has directed the Parent to Parent projects at the Beach Center on Families and Disability at The University of Kansas. Her research with and for parents who are participating in Parent to Parent programs has added to the descriptive and evaluative information that is now available on Parent to Parent. In addition to her research on Parent to Parent, Betsy also serves as a national consultant for those who are interested in starting or expanding a local or statewide Parent to Parent program in their area and as a facilitator for representing and meeting the national needs of local and statewide Parent to Parent programs and others with a commitment to comprehensive family-centered family support services. Although neither of Betsy's two daughters has a disability, Betsy had a very close relationship with her cousin, Jamie, who had epilepsy and cerebral palsy. Jamie's friendship and his special needs helped to determine Betsy's professional career path.

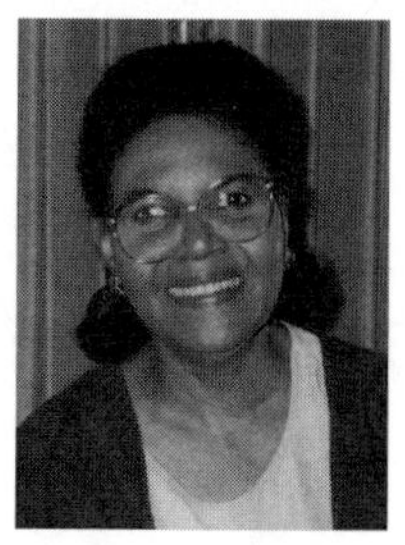

Florene Stewart Poyadue, M.A., is an award-winning master teacher, counselor, registered nurse, and mother of four children—one of whom, Dean, has special needs. She founded Parents Helping Parents, Inc., a nonprofit family resource center now recognized by the Maternal and Child Health Bureau as a national model. Parent leaders and professionals from foreign countries have consulted with her about developing Parent to Parent programs in their homelands. With Kaiser Permanente as partner, she developed a method for cultivating family-centeredness in managed health care. An internationally acclaimed keynote speaker and consultant with more than 25 years of experience, she also has traveled throughout the United States of America and Canada helping others solve problems and create service systems. Her alma mater, Santa Clara University, awarded her an honorary doctorate in public service before she delivered its 1993 commencement address; and the state of California named her a Woman of the Year in 1991.

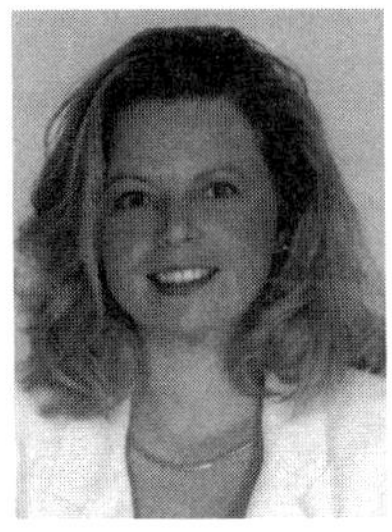

Jane Leora Young is a freelance writer and has more than 100 published articles in various publications. She received her associate degree in liberal studies and a certificate in writing social commentary from Pennsylvania State University. She earned her bachelor's degree in communications from Columbus University. Jane has worked with Parent to Parent of Pennsylvania for 5 years and has more than 10 years of personal experience working with individuals with autism and attention-deficit/hyperactivity disorder. She published a children's book, *This Is the Story About a Boy Named Zack* (Minuteman Press, 1997), which is centered around illustrations that her son with autism created, and a poetry book, *Monday Morning* (Sterling House Publishers, 2000), which explores the sorrow, joy, and acceptance of having a child with special needs. She is working on a series of reworked fairy tales that feature individuals with disabilities and a book that discusses the world of disability when it affects a middle-class family. Jane is active in local, statewide, and national support groups, including the Advisory Board on Autism and Related Disorders (ABOARD), the Autism Society of America, and Supporting Autism and Families Everywhere (SAFE). She is a public speaker on autism, communication needs, and siblings. She plans to continue her research, writing, speaking, and teaching in the hope that she can improve the lives of individuals with disabilities. Jane resides in Huntington Mills, Pennsylvania, with her husband, Rodney, and their three sons, Eddie, Zachary, and J.R.

Foreword

We write in two capacities. First, we write as parents of a young man, J.T., who has cognitive and emotional disabilities. We have long recognized the comfort and power of support from other parents in our own family life. Other parents have inspired us, contributed creative ideas for community inclusion, and shared both the laughter and the tears associated with having a child with a disability. We have been amazed at the strength of the parent bond, especially as we have traveled to other countries and interacted with parents whose language is not even understandable to us and for whom our language is equally mysterious. Despite the language barrier, we have experienced camaraderie that can come only from shared experience. We know in our heads and in our hearts that parent to parent support creates a universal bond.

Second, we write in our professional roles as co-directors of the Beach Center on Families and Disability at The University of Kansas in Lawrence. Here, we are fortunate indeed to have a collaborative partnership with Parent to Parent, one that has grown since 1988. We have conducted research, and we are always engaged in program development with the Parent to Parent network, to ensure that the very best practices of participatory action research are put into place. Participatory action research emphasizes an equal partnership between parent leaders and researchers so that research will be a means to an end. The end is to strengthen the national Parent to Parent network and families who have children with disabilities.

Historically, our good fortune derives from, and we gratefully acknowledge, the leadership of two people who, in their roles at the U.S. Department of Education, were instrumental in linking Parent to Parent and the Beach Center. Our first project officer, Naomi Karp, asked us to conduct research and program development with the Parent to Parent network. Patricia McGill Smith, who at the time was the Associate Assistant Secretary of the Office of Special Education and Rehabilitative Services, had been an early participant in Parent to Parent programs in Nebraska and helped target federal funds for our partnership with Parent to Parent. Thus, a portion of the work reported in this book resulted from Naomi's and Patty's efforts as "advocates" within the U.S. Department of Education.

Another element of our good fortune is less easy to identify by named people. That is because we have been graced by the generosity of literally hundreds of leaders within the Parent to Parent movement. These extraordinary people have been our partners in designing and implementing research and using the results of the research for Parent to Parent. To be a partner, these individuals opened their hearts and minds, allowed us to enter into those precious spaces, and thereby assured us not only that our research with them would have an authentic ring but also that they regarded us worthy of their trust and efforts.

We commend our colleagues and the authors of this book—Betsy Santelli, Florene Stewart Poyadue, and Jane Leora Young—for the superb job that they have done compiling family stories, program strategies, "how-to" tips, and extensive resources into this invaluable handbook for parents throughout the world. This book represents the essence of collaboration in every step, from the initial vision for the book through its completion.

We especially celebrate the fact that the information in this book will serve as a catalyst for more Parent to Parent relationships and programs; the end result will be enhanced quality of life for families who have children with disabilities. Parent to parent support is at an all-time high in the United States of America, but we know that it has not even begun to reach a saturation point in terms of what is possible. As you read this book—whether you are a new parent who is just beginning the journey of disability or a veteran parent who has accumulated wisdom that can only come from experience—we urge you to enlarge the "figure-8s" of the Parent to Parent movement.

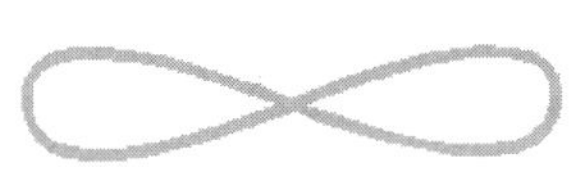

Figure-8s are unbroken loops of reciprocal support between two people in which the receiver becomes the giver. This is exemplified in the following excerpt from a parent in our research study:

When our son with Down syndrome was born 3 years ago, my husband and I were shocked and devastated. We called our Parent to Parent program, which supplied us with invaluable information, as well as sent a "support couple" to talk with us. It was important to us to meet with the couple—not just the mother—since my husband takes as much responsibility for caring for our children as I do. Also important was that we were matched with a couple whose child also had been through open heart surgery (our son had major heart defects). The couple that our Parent to Parent program sent to help us were such warm, optimistic, "normal" people—they gave us hope. About a year later, my husband and I were trained by our program to be support parents. The Parent to Parent office has many requests for visits from both father and mother. My husband was one of the very few men willing to go through formal training. I also have found that support for non–English speaking families is hard to come by. It has been satisfying to me to be able to serve the Spanish-speaking community.

May you build figure-8s in your own life and in the lives of other families who have a child with special needs. Building this reciprocity is the essence of creating the kind of society in which we are all fully nurtured.

Ann and Rud Turnbull
Beach Center on Families and Disability
The University of Kansas, Lawrence

Dear Parents and Professionals,

It gives us great joy that this book has been written! Congratulations to all of the parents and professionals who have worked so hard to gather the information, conduct the research, organize the stories, and capture the essence of Parent to Parent. Sharing experiences, strengths, and hope is the hallmark of the Parent to Parent philosophy. And the information shared in *The Parent to Parent Handbook: Connecting Families of Children with Special Needs* not only showcases the tremendous success and positive outcomes of years of collective action, it is a special resource for anyone who lives or works with children with disabilities or special needs.

Parent to Parent programs will continue to change lives throughout the world because they are based on a universal value that families can face difficult challenges and turn them into positive forces. The phenomenal growth of Parent to Parent since 1975 speaks to this truth in a powerful way. *The Parent to Parent Handbook* will help both parents and professionals move forward with confidence and assurance in understanding the family experience and in developing Parent to Parent programs of their own—an everlasting testimony to the strengths of those caring for children with disabilities.

As members of the program development team for one of the earliest Parent to Parent programs, the Pilot Parents Program, we know well that meeting parents of other children with disabilities can help families find their way out of isolation, frustration, and hopelessness. We firmly believe that parents help other parents understand that having a child with a disability is not the end but a challenge to begin. And parents do not have to begin alone—experienced supporting parents in hundreds of Parent to Parent programs nationally are available as reliable allies.

We wish you well on your journey—your efforts on behalf of families who have children with special needs will be supported by the experience and commitment of the parents and professionals you will meet in the pages of this book; your efforts will be treasured by those who follow in your footsteps. God bless all who have been or will be a part of Parent to Parent.

Frances E. Porter   Shirley Dean   Patricia McGill Smith

Preface

This is a book about a very particular kind of support for parents who have a child with special needs—parent to parent support. Parent to Parent programs offer a parent the chance to be connected one-to-one with another parent who knows firsthand about the feelings and realities that come with having a child with a disability. There are hundreds of Parent to Parent programs in the United States of America, as well as in countries around the world, that have been matching parents since 1975.

Although information about parent to parent support has been available through a few longstanding Parent to Parent programs, resources for those wishing to start or expand a program and research-based information about parent to parent support has only been available since 1990. However, because there is not a national Parent to Parent organization to collect information and compile resources, those with an interest in Parent to Parent don't know where and how to start. This book is our collective effort to provide not just a starting point but a thorough review of the history, characteristics, and research-based efficacy of Parent to Parent, along with step-by-step guidelines for starting and securing the future of a Parent to Parent program. We have included and are grateful for the many individual family and program stories that are the foundation of the book.

We have benefited immensely from not only our own partnership as co-authors but also from our differing perspectives—a family researcher at the Beach Center on Families and Disability at The University of Kansas; one of the co-founders of a veteran and highly successful Parent to Parent program (Parents Helping Parents in Santa Clara, California) and a national leader in the field of family support; and a parent of a child with autism who began her journey without support and now coordinates a local Parent to Parent program in Pennsylvania. Although we each have had our own unique experiences with Parent to Parent that we believe add to the richness of the chapters, we share a commitment to the importance of parents helping other parents. The strength of our own partnership has been increased a thousand-fold by the contributions of the many Parent to Parent program directors and families to whom you will be introduced throughout the book.

If you are a parent of a child with special needs reading this book, you will find comfort in knowing that your feelings are shared by other parents and that Parent to Parent offers an effective way to connect with other parents for emotional and informational support. If you are a service provider, you will learn the importance of helping parents to connect one-to-one with other parents who share their experiences and of advocating for including parent to parent support in your community's comprehensive family support services. If you are a student preparing to work for and with families who have children with special needs, or if you are a faculty member involved in preservice education, you will see how you can seek out parents as teachers and incorporate the principles of parent to parent support into your own education. If you are a policy maker involved in developing or enhancing family support policy, you will appreciate that an essential strategy for providing for the needs of children with disabilities is to ensure that their parents are supported.

The foundation of Parent to Parent is the one-to-one partnership between two parents who share similar family and disability issues. The success of Parent to Parent is derived from its contributing partners and reliable allies—the parents whose energy, heart, and soul form the basis of the unique support they provide to other parents through Parent to Parent programs; the service providers who embrace parents as full and equal partners and support the development and the work of Parent to Parent programs; students and professors who benefit from and involve parents as community faculty members to promote family-centered care; and policy makers who celebrate and advocate for financial and legislative support for the contributions parents make to the system of comprehensive support for families who have children with special needs. We hope this book will add to the strength of these partnerships and that these collaborative efforts will sustain and enhance Parent to Parent as a national resource.

Sometimes when I just glimpse my son I see,
The little ol' boy that was to be,
Damn chromosome!
Three years have flown for you and me,
And now with wiser eyes I see,
You are the boy that was to be.
WELCOME HOME!

—Florene Stewart Poyadue

Acknowledgments

Although only three co-authors are listed on this book, there are many people who have contributed in immeasurable ways. Without the visions of Parent to Parent program directors nationally and the hopes and dreams that parents have for their children with special needs, there would be no Parent to Parent programs and hence no need for a book about Parent to Parent. We gratefully acknowledge all of those with the vision, the hopes, and the dreams—you pointed the way. We especially want to recognize and express our appreciation to our editorial advisory board of Parent to Parent leaders who, through countless conference calls, helped us to frame the content of the book and then submitted written materials sharing their personal and professional experiences as directors of Parent to Parent programs with us.

We celebrate the wisdom and the experiences of the parents of children with special needs whose stories are the foundation of this book: Catherine and W.C. Hoecke, Jane and Rodney Young, Catherine and Richard DuBow, and Maria and David Hislop. We believe that their family stories will be an inspiration and a comfort to so many other families who travel with them. We also thank the families whose stories we were not able to include in the book for their unique contributions to the development and feel of each chapter. In a similar way, the program development stories of many Parent to Parent programs serve as the basis for the recommended practices described in each chapter.

We also pay special tribute to Ann and Rud Turnbull, co-directors of the Beach Center on Families and Disability at The University of Kansas; Naomi Karp, former project officer for the Beach Center from the Office of Special Education and Rehabilitative Services at the U.S. Department of Education; and Patricia McGill Smith, former director of the National Parent Network on Disabilities, for inaugurating the research partnership between Parent to Parent and the Beach Center. As a writing team, we benefited immensely from the editorial talents of many at Paul H. Brookes Publishing Co. We especially thank Theresa Donnelly, Heather Shrestha, and Deb Mills.

When a book is as collaborative an adventure as this one, we know that we have not acknowledged everyone. Please forgive our omissions. Just as Parent to Parent benefits from the individual and often unacknowledged contributions of many, so too this book benefits from the gifts of many. Your generosity is what Parent to Parent is all about.

BETSY

In addition to all of my wonderful previously acknowledged Parent to Parent friends, I would like to thank Ann and Rud Turnbull for giving me the opportunity to coordinate the Parent to Parent research at the Beach Center that has helped Parent to Parent become more widely available and more credible as a national resource for families and to continue to network with Parent to Parent leaders to answer the many *so what* questions generated by the research. And to my family—my husband, Jim, and my daughters, Maren and Tami—thank you for your patience and enthusiastic support even as the book adventure seemed to stretch on and on! Your collective belief in the project, in its importance, and in me are gifts of the highest order. To those in my family who have been touched by disability—Sherleigh and John Pierson; Sherleigh's son, Jamie, who had cerebral palsy and epilepsy; my mom, Maxine Brown, who was their reliable ally long before Parent to Parent programs were available; my nephew, Steve Ische, who had cystic fibrosis; and his parents, Sue and Mike Ische—you were and are my teachers and the source of my passion and commitment.

FLORENE

I would like to thank Georgette and Roy Strohm, Mary Ellen and Bruce Peterson, Eddie and Lavelle Souza, and all of the past staff and board members of Parents Helping Parents. They each individually and collectively worked with me to grow Parents Helping Parents into a dynamic model worthy of inclusion in this book as an example of a quality Parent to Parent program. They and all of the thousands of children and families who trusted me to serve them provided me with numerous opportunities for learning. My gratitude goes to many professionals as well, and especially my professors at San Jose State University and Santa Clara University, who have guided my formal and informal education through their support, friendship, encouragement, and respect for my thoughts, ideas, and opinions. They enhanced in me the spirit of "can do." A special thank you goes to Elayne Bagwe and Gita Dedek who had the vision to start a visiting parent program called Parents Helping Parents. A very special thank you goes to my family who, as always, has been my inspiration, my rock, and my shield during the writing of this book. My husband, Octave, my children—Turhan, Keith, Jill, and Dean—all provided time, encouragement, and suggestions when the words just did not seem to flow. Octave, better known as "Sweetie" to most of the world, proved to be a great "research assistant"—locating persons, places, and things when I just couldn't stand to search another minute. Thank you Jay Quinn, Antonia Symone, Aidan Gabriel, Alexandra, and Donovan—my grandchildren. Your smiling faces provided the much needed relief just when I needed it the most and reminded me of the importance of support for children and families.

JANE

I would like to give credit to my three sons—Eddie, Zachary, and J.R.—who changed the focus of my life and made me believe in a new kind of dream. Thanks goes to my husband, Rodney, whose unfailing support sustained me and made all of us remember fun. And last, thank you to old and new friends in the Parent to Parent of Pennsylvania network who gave me the confidence to continue forward.

PARENT TO PARENT EDITORIAL ADVISORY BOARD

Thanks to the following Parent to Parent program directors who served on the Parent to Parent Editorial Advisory Board:

Kathy Brill, Parent to Parent of Pennsylvania
Veronica Brown, Parent Information Network of Kentucky
Beverly Crider, formerly with the Family Support Network of Michigan
Nancy DiVenere, Parent to Parent of Vermont
Elizabeth Fletcher, formerly with Parent to Parent of Virginia
Shirley Geissinger, Family Support Network of North Carolina
Connie Ginsberg, The Family Connection of South Carolina
Diane Klemm, formerly with Statewide Parent to Parent of New Jersey
Tanya Baker McCue, Parents Reaching Out
Donna Olsen, Indiana Parent Information Network
Bev Parry, Parent to Parent of New Hampshire
Kathie Peterson, formerly with HOPE Parent Network
Mary Slaughter, formerly with RAISING Special Kids
Patricia McGill Smith, formerly with the National Parent Network on Disabilities
Cathy Spraetz, formerly with Parent to Parent of Georgia
Maryellen Sullivan, Parent to Parent of New Hampshire
Sallie Van Curen, Parents Reaching Out
Linda Williams, formerly with Parent to Parent Support of Washington

The Parent to Parent Handbook

I

Learning About Your Child's Disability

1

Unexpected Feelings

The Emotional Side of the Experience

"We do not succeed in changing things according to our desire, but gradually our desire changes."

—Marcel Proust

Welcome to Holland

I am often asked to describe the experience of raising a child with a disability—to try to help people who have not shared that unique experience to understand it, to imagine how it would feel. It's like this. . . .

When you're going to have a baby, it's like planning a fabulous vacation trip—to Italy. You buy a bunch of guide books and make wonderful plans. The Coliseum. The Michelangelo David. The gondolas in Venice. You may learn some handy phrases in Italian. It's all very exciting.

After months of eager anticipation, the day finally arrives. You pack your bags and off you go. Several hours later, the plane lands. The stewardess comes in and says, "Welcome to Holland."

"HOLLAND?!?" you say. "What do you mean, Holland?? I signed up for Italy! I'm supposed to be in Italy. All my life I've dreamed of going to Italy."

But there's been a change in the flight plan. They've landed in Holland and there you must stay.

The important thing is that they haven't taken you to a horrible disgusting, filthy place full of pestilence, famine and disease. It's just a different place.

So you must go out and buy new guide books. And you must learn a whole new language. And you will meet a whole new group of people you would have never met.

It's just a different place. It's slower-paced than Italy, less flashy than Italy. But after you've been there for a while and you catch your breath, you look around . . . and you begin to notice that Holland has windmills . . . Holland has tulips. Holland even has Rembrandts.

But everyone you know is busy coming and going from Italy . . . and they're all bragging about what a wonderful time they had there. And for the rest of your life, you will say, "Yes, that's where I was supposed to go. That's what I had planned."

And the pain of that will never, ever, ever, ever go away . . . because the loss of that dream is a very very significant loss.

But . . . if you spend your life mourning the fact that you didn't get to Italy, you may never be free to enjoy the very special, the very lovely things . . . about Holland.

—Emily Perl Kingsley, © 1987

EMOTIONAL ADJUSTMENT TO THE DISABILITY EXPERIENCE

Parents who have children with disabilities, an ongoing medical condition, or other special needs find out about their child's condition in different ways and at different times. Some families know immediately about their child's diagnosis, whether at birth or later in life, whereas others struggle for years to find a diagnosis. Despite the differences in each family's situation, many of the feelings that each family experiences are the same—shock, denial, anger, sadness, guilt, confusion, and loneliness—yet they also feel hope, peace, and love.

Whether you have just discovered that your child has a disability or you have known about your child's disability for years, the joys and sorrows that come with caring for a family member with a disability, an ongoing medical condition, or other special needs probably were not experiences that you imagined or expected for you and your family. You had your own visions about what parenting your child was going to be like and how you were going to feel. You had visions based on what you knew and saw around you; visions based on your own hopes and dreams for your child; visions that didn't include disabilities. And then, whether at the birth of your child or later in your child's life, you learned about his or her disability. You are on a different journey now. But you do have company, and the experiences of other parents of children with disabilities can be a source of strength and direction.

A Family from South Carolina

Catherine and her husband, W.C., had been married for 5 years before they had children. They had carefully considered their decision to have children, and they knew that the time was right. A midwife would be working with them to ensure that their infant was born in the most natural of ways. This first pregnancy was an exciting time for them—they dreamed vividly about first steps, preschool, trips to the zoo, and music lessons. But these dreams were interrupted by the unexpected.

How do you enjoy a situation that you thought you would never find yourself in? How do you cope with the fact that your child has a lifelong disability? You may feel overwhelmed, to say the least.

That's where we were the day Karl was born. Although the birth went well, a few minutes later the midwife laid Karl in my arms and said, "It is my firm belief that Karl has Down syndrome." She showed us some of the physical indications and said that she would need to get verification from a doctor, but she wanted to be honest with us from the start. Not only were we in shock from the pain and trauma of childbirth, but now we were dealing with an unexpected reality. The midwife, who had become our friend during the pregnancy, offered a prayer for us—thanking God that Karl had been given two wonderful parents and pointing out that Karl would be our teacher in many ways. We still get strength from that prayer—it was exactly what we needed at that moment. When the hospital neonatal specialist confirmed the diagnosis of Down syndrome, he made a special point of reminding us that Karl was first and foremost an infant and that for the next few years his needs would be like those of any infant. We found her prayer and his words to be reassuring. We were relieved to know that for a while Karl would be just like any other infant. We would have time to get used to the reality that Karl had Down syndrome.

Later that day the neonatal specialist told us about The Family Connection, a Parent to Parent program in our area. She said that, with our permis-

sion, The Family Connection could match us with another parent who had a child with Down syndrome and had been through this experience, too. We accepted the offer even though we were nervous about having a stranger enter our lives when we were both feeling vulnerable. Within hours, Jean, a supporting parent and the mother of Nate, was in our hospital room. She was low-key—just a typical mom doing typical things with her family. She showed us pictures of Nate—he looked content and happy—and we found ourselves thinking that maybe things weren't so different after all. Jean gave us hope that life and family go on, and in the following months she regularly encouraged and listened to us. She helped us begin to create new dreams for Karl and for our family.

LOSS OF THE DREAM

As parents prepare for parenthood, they have dreams about their child and about what life will be like for their son or daughter as he or she grows up—everything from who the child will look like and what his or her favorite hobby will be to speculation about the life choices their son or daughter will make down the road. When parents learn that their child has a disability, an ongoing medical condition, or other special needs, regardless of when and how they learn it, they experience grief similar to that experienced when a loved one dies. They grieve for the loss of the child they dreamed about, the child they envisioned as they anticipated adding children to their family. When parents grieve it is for the loss of a dream. An intense emotional period comes with this loss, and although painful, it does help parents cope.

If you are a parent whose lost dream came suddenly and unexpectedly, you may be surprised at the intensity of your feelings—the depth of your sadness may be something you have never experienced before. Perhaps you are a parent who has known in your heart that something was wrong with your child for months or years. Even though you had your suspicions, you may be surprised that you still find that the confirmation of your hunches is a shattering experience. In either instance you are being required to replace a dream with an uncertain vision of what life will bring for your child and your family.

SHOCK AND PANIC

For most parents the loss of the dream is unanticipated and comes as a shock, especially if your child's disability is discovered at the end of an exhausting labor and delivery experience, as it was for Catherine and

W.C. Parents have a range of emotional reactions as they respond to the shock of their child's disability. Some parents may cry or scream at the medical personnel who inform them of their child's status; others may feel numb and seem removed from their new reality. Sometimes parents need to make important medical decisions right after the disability is discovered, but the intensity of the shock leaves them feeling so overwhelmed and anxious that they find it difficult to remember the information being shared with them and to make plans. It is important for professionals and parents to understand that these feelings and behaviors are natural and common responses to receiving difficult and unexpected news. Although the medical concerns of the child must be met, equal time and attention should be given to meeting the emotional needs of family members. For some parents the opportunity to talk to another parent who has *been there* is one way of supporting their emotional needs.

A Family from Georgia

Twins had never figured into Cathryn's dreams, but with a clear ultrasound revealing two infants, she and her husband, Richard, began to prepare—two cribs, two quilts, two infant seats, and a lot of diapers. Her pregnancy continued uneventfully, and she went into labor 2 weeks early.

The delivery room was full of people—this was my first realization that twins were considered high risk. Gregory was delivered easily, but Daniel's birth was difficult, so we were all relieved when he was delivered and looked fine. Both infants were taken to the nursery to be examined, and I went to the recovery room. Soon a nurse brought Gregory to me, and I spent those first minutes getting to know my son. I was so absorbed that only Richard wondered where Daniel was. He went to look in the nursery window, and when the nurses noticed him they closed the blinds. Something was wrong with Daniel.

Daniel had been injured by the use of forceps, and the pressure from the internal bleeding was causing seizures and brain damage. A blur of doctors, specialists, nurses, and social workers came through the hospital room to talk to us about Daniel, but their words seemed foreign, and we were in such a daze that we couldn't remember what they were saying. I do remember noticing that all of the other rooms on the maternity floor had banners, balloons, and pictures of the infant on the door. Our door was bare. To this day I regret that our joy over one infant was colored by our uncertainty and fear about the other.

After nearly a week in the hospital, Gregory and I went home and Daniel was transferred to the neonatal intensive care unit (NICU) of a pediatric hospital. Ten days later Daniel came home—with an apnea monitor and nurses who were with us 24 hours a day. Although the nurses were helpful, this was a stressful time for us. There were so many people in our apartment that we had no privacy. We didn't feel free to argue, cry, or comfort each other, so we became angry and distant.

Gregory and Daniel were our parents' first grandchildren. We put up a brave front so they wouldn't worry about us, and we kept our feelings to ourselves in an effort to protect them. Most of our friends had no experience with disabilities, so they felt uncomfortable and stayed away. Some would say that we were brave, special, or chosen by God to raise Daniel. We didn't feel any of those things as we struggled to keep our heads above water. Isolation compounded our sense of loss. I fantasized about running away and abandoning my family. I even imagined Daniel dead.

When Daniel was 4 months old, his pediatric neurosurgeon told me about Parent to Parent of Georgia. I called right away and a supporting parent called me back the next day. We talked for nearly 2 hours. It was a relief to be able to express my feelings openly and honestly—even the ones I was ashamed of. I was afraid, exhausted, lonely, and angry. None of this came as a surprise to the woman on the telephone, and her understanding and support enabled me to begin to deal with my emotions and to start looking outside of myself. I began to learn about disabilities and to explore the services available in our community.

DENIAL

One of the first reactions for many parents after finding out that their child has a disability is *denial*—the sense that this cannot be happening and that there must be some mistake. Parents may refuse to talk about their child's situation, even to the point of resisting medical advice. Other parents react by keeping themselves busy with other life activities so that they will not have time to focus on the disability-related challenges that are painful. On the surface, these responses make it seem as if parents do not care about their child or about getting medical care, when in actuality parents are buying themselves the time they need to understand their new reality and acknowledge their own feelings.

The introduction to a disability came with such force and immediate medical concerns for Cathryn and Richard that they were forced to participate fully in their new world. The presence of nurses 24 hours a day and the brave front they felt they had to show to others meant that they had no time or space to focus on their own emotional needs. The daze they experienced was, in fact, a part of their denial. There was so much going on in their lives that was painful and overwhelming that Cathryn imagined herself running away in an effort to deny their new reality.

No parent experiences denial in the same way or for the same amount of time. You may find that your ears refuse to hear what the professionals are telling you about your child and your eyes are blind to the evidence being presented to you. You may even find yourself talking to others about your child and not mentioning the disability.

Denial serves an important purpose if you are a parent of a child with special needs. Although you may feel full of doubt, helpless, or argumentative, and you may refuse to talk about your child's situation or do things that others are encouraging you to do, denial buys you time and shelters you from having to deal with too much too soon. The denial that you experience is shielding you from the initial impact of your shattered dreams, giving you time to discover your own inner strengths and allowing you time to find people and resources who can help you. Feelings of denial are a healthy and helpful response to a life-changing experience, but if they last too long, they can interfere with the steps you will need to take to begin to feel more comfortable with your child's disability.

SADNESS AND DEPRESSION

No one can describe all of the anguish that parents feel when they learn of their child's disability or special needs except for another parent who has been there. And even when they do understand, you may find that after a brief respite, despair washes over you again, triggered by reminders of your new reality—seeing an infant without a disability, friends who don't call or stop by, and people who tell you how strong you are and how well you are coping. Cathryn remembered a wave of sadness that was triggered when she noticed that all of the other rooms on the maternity floor had balloons on the door and pictures of the infant while their room did not.

Depression may accompany your sadness and take over as you wrestle with thoughts such as, *Why should I even try because nothing can change what has happened?* You may feel so exhausted by these thoughts that you find it difficult to drag yourself through each day. Physical symptoms—a lump in your throat, a knot in your stomach, difficulty catching your breath—may make you wish you could crawl into bed and pull the covers over your head. Faced with the loss of the child you expected and with the presence of a new reality, it is not surprising that you find it hard to imagine that things will get better and you wonder how you will be able to manage on behalf of your child. These are frightening, sad, and depressing feelings of hopelessness and helplessness. Because these are terrifying feelings, it is hard to believe that depression is a normal and necessary part of the grieving and adjustment process. Acknowledging and working through the sadness that accompanies personal loss is an important part of the adjustment process. Many parents find that talking to another parent who has had these same feelings helps them to deal with their own feelings.

A Family from California

David and Maria met in Spain, Maria's native country, where David was studying Spanish, and within a year they were married. They moved back to the United States, built a home close to David's parents, and began their own family. This was not an easy road for them, however, as Maria had a series of miscarriages and lost their daughter Teresa at 25 weeks.

Two years after Teresa died, I could not think of living in our beautiful house without a child. We became pregnant again, and this time we did everything that we could do to ensure success. We had a doctor that we liked, and he knew about our past experiences, so we were optimistic for the best results. My dreams were filled with visions of our child bringing life to our home.

By my 29th week I started to have contractions, and 1 day later our daughter, Lucia, was born. Weighing $2\frac{1}{2}$ pounds and measuring 15 inches long, Lucia was rushed to the NICU, where she was placed on a respirator and connected to all kinds of tubes. The doctor told us that because she was premature we would have to wait and see whether she would survive. Little did we know that Lucia's birth was only the first of many challenges she would face in the NICU—cardiac arrest on the second day of her life, lung damage from the respirator, seizures, hydrocephalus that required a shunt, and a rare fungal infection in her brain that meant that Lucia, at 3 weeks of age, needed to have surgery on the front right lobe of her brain. There was not a day when we did not receive bad news. We had no control over what was happening to our family.

Finally, after weeks in the NICU, Lucia was able to come home. Despite all of the medical intervention that Lucia had while in the NICU, she came home with serious physical and intellectual disabilities. We were told that she was not doing well and that she would be a burden in our life. One doctor advised us to put Lucia in an institution. We were furious, but we also were terrified and wondered what tomorrow would bring.

As we were leaving the hospital, the discharge nurse told us about Cali-

fornia Children's Services, where we found a doctor who followed Lucia's progress until she was 2 years old. When we had an official diagnosis of cerebral palsy, I contacted our local United Cerebral Palsy agency. Through this agency I met helpful professionals and connected with other parents whose children also had cerebral palsy.

FEAR

Parents may have many fears—for their child, for other family members, for themselves, and for their family as a whole. For some parents an underlying fear may be whether they will be able to love their child with a disability—whether that bond will be there. And then, particularly if their child has some complex medical concerns or significant disabilities as Lucia did, there is the fear about whether they will be able to take care of their child.

People often fear the unknown. Until a diagnosis is clear, parents worry that their child's disability will be worse than they imagined. You may find yourself imagining all kinds of realities that may never happen, but until you have more information you fear a bleak future. You may worry about bad news that you will get in future medical appointments and whether your child will be able to attend school with his or her peers. You may have financial worries that you didn't have before—what if your child's medical expenses are more than your insurance company will pay for? What if you can't find in-home care for your child and have to quit your job, thus reducing your family income? What if your child doesn't have any friends? Will you be strong enough to handle the challenges that the future may bring? These fears are natural, and you will find that as you learn about your child's disability and gain confidence in your ability to cope, your fears will begin to diminish over time. Connecting with other parents who have had the same fears can be comforting and reassuring.

ANGER

For many parents anger is the most difficult emotion because it may be so intense that it touches anyone within reach—medical personnel, spouses, other children, friends, and co-workers. As you begin to adjust to your child's disability, you are dealing with a myriad of emotions—a sense of loss, feelings of injustice, personal guilt, and feelings of incompetence, helplessness, and hopelessness. Anger is usually secondary to these feelings and is the only one that is directed toward others. In your anger you may find yourself searching for chances to blame others. At any time anyone may say or do something that will trigger your anger, and you may lash out at them in surprising ways. Maria remembers the rage she experienced when the pediatric neurologist told her that Lucia would be better off in an institution. Although her anger was directed at the doctor, she was angry at the system for not providing information about other options that might exist for Lucia.

Unfortunately anger can be difficult for others to bear, and it is the emotion that is least likely to be accepted by those around you, including family and friends. Parents who get angry with others may be rejected by the very people who otherwise might be supportive of them. But conversely, when anger is not expressed, it may be internalized and consume energy that could be used to find new directions and supports. When parents are encouraged to recognize their anger as natural and common, then they can express and acknowledge their anger and begin to move on.

A Family from Pennsylvania

Jane and her husband, Rodney, are parents of three boys, Edward, Zachary, and J.R. Their middle son, Zachary, has autism. Jane remembers yearning for the parent support she now facilitates for others.

Zachary's birth was easier than my first pregnancy, and I remember enjoying the whole process and feeling relieved that we had a healthy infant. When we brought Zachary home, I promised myself that I would not compare my sons with each other. They were close in age, and I wanted them to feel special and unique. I felt certain that I could contribute to their individuality because I was going to be a full-time mom.

Over time I began to notice that Zachary would not let anyone hold him but me—but I convinced myself that he and I had a special bond. Zachary also was extremely quiet—but I told myself that he was content because I was always there for him. He hated strangers being nearby—but I thought he was shy. As the months passed I noticed (and rationalized) other behaviors—his need for routine was just his own individual style of independence; his interest in lining up objects reflected his orderly approach to life. The list went on, but I convinced myself that everything was fine. There was no need to acknowledge my concerns—not just yet.

But by the time Zachary was 2 years old, I knew something was not right. And although I had promised myself that I would never compare my two boys, I found myself doing just that. I began to feel nervous and guilty at the same time. I noticed that Zachary's early babbling was not developing into words. He preferred to play alone in a corner. He did not respond to his name, but he would come running to me if I put on his favorite tape. I began searching for answers in conversations with his doctor, my friends, and my older son's teacher. At this point no one seemed to think his behaviors warranted my concern, and I allowed myself to be pacified by their opinions.

But then at $2\frac{1}{2}$, Zachary began to run away, and despite our efforts to keep him close to home, one day we couldn't find him. We called our neighbors, the police, and the fire department for help. As I was explaining the situation to all of these community members, the flood of emotions I had been trying to suppress overwhelmed me—I could no longer deny that there was a problem. When my husband found Zachary, unharmed nearly 2 miles away, we were both filled with relief, but also emotionally wrenched. At that point we started another search—the hunt for a diagnosis.

For 2 years we navigated unfamiliar terrain—we met with numerous doctors, and Zachary endured endless tests. Finally we found our answer—autism. Although this was a diagnosis we knew little about, I was relieved that day because at least we knew something.

My initial relief gave way to other feelings. I found myself waking up in the middle of the night, jolted awake by feelings of panic and terror. How were we going to manage? What kind of life could we create for Zachary? Will he have friends? What kind of adult will he be? Will someone always be there for him? I was so frustrated that this had happened to Zachary and to us. I had done all of the right things during my pregnancy. Was there something I missed? I was angry at the pediatricians who had ignored and dismissed my concerns about Zachary. I was angry at the pediatric neurologist who gave my son a life sentence at age 3, telling us that Zachary would need to be placed in a residential setting. Why wasn't there more information to help us do the best we could for Zachary? Guilt joined my feelings of frustration. Was there anything I could have done differently?

Then came regret—the sadness deep in my soul that came from knowing that Zachary would not be like other children. I began to realize that Zachary would have challenges that other children don't face, at least not to the same degree—the uncertain stares, isolation, never having a best friend, or never being picked for the little league team. I grieved for our whole family because our lives would never again be the same.

ANXIETY

The loss of a dream for their family forces parents to make changes within themselves to match the changes in their new environment. Attitudes, priorities, beliefs, values, and day-to-day routines undergo significant changes—and these changes require a lot of energy. You may find that your own anxiety is a source of energy that helps you to make the changes that are required when you have a child with special needs. You may feel as though you are operating at a frenzied pace because there is so much to think about and do on behalf of your child. New realities need to be faced and addressed, and your anxious feelings will provide you with the energy that you need. Although your anxieties may make you feel tense, this inner energy serves an important purpose.

Some people may see your anxiety as inappropriate and may urge you to calm down or relax—to take things slower. But ignoring or not acting on your anxieties may actually keep you from making the changes that are being required of you. For Jane, her anxieties about Zachary's development and his behaviors helped her to begin to search for answers by talking with doctors, friends, and her older son's teachers, which led to the diagnosis. You may find that your anxiety is the catalyst for talking with other parents who have children with disabilities—parents who will understand your anxious feelings. In addition, your anxieties provide you with energy to address new questions and to advocate for your child.

GUILT

In many cases the causes of a disability are not clear, and questions such as, *Why did this happen to our child?* cannot be answered easily. Nevertheless, parents feel a need for answers. As they look for answers, parents may wonder what they might have done to cause the problem and blame themselves. Jane recalls looking back over her pregnancy and wondering if there was something she should have done differently so that Zachary's autism wouldn't be a part of their new reality. Should she have eaten differently or not taken those decongestants when she had that bad cold? Did she drink too much coffee? Should she have exercised more? Less?

With the current emphasis on the prevention of disabilities, it is no wonder that parents grapple with feelings that they may have inadvertently caused their child's disability. The media are full of speculative ideas about what might cause various disabilities—everything from over-the-counter medications to diet, stress, age, genetic influences, or amniocentesis—and yet the causes of most disabilities are not easily identified. This ambiguity gives parents the room to blame themselves. Sometimes parents react to their feelings of guilt by looking into their past and expecting to find a single horrible act that caused it all. Some parents figure that they must have done something to deserve this new reality and now they are paying for it. Their feelings of guilt may be manifested in spiritual or religious interpretations of blame and punishment—that somehow they committed a sin and are now paying for it. Some parents may find themselves revisiting the event countless times and feeling overwhelmed with *if only* thoughts. But for most disabilities, no matter how hard you search, you probably never will find such a cause.

If you are a parent and are blaming yourself for your child's disability, you should remember that the cause of most disabilities is beyond your control. Most disabilities happen independently of anything parents do or don't do during the pregnancy and childhood. This reality may not be enough to keep you from questioning yourself and wondering whether you should have done something different along the way. Even if your child's disability resulted from an accident that you feel responsible for, you may find some peace in remembering that no parent can shelter a child from every possible danger. It may be reassuring to know that other parents have asked themselves the same questions and felt the same pain. Your feelings are a normal part of the adjustment process. Sharing your feelings with other parents who understand because they also have wondered about these same questions will help you to acknowledge your concerns and to feel less alone.

MOVING TOWARD ACCEPTANCE AND APPRECIATION

Despite these common and well-documented responses to the losses that come with learning that their child has a disability, no two parents will experience these emotions in the same way. Some parents may know each feeling and experience it intensely, whereas others will know only some of these feelings. Each parent will follow his or her own sequence and may experience these feelings many times throughout his or her life, although less intensely. There is no right or wrong response, and your path through these experiences will be uniquely yours. Other parents who have shared your experiences can encourage you to remember that your feelings are normal and that you are not alone. As you begin to understand these feelings as common and necessary, you will develop coping strategies and a sense of appreciation. Connections with and support from other parents will help you on your journey. Families grow to appreciate the unique individual that their child with special needs is and all that he or she has added to their lives.

SUMMARY

The emotional adjustment to having a child with a disability varies from parent to parent and from day to day, and the feelings are often re-experienced in new and old ways as the child moves through life's transitions. Being familiar with these feelings and understanding that they are normal reactions may make them less overwhelming. Talking with others who have experienced these same feelings also is helpful.

Fortunately there are many opportunities for parents to be supported in their emotional adjustment. As was true for Catherine and W.C., Cathryn and Richard, Maria and David, and Jane and Rodney, many parents discover how important it is to connect with another parent who knows firsthand about the feelings they are experiencing. The understanding of another parent who has experienced the emotions that come with learning that your child has special needs is more valuable than any other support.

RESOURCES

Batshaw, M.L. (1997). *Children with disabilities* (4th ed.). Baltimore: Paul H. Brookes Publishing Co.

Batshaw, M.L. (2001). *When your child has a disability: The complete sourcebook of daily and medical care* (Rev. ed.). Baltimore: Paul H. Brookes Publishing Co.

Berube, M. (1996). *Life as we know it: A father, a family, and an exceptional child.* New York: Pantheon Books/Random House.

Duffy, S., McGlynn, K., Mariska, J., & Murphy, J. (1990). *Acceptance is only the first battle* (2nd ed.). Missoula: Montana University Affiliated Rural Institute on Disabilities.

Featherstone, H. (1980). *A difference in the family: Life with a disabled child.* New York: Viking-Penguin.

Fialka, J. (1997). *It matters: Lessons from my son.* Huntington Woods, MI: Author. (Available from the author, 10474 LaSalle, Huntington Woods, MI 48070, [248] 546-4870, ruaw@aol.com)

Gill, B. (1993). *Changed by a child: Companion notes for parents of a child with a disability.* New York: Doubleday.

Marsh, J.D.B. (Ed.). (1995). *From the heart: On being the mother of a child with special needs.* Bethesda, MD: Woodbine House.

May, J. (1992). *Circle of care and understanding: Support programs for fathers of children with special needs.* Bethesda, MD: Association for the Care of Children's Health.

McAnaney, K.D. (1992). *I wish: Dreams of realities of parenting a special needs child.* Sacramento: United Cerebral Palsy Association of California.

Meyer, D.J. (Ed.). (1995). *Uncommon fathers: Reflections on raising a child with a disability.* Bethesda, MD: Woodbine House.

Miller, N.B. (1994). *Nobody's perfect: Living and growing with children who have special needs.* Baltimore: Paul H. Brookes Publishing Co.

Poyadue, F.S. (1978). *Fleeting moment.* Santa Clara, CA: Parents Helping Parents, Inc.

Poyadue, F.S. (1998). *The modern art of caring for families.* Santa Clara, CA: Parents Helping Parents, Inc.

Simons, R. (1987). *After the tears: Parents talk about raising a child with a disability.* Orlando, FL: Harcourt Brace & Co.

Weinhouse, D., & Weinhouse, M. (1994). *Little children big needs: Parents discuss raising children with exceptional needs.* Niwot: University Press of Colorado.

ORGANIZATIONS

Books on Special Children, Post Office Box 305, Congers, NY 10920; telephone: (914) 638-1236; fax: (914) 638-0847; e-mail: bosc@j51.com. Books on Special Children has an annotated list of books and articles on special-needs topics.

Disability Bookshop (Twin Peaks Press), Post Office Box 129, Vancouver, WA 98666; telephone: (360) 694-2462; fax: (360) 696-3210; e-mail: 73743.2634@compuserve.com. The Disability Bookshop will try to find any special-needs book a customer is looking for. The Bookshop's catalog costs $5.

Special Needs Project, 3463 State Street, Suite 282, Santa Barbara, CA 93105; telephone: (800) 333-6867; fax: (805) 683-2341. The Special Needs Project has a catalog (*Good Books About Disabilities*) of books for adults and children on disability issues and also will attempt to locate specific books that they do not carry.

2

New Challenges and Information

The Logistical Side of the Experience

"The family is the association established by nature for the supply of man's everyday wants."

—Aristotle

Families meet the needs of each family member as well as the needs of the family as a whole. They accomplish many tasks on behalf of family members and play a critical role in caring for the family's physical and emotional well-being. Families provide love and affection and nurture each other's self-esteem. They meet the financial and daily care needs of the family as a whole. Families teach and support each other, providing a safe place to learn about social relationships and participation in society. Members of the family interact with each other in different ways—parents with each other, parents with children, siblings with each other, and the family as a whole with members of the extended family and the community.

For families who have a child with a disability, the extra caregiving responsibilities often have an impact on the other activities of the family. Regardless of how and when a diagnosis is made, each member of your family is making adjustments in how family activities are carried out and how interactions with other family members occur. These adjustments and new realities are the logistical side of the experience.

Catherine and W.C.—Living from Day to Day

When we came home from the hospital with Karl, we came home not only with Karl but also with a lot of instructions from the hospital staff on how to take care of Karl's medical needs. Karl had jaundice, and for the first several days at home he needed to sleep under a fluorescent light. To protect his eyes from the fluorescent light, we had to tape a mask over his face to cover his eyes throughout the night. Thank goodness for the volunteers from our church, who took 4-hour shifts to watch Karl to be sure his eyes were protected as he slept and to help us get the sleep we so desperately needed. But you know, even though we appreciated the relief shifts at night, we also yearned to have the privacy we needed as a couple to begin to get used to our new reality.

My mom came to help out, and her presence was very reassuring. Karl was our first child, and we really had no idea how much help we needed—as first-time parents and as providers for Karl's special needs. Because my mom was there, we had an extra set of hands as we learned to manage our new responsibilities. Together we learned to cross Karl's hands over his chest while we were feeding him to help firm his muscle tone, together we made the daily trips to the doctor to have his blood tested to check his bilirubin levels, and together we cried—fearing for what the future would bring for Karl and for us. We wondered if we were up to it all.

One of our biggest challenges was dealing with our different perspectives about caring for a child with special needs. Until we recognized that we each had our own way of thinking about Karl's disability and that our perspectives were okay, we found ourselves being impatient with each other over our different dreams and expectations for Karl.

Jean, our supporting parent, helped us so much through those early weeks and months. Without Jean it would have taken us a lot longer to learn about early intervention and that Karl could begin to benefit from home-based services right away. With Jean's encouragement we explored our options, and at 6 weeks of age Karl started receiving early intervention services in our home. Jean also shared a notebook that listed other services for children with disabilities and their families. We remember thinking how incredible Jean's timing was—she knew how overwhelming those first few weeks are, and she waited until we had our feet on the ground before sharing this wonderful resource with us. By the time she did, we were ready for it and we devoured it cover to cover and used it to keep all of our medical records together.

W.C. and I had to rethink our professional lives and how to balance those with Karl's needs. For the first several months, I was able to stay at home with Karl during the day. After the first 3 months, W.C. returned to graduate school and I went back to work. Yet our schedules permitted us to keep Karl at home and manage routine feedings. After several months of juggling work and school demands, finding baby sitters who were willing and comfortable taking care of Karl, coordinating trips to the doctor (he was being seen regularly by not only our family practitioner but also an ear, nose, and throat specialist; an eye doctor; a cardiologist; an orthopedist; a homeopathic specialist; and a physical therapist), and being there for Karl when he was sick or receiving in-home therapies and early intervention services, I decided that I needed to stay home to oversee all of these aspects of our lives, and especially to follow through on his therapies. It was a difficult decision because we were also facing a lot of unanticipated medical bills, but we knew it was the right decision for Karl.

Our church community continued to be an important resource for us. Although we appreciated the support that came in many ways (the nighttime shifts, casseroles brought to our house, the best wishes of well-meaning friends), we also recognized that the schedule of activities we had built to meet Karl's needs left us with little time for relating as a couple. Fortunately, an elder in our church sensed the growing isolation and stress we were feeling, and through a financial gift he made it possible for us to go out once a week.

When Karl was 2 years old, his brother, Franklin, was born, and 2 years later Anna joined our family. After each child we began piecing together a family schedule—one that would support the growth and development of all of our children, as well as our own adult needs.

For the most part Karl and Franklin are good friends, although Franklin sometimes finds it hard to understand why Karl gets so much attention from the therapists and he doesn't. And even though Franklin is beginning to realize Karl's limitations and adapts his play easily to accommodate them, I know that soon I will have to explain Karl's disability to Franklin and later to Anna. I worry not only about how Karl's disability will affect him as he gets older but also how it will affect his brother and sister. Will my children be good friends, and will they each have friends of their own?

We have been lucky that a local church has a wonderful fully inclusive preschool that Karl and Franklin attend 3 days a week. Next year, Karl and Franklin will participate in the K-4 class together, and I will do some home schooling so hopefully Karl will be ready for kindergarten. I sure am glad that Jean has had experience in working with her son's schools. I expect to be learning a lot from examples of wonderful working relationships between parents like Jean and their school districts.

EMOTIONAL AND SOCIAL NEEDS

Meeting Emotional Needs

Everyone needs to feel accepted and loved for who they are, and families are an important source of this affection. The intimacy of the living environment that parents share with their children means that parents have a unique opportunity to send their children messages of unconditional love. Because children carry these early messages about their value and self-worth with them throughout their lives, the role that parents play in providing affection and nurturing self-esteem is critically important. As a parent of a child with a disability, you may feel that the extra time you devote to meeting the special needs of your child is taking away the time for you to respond to the affection needs of your other children. It is a delicate balancing act faced by all parents who have children with special needs.

Brothers and sisters without disabilities may interpret the time and attention that parents give to the sibling with a disability to mean that they are not as important in the eyes of the parents. Or, they may wonder if their brother or sister's disability is somehow their fault. Although Franklin and Anna are still young, Catherine worries some about how having Karl as their sibling will affect their own self-esteem and about the quality of the relationship they will have with Karl as they all grow up. Most parental concerns about siblings are unfounded, as siblings tend to grow up to be just fine—more mature and caring than their peers. When siblings have a chance to connect with other siblings who have brothers or sisters with special needs, they often find it reassuring to find that they are not alone with their feelings. The Sibling Support Project—a national resource that offers interactive group activities called *Sibshops*—creates wonderful opportunities for siblings to connect with other siblings (see Chapter 3).

You also may find that because you spend so much time taking care of the disability-related needs of your child with special needs, you don't have much time left to foster your child's self-esteem. Your child may experience self-esteem issues as he or she grows up and begins to deal with the challenges that the disability presents and the realization that other children do not have these same challenges. For example, he or she may feel rejected by peers who find it hard to look beyond the disability or may begin to resent that sports activities at school don't include those who use wheelchairs. So, it is important that families (and professionals) recognize and affirm the strengths and positive contributions of every member of the family. By spending a few minutes a day in one-to-one activities with each child in the family, you can help them to feel loved and valued.

You may even find that your own feelings of self-worth are affected. As parents begin to care for their child with special needs and deal with the many logistical realities, many wonder if they will be able to do a good job at something they feel so unprepared for. Feelings of guilt and fear are a natural part of the adjustment process that you read about in Chapter 1, but they may make parents emotionally vulnerable. Sometimes connecting with another parent who knows those same feelings is helpful. When parents feel nurtured and supported, they are better able to nurture and support their children. Parent to Parent programs are founded on this principle and support children with disabilities by making sure that their parents are supported.

Meeting Social Needs

The social relationships that people enjoy with each other begin with relationships within the family. As parents interact with their infants, they teach them when to talk, when to listen, how to share, how and when to express feelings, how to be polite, and how to be playful. The interactions that siblings have with each other also shape the friendships that they will have with other children as their worlds expand. Within the family, children have opportunities to learn about and practice social skills that will be used in countless interactions in every aspect of life.

When a child has a disability, the nature of that disability may affect the quality of the social relationships the child will have with others. A child with autism may not be comfortable making eye contact with others, whereas a child who has a hearing impairment may use sign language instead of verbal communication. For some children with severe cognitive delays, communication may be accomplished through touch rather than speech. Parents of children with Down syndrome may worry that their children will be too trusting or misread overtures from others. Parents and siblings can model appropriate social responses for the child with special needs in a familiar and comfortable setting. Through the social interactions that happen within a family every day, each member of the family develops a unique social relationship with the others and learns how to make social connections outside of the family. Family members also are in a wonderful position to show others how to relate to the family member with a disability.

You also may be concerned that your child's disability will stand in the way of the friendships with other children, which are such an important part of life. Catherine and W.C. noticed that Karl was not invited to neighborhood birthday parties, and Catherine described their efforts to facilitate friendships for Karl as a "real struggle." Although Karl and Franklin participate in a neighborhood play group, natural opportunities for friendships to develop are scarce. Many parents find creative ways to support budding friendships and encourage new ones, and often these solutions are suggested by other parents. Some parents strive to make their child's wheelchair or walker look more like a piece of play equipment by substituting brightly colored handle grips or decorating it with colored lights at holiday times. These unique modifications spark an interest, and when other children come closer to look, a relationship often begins. Other parents participate in disability awareness activities in their child's classroom—introducing various disabilities through puppets and fostering a discussion about how the similarities that exist among all children are greater than the disability-related differences. This dialogue often paves the way to new friendships.

In addition to supporting your child's friendships, having fun together through leisure activities, although perhaps not critical to the survival of the family, offers family members time to nurture their own interests and interact socially with others. There are many kinds of recreational activities—indoor, outdoor, and participatory—to meet the different interests of each family member. How you participate in recreational activities will depend in part on the nature of your child's disability and the recreational choices in your community.

Fortunately, finding inclusive recreational activities is becoming easier as community leaders recognize the value of community events and programs for children with special needs and their peers without disabilities. Much of the progress made has been the result of proactive parents. Legislation requiring accessibility for people with disabilities means that many of the physical barriers have been removed. The wider availability of inclusive community events and programs and greater accessibility, however, does not necessarily mean that a child with special needs will be welcomed with open arms.

Jane, Rodney, and Zachary—Getting There Gradually

The fact that autism is a hidden disability has sometimes made our lives more difficult than if Zachary's disability were readily apparent. When we are in public places with a lot of noise and people, such as a grocery store or a school event, Zachary often screams uncontrollably because he is overly sensitive to noise. People stare at us, and I can tell they are wondering why we can't control our son. Once when we went to an amusement park and received a special disability pass, people accused us of lying about Zachary's disability because he looked just fine to them. Sometimes it is easier not to go out as a family because we are never sure how Zachary will act and how others will respond to him and to us.

Because Zachary's behavior is so unpredictable, we have a hard time finding baby sitters. Our friends tell us that they would like to help out, but they aren't comfortable taking on the responsibility of watching Zachary. My great-aunt and great-uncle help out some, and my mother-in-law always takes the kids on the Fourth of July so that we can celebrate our anniversary. We really don't have much close family around, so we stay at home a lot.

Fortunately, Zachary is eligible for Supplemental Security Income (SSI), and we have chosen to use some of those funds to make it possible for Zachary and his two brothers to enjoy some recreational activities at home. We have a swimming pool that the boys really love, and Zachary has his own computer with software designed to accommodate his special needs. Zachary has always loved to draw, so we bought him an easel.

We're lucky that for the most part Zachary and his brothers get along pretty well. When Eddie and Zachary were younger, Eddie used to ask me why Zachary would sit with his face to the wall instead of playing with him, but Eddie seems to understand Zachary's different style. When Zachary does interact with others, he often is the follower. As the younger brother, J.R. loves it that Zachary will follow him around—not too many older brothers will do that!

For a while an occupational therapist and a speech-language therapist came to our house to work with Zachary, but Zachary would run away or refuse to cooperate. When he did a little better in a small parochial classroom with 10 children, we hoped that he could make it in the public schools. But it didn't take us long to find out that public schools are too chaotic and noisy for him. His second-grade classroom was right next to the cafeteria, and Zachary simply couldn't handle the noise as the children came and went during the three lunch periods. And the school bell threw him completely out of control. I thought perhaps that I could home-school Zachary, but with J.R. still at home, it was too much. Reluctantly, we put him in an alternative school that is part of our school district but serves only children with disabilities. We don't feel good about segregating Zachary, but for the first time his learning needs are being met.

At a Parent to Parent seminar, I met Denise, another mom who has a child with autism. We bonded at the seminar, exchanged telephone numbers, and although we weren't formally matched because Parent to Parent was just getting started in our area, my friendship with Denise helped me accept the position of coordinator for our new Parent to Parent program. I knew what life had been like without Denise, and then how much better it was with her as my reliable ally, and I wanted to be sure that other parents had the same opportunity to be connected.

FINANCIAL NEEDS

Families work to ensure that money is available to take care of the basic life needs of food, shelter, and clothing for each family member. In addition to these basic expenses, you may need to pay for extra medical appointments and treatments, as well as medications, special equipment or foods, structural adaptations to your home, or a car or van with a wheelchair lift. You may find that the presence of a disability within the family affects both the capacity of your family to earn an income and how the funds available to your family are spent. Karl's need for different kinds of therapy and multiple medical appointments eventually meant that Catherine needed to quit her job so that she could stay home to coordinate Karl's demanding schedule of activities. Although Karl's therapy and medical treatments were an important priority for the family, there was no question that the reduced family income had to be stretched even further. Many parents discover that maintaining full-time employment is hard because it is so difficult to find qualified child care for children with special needs and so many appointments need to be kept with doctors and therapists.

Although some families find that the special needs of their child are covered by their private insurance provider, the number of children with special health care needs whose parents can keep them insured under the family's health insurance plan has been declining every year. Many families find that they cannot get private insurance for their child with a disability because of the child's preexisting condition, because clauses in the insurance policy exclude the very benefits that the child needs, or because the deductibles and co-payments are too high. Other families discover that their child's medical needs are so severe that even when they are covered by private insurance, the amount of coverage provided is not sufficient.

Your family may be eligible for financial support to supplement your insurance or to pay for medical care and services that your child with special needs may require. For example, *SSI* is an income assistance program administered by the federal government that provides direct cash payments to people with disabilities whose income and resources are below specified levels. *Medicaid* is a medical assistance program for low-income individuals, including children with disabilities, and most children who are eligible for SSI also are eligible for Medicaid (and some children qualify for Medicaid benefits even when their parents' income is higher than the specified levels). Many states have passed legislation to help families of children with disabilities address their financial concerns, but you may need to be persistent to get the answers you need. Here are some tips:

- Ask the professionals who are providing services to your child (e.g., doctors, nurses, social workers, therapists, teachers) about available sources of financial aid.
- Remember that each state has different state-level agencies that coordinate the provision of services to children with disabilities or special health care needs.
- Contact the disability organizations in your community.
- Get in touch with Family Voices, a national organization for families that works to ensure that families are fully informed about financial support and health care issues related to their child's disability or chronic illness (see Chapter 3).
- Follow up on all leads. Although applying for various types of financial assistance involves paperwork, sometimes the extra effort does result in supplemental funding that can help to pay for your child's medical bills.
- Check with other parents who have children with special needs—their tips will be particularly relevant.

DAILY CARE AND MEDICAL NEEDS

Meeting Daily Care Needs

Families work together to set schedules and meet the daily care needs of family members—cooking meals, maintaining and cleaning the family home, transporting family members, and obtaining necessary medical care. When a family member has a disability, there may be specific daily care needs on top of those already being met by the family. For instance, some children with disabilities require a special diet or special feeding procedures; therefore, the daily task of cooking meals is no longer as simple as it once was. Because Zachary was sensitive to the feel and taste of food, as well as to touch, Jane needed to modify meals for him. In your family there may be special equipment (perhaps a wheelchair or a mist tent over the bed) that needs to be maintained and cleaned. If your child uses a walker or a wheelchair, transportation can become more of a challenge. You will need extra time and energy to transport not only your child but also the supportive equipment—and your child's disability and the services being received may mean that your family is doing more transporting.

Meeting the day-to-day care needs of children with disabilities and still being responsive to the needs of other family members is an awesome responsibility—one from which all parents need a break. But finding alternative care providers who are comfortable caring for a child with special needs is difficult at best. And yet all parents need some time for themselves during which they are completely relieved of the caregiving responsibility. A mother who found a wonderful live-in caregiver to stay with her child with a chronic illness while the rest of the family spent a week at the beach explained:

> The week that our family stayed at the beach was the most wonderful gift. . . . It gave us the opportunity to stand outside the situation and view it from a distance. It enabled us to review what had gone on before, to put things into perspective, think, and plan. We were also physically restored, and were able to go on with much more strength . . . caring for our daughter. (Ambler, 1996, p. 2)

There are different kinds of child care, and the kind of child care you look for will depend on your child's disability, the cost of the care, and how long you need it. If your child needs close supervision but does not have complex medical needs, then perhaps a relative, family friend, or neighborhood baby sitter might take care of your child. Sometimes parents of children with special needs establish an informal babysitting co-op for trading child care services among themselves.

Established child care centers are gradually becoming more inclusive of children with special needs, but too often child care centers are not prepared (in terms of staff or equipment) to take children with disabilities. Although the Americans with Disabilities Act (ADA) of 1990 mandates full access to child care for children with disabilities, the law also provides for flexibility when the needs of the child are complex. Parents often find that they need to be resources for child care providers to ensure that the care their child with special needs receives is the best it can be.

Respite care, a system of temporary child care for children with special needs, is another option for parents. Usually, respite care providers have received some specialized training in caring for children with disabilities and special health care needs, and they can provide care for just a few hours or for several days or weeks at a time. Respite care, however, is not designed to be a long-term child care solution for a parent who decides to return to work—but it can be a solution for temporary child care needs. To find out more about respite services in your community, check with agencies that are providing services to children with disabilities and their families. The National Respite Locator Service maintains a database of respite care providers and can put you in touch with providers in your area (see the list of resources at the end of this chapter).

Meeting Medical Needs

Your child's medical needs may mean that there are different medical providers in your lives—pediatricians, surgeons, therapists, nutritionists—with each of them giving you information related to their specialty area and suggesting various courses of treatment. Many parents find it challenging to sort through and organize all of the information related to the medical needs of their child with a disability, as well as to juggle the suggested treatment plans while being the source of comfort for their child. It can quickly feel overwhelming. Parents who have had experience in this area share the following tips:

- Develop a system for keeping all medical records together (perhaps a three-ring binder). Dividers within the binder can be used to separate information from each specialist.
- Keep a log of all conversations that you have with providers (e.g., telephone, e-mail, fax) in your binder; include dates and times, names and contact information, the outcome of each contact, follow-up that is required, and who will do it and by what date.
- Keep a roster of the telephone and fax numbers of the professionals you are dealing with in the front of the binder so that you don't have to look up numbers each time you want to call.
- Ask for and keep copies of medical records and diagnostic information.
- Ask medical staff to show you (and other family members involved in the care of your child) how to use any special equipment that your child needs. Find out how you can get technical assistance *after hours* or how you might speak with other parents whose children are using the same medical equipment to learn more.
- Find out what you can do to make a hospitalization experience less scary for your child.

EDUCATIONAL NEEDS

Families play an enormous role in the education of their children—as their children's first teachers and as their educational partners and advocates. Families have legal rights to early intervention services for children with special needs from birth to 3 years of age and special education programs for children ages 3–21. These rights are granted and protected by the Individuals with Disabilities Education Act (IDEA) Amendments of 1997.

Part C of IDEA mandates that all infants and toddlers with or at risk for developmental delays are eligible for early intervention services (until their third birthday). Early intervention services may include any and all of the following: special instruction, speech-language pathology and audiology, occupational therapy, physical therapy, psychological services, family training, counseling, service coordination, medical services for diagnosis and evaluation, early identification, screening, assessment services, health services, vision services, assistive technology devices and services, transportation, and related costs necessary to receive services. Early intervention services must be planned for by a multidisciplinary team, including parents, that jointly develops a written plan of services called the individualized family service plan (IFSP). Early intervention services must be provided by qualified people in natural environments (e.g., family home, child care center). Early intervention therapists supply important and specific supports and often have suggestions for additional therapy activities at home.

Under Part B of IDEA, children ages 3–21 who have developmental delays, mental retardation, autism, emotional disturbance, or learning disabilities, as well as those with vision, hearing, speech, orthopedic, or other health impairments, are eligible for special education and related services (services that *enable* a child to benefit from special education services). These services include transportation, speech-language and audiology services, psychological services, physical and occupational therapy, recreation, early identification and assessment, counseling, medical services for diagnostic and evaluation purposes, school health services, school social work services, and parent counseling and training. Special education and related services must be provided in the least restrictive environment, allowing the child to be educated with his or her peers without disabilities. As in early intervention, parents are invited to participate on a multidisciplinary team to develop the written plan of educational services called the individualized education program (IEP).

New challenges sometimes begin when children with disabilities turn 3 years old and they and their families make the transition out of early intervention services. Sometimes the educational services provided by the schools are less family centered than the services provided by the early intervention program. Although IDEA requires school districts to provide appropriate educational services to children with disabilities in the least restrictive environment, there is still a lot of variability in the quality of these services.

Many parents find that they must be proactive in their partnerships with school personnel to ensure that the educational rights of their children with disabilities are fully met. And many parents are recognizing that other parents are their best allies in this process. Parent advocates who have received training in special education law understand what the law means for parents who have children with disabilities, and they know how to interpret the law so that it is meaningful for new parents. Here are some tips that you might find helpful as you work with educational professionals to develop the best possible educational options for your child:

- Strive for partnerships with professionals that are characterized by mutual respect, trust, and openness, with information being shared equally among all partners.
- Celebrate the expertise that all members of the educational planning team bring to the process.
- Ask for explanations for any terms that you don't understand.
- Consider taking notes during the meeting so that you will have a record of the discussions and the decisions.
- Prepare for the meeting by writing down any questions or concerns that you would like the team to address during the meeting.
- Let professionals know if you are concerned about their recommendations for your child.
- Consider how suggested home activities will fit into your family schedule.
- Think about what role you want to play as you partner with professionals around your child's educational needs.

For more information about the education and legal rights of children with special needs and their families, you may want to contact the Parent Training and Information Center (PTI) in your state (see Chapter 3 and Appendix C).

PLANNING FOR THE FUTURE

Preparing each family member for the future is another important function that families play, and families work hard to ensure that their family members have every opportunity to succeed and enjoy life as adult members of society. This is a challenging role for any family, but one that may be even more challenging when a child has special needs. Fortunately, since 1980 options for adults with disabilities to participate more fully as contributing members of society have expanded.

Parents of young children with special needs often are so focused on meeting the present-day needs of their child and family that thinking about what the future may hold and how to prepare for that future is sometimes hard to do. And although IDEA requires that school personnel, parents, and adolescent students with disabilities begin to plan for the student's transition from school to postschool environments (e.g., employment, supported or independent living, additional training), there are many ways parents can foster self-determination and independent living skills beginning when the child is quite young:

- Allow your child to make choices. Parents can help children make appropriate choices by giving them controlled options.
- Share your belief in the importance of fostering self-determination skills with the providers or community leaders who also are interacting with your child.
- Ask your child about his or her hopes and expectations for the future.
- Talk with the professionals who are providing services to your child about including opportunities for your child to develop and practice the daily living skills that will help him or her to live as independently as possible as an adult.
- Remember that the home, school, and community all provide opportunities for children to learn, make choices, and solve problems.

Planning the transition from school to adult life is required by law to begin once a student reaches 14 years of age, and this transition planning is a part of the student's IEP. These transition services are intended to prepare students to make the transition from the world of school to the world of adulthood, and students with disabilities and their families are invited to take an active role in this transition planning. As a child with special needs nears the age of 18 (the age of majority), depending on the nature and severity of his or her disability, parents also may need to resolve the issue of who will serve as the legal guardian if the child is not capable of doing so and may need to take the legal steps required to establish a conservatorship after the age of 18. The legal conservator, parents, or nonrelated individual will have authority to advocate for and make decisions on behalf of the child. You will need to consult an attorney. Many parents find it helpful to talk with other parents whose sons or daughters with special needs are a few years older about how they managed all of these transitions, including Medicare, health care, and Social Security services.

When a child with a disability reaches the age of 21, entitlement to public education ends, and young people and their families are faced with many decisions about the future. Instead of dealing with the school district and its familiar procedures and acronyms, families of young adults with disabilities may begin to deal with vocational rehabilitation and independent living systems with new procedures and acronyms. Be sure to check with your state vocational rehabilitation agency to learn about the medical, therapeutic, counseling, education, training, and other services they may provide to prepare people with disabilities for work. Goodwill Industries can be another source of support, information, training, job development, and job coaching. Also, local junior colleges (community colleges) are creating and offering education beyond high school for transitioning to independent living. The Transition to Independent Living program at Taft College can be a source of information about these types of programs. (You can contact Taft College at the following address: 29 Emmons Park Drive, Taft, CA, 93268; telephone: [661] 763-7700; fax: [661] 763-7705.)

Supported living and employment opportunities for adults with disabilities are getting better as disability policy moves from funding institutional settings to funding community-based supports. An increasingly available option for parents and their adult family members with special needs is for families to receive funds for establishing and coordinating adult services rather than to have the funds go to agencies. Families are beginning to discover that with these funds they can create the kind of living environment that they and their adult family member envision. Some adults with disabilities are living in their own homes, perhaps with chosen housemates; working in regular jobs, perhaps with a job coach; and participating in social and community activities just as people without disabilities do. Be sure to talk with providers and other parents about how you might gain access to and creatively use this individualized funding.

Another aspect of planning for the future that is difficult for parents of children with special needs is planning for the care of your family member with special needs when you are no longer able to do so. Where and how will he or she live, and will there be enough money to sustain a quality life? Parents need to be aware of many legal issues regarding estate planning and developing a will to offer your child with special needs the greatest possible protection. Talk with other parents to learn about their strategies and where you might find a lawyer who specializes in estate planning, special trusts, and disability law. There are ways to provide added financial assistance without losing government assistance.

SUMMARY

Families nurture the growth, development, and well-being of each family member, and every family has its own set of joys and challenges that makes their situation unique. When a child has a disability, there are many emotional adjustments, but there also are a lot of changes to the daily life as families learn to carry on the work of their family in new and different ways in response to their child's disabilities. Parents don't have to take on these emotional and logistical challenges alone, however. There are different family support opportunities, formal and informal, available to families that are caring for family members with special needs. Chapters 3 and 4 give you a broad introduction to these support resources and then introduce you to a special kind of support—parent to parent support.

Celebrating Holland—I'm Home

I have been in Holland for a while now. It has become home. I have had time to catch my breath, to settle in and adjust, and to accept this different trip than I'd planned.

I reflect back on those years when I first landed in Holland and remember clearly my shock, my fear, my anger. In those first few years, I tried to get back to Italy as planned, but Holland was where I was to stay. Today, I can say how far I have come on this unexpected journey, how much I have learned about Holland. But it has been a journey of time.

I worked hard. I bought new guidebooks. I learned a new language, and I slowly found my way around in Holland. I met others whose plans had changed like mine and who could share my experience. Some of these fellow travelers had been in Holland longer than I and were seasoned guides, assisting me along the way. Many have encouraged me and have taught me to open my eyes to the wonder and gifts to behold in this new land. We supported one another, some have become very special friends, and I have discovered a community of caring. Holland isn't so bad.

I think that Holland is used to wayward travelers like me and has become a land of hospitality, reaching out to welcome, assist, and support newcomers. Over the years, I've wondered what life would have been like if I'd landed in Italy as planned. Would life have been easier? Would it have been as rewarding? Would I have learned the important lessons I benefit from today?

Sure, this journey has been challenging and at times I would (and still do) stomp my feet and cry out in frustration and protest. And, yes, Holland is slower paced and less flashy than Italy, but this, too, has been an unexpected gift. I have learned to slow down and look closer at things, with a new appreciation for the remarkable beauty of Holland. I have discovered that it doesn't matter where you land. What's more important is what you make of your journey and how you see and enjoy the very special things that Holland has to offer. I have come to love Holland and call it home.

Yes, I landed in a place I hadn't planned. Yet I am thankful, for this destination has been richer than I could have imagined!

—Cathy, a parent of a child with special needs

REFERENCES

Ambler, L. (1996). *Respite care.* Washington, DC: National Information Center for Children and Youth with Disabilities.

Americans with Disabilities Act (ADA) of 1990, PL 101-336, 42 U.S.C. §§ 12101 *et seq.*

Individuals with Disabilities Education Act (IDEA) Amendments of 1997, PL 105-17, 20 U.S.C. §§ 1400 *et seq.*

RESOURCES FOR PARENTS AND PROVIDERS

Anderson, W., Chitwood, S., & Hayden, D. (1997). *Negotiating the special education maze: A guide for parents and teachers* (3rd ed.). Bethesda, MD: Woodbine House.

Beckman, P.J., & Boyes, G.B. (1993). *Deciphering the system: A guide for families of young children with disabilities.* Cambridge, MA: Brookline Books.

Callahan, M.J., & Garner, J.B. (1997). *Keys to the workplace: Skills and supports for people with disabilities.* Baltimore: Paul H. Brookes Publishing Co.

Cantor, J.A., & Cantor, R.F. (1995). *Parent's guide to special needs schooling: Early intervention years.* Westport, CT: Greenwood.

Capper, L. (1996). *That's my child: Strategies for parents of children with disabilities.* Washington, DC: Child & Family Press.

Chandler, P.A. (1994). *A place for me: Including children with special needs—early care and education setting.* Washington, DC: National Association for the Education of Young Children.

Ferguson, T. (1996). *Health online: How to find health information, support groups, and self-help communities in cyberspace.* Reading, MA: Addison Wesley Longman.

Gorn, S. (1997). *What do I do when? The answer book on individualized education programs.* Horsham, PA: LRP Publications.

Hallowell, E. (1996). *When you worry about the child you love.* New York: Simon & Schuster.

Johnson, B.H., McGonigel, M.J., & Kaufmann, R.K. (1991). *Guidelines and recommended practices for the individualized family service plan* (2nd ed.). Bethesda, MD: Association for the Care of Children's Health.

Leff, P.T., & Walizer, E.H. (1992). *Building the healing partnership.* Cambridge, MA: Brookline Books.

Lowe, P. (1993). *Care pooling: How to get the help you need to care for the ones you love.* San Francisco: Berrett-Koehler Publishers.

Pierangelo, R., & Jacoby, R. (1996). *Parents' complete special education guide.* Upper Saddle River, NJ: Prentice Hall.

Rosenfeld, L.R. (1994). *Your child and health care: A "dollars & sense" guide for families with special needs.* Baltimore: Paul H. Brookes Publishing Co.

Spiegle, J.A., & van den Pol, R.A. (1993). *Making changes: Family voices on living with disabilities.* Cambridge, MA: Brookline Books.

Sullivan, T. (1995). *Special parent, special child.* New York: G.P. Putnam's Sons.

Wilson, N.O. (1994). *My child needs special services: Parents talk about what helps. . . . and what doesn't.* Bedford, MA: Mills & Sanderson.

RESOURCES FOR CHILDREN

Booth, Z. (1996). *Finding a friend.* Mount Desert, ME: Windswept House Publishers.

Buehrens, A., & Buehrens, C. (1991). *Adam and the magic marble.* Duarte, CA: Hope Press.

Bunnett, R., & Sahlhoff, C. (1992). *Friends in the park.* New York: Checkerboard Press.

Caffrey, J.A. (1997). *First star I see.* Fairport, NY: Verbal Images Press.

Derby, J. (1993). *Are you my friend?* Scottdale, PA: Herald Press.

Duncan, D. (1994). *When Molly was in the hospital: A book for brothers and sisters of hospitalized children.* Windsor, CA: Rayve Productions.

Exley, H. (1984). *What it's like to be me.* New York: Friendship Press.

Gehret, J. (1992). *I'm somebody too.* Westport, NY: Verbal Images Press.

Hodges, C. (1995). *When I grow up.* Hollidaysburg, PA: Jason & Nordic Publishers.

Kent, D., & Quinlan, K.A. (1996). *Extraordinary people with disabilities.* Danbury, CT: Children's Press.

McCarthy-Tucker, S. (1993). *Coping with special-needs classmates.* New York: Rosen.

McConnell, N.P. (1993). *Different and alike* (3rd ed.). Colorado Springs: Current.

Meyer, D., & Vadasy, P.F. (1996). *Living with a brother or sister with special needs: A book for sibs* (2nd ed.). Seattle: University of Washington Press.

Meyer, D.J. (1997). *View from our shoes: Growing up with a brother or sister with special needs.* Bethesda, MD: Woodbine House.

Smith, S.L. (1994). *Different is not bad, different is the world.* Longmont, CO: Sopris West.

Stein, S.B. (1991). *About handicaps: An open family book for parents and children together.* New York: Walker & Co.

Westridge Young Writers Workshop. (1994). *Kids explore the gifts of children with special needs.* Santa Fe, NM: John Muir Publications.

DISABILITY RESOURCES ON THE INTERNET

Disability Resources, Inc., 4 Glatter Lane, Centereach, NY 11720-1032; telephone: (516) 585-0290; http://www.disabilityresources.org. Provides links to the best disability resources on the web, including national and international sites, documents, databases, and other informational materials.

Exceptional Parent Magazine Search and Respond, 555 Kinderkamack Road, Oradell, NJ 07649-1517; telephone: (201) 634-6550; http://www.eparent.com. Provides information and connections with other parents for parents of children with special needs.

Family Village, 1500 Highland Avenue, Madison, WI 53705; telephone: (608) 263-5973; TDD: (608) 263-0802; fax: (608) 263-0529; http://www.familyvillage.wisc.edu. Provides information about disabilities and links to resources, and facilitates connections among parents who have children with disabilities.

Information About Early Intervention, http://www.nectas.unc.edu. NECTAS is a federally funded project that provides information about 1) recommended practices in early childhood services for young children with disabilities, 2) national early childhood policies, and 3) early childhood research. The mission of NECTAS is to improve services and results for young children with disabilities and their families.

Information About IDEA, http://www.ideapractices.org, http://www.ed.gov.offices/OSERS/OSEP. Provides information about the Individuals with Disabilities Education Act (IDEA) and recommended practices.

MUMS: Mothers United for Moral Support, 150 Custer Court, Green Bay, WI 54301-1243; telephone: (877) 336-5333 (parents only); (920) 336-5333; http://www.mums@waisman.wisc.edu/~rowley/mums. Helps to match parents whose children have similar disabilities and to support the development of disability-specific support groups.

Our-Kids, http://rdz.stjohns.edu/library/support/our-kids. An on-line support group for parents and others worldwide who care about children with disabilities or delays. It was founded by parents for parents, and the material that can be accessed from the web site was contributed by parents.

FEDERAL GOVERNMENT AGENCIES

Administration on Developmental Disabilities, U.S. Department of Health and Human Services, Room 329D, Humphrey Building, Washington, DC 20201; telephone: (202) 673-7678.

Office of Special Education Programs, Office of Special Education and Rehabilitative Services, U.S. Department of Education, 330 C Street, SW, Switzer Building, Washington, DC 20202; telephone: (202) 554-7699.

Office of Vocational and Adult Education, U.S. Department of Education, 4090 MES, 400 Maryland Avenue, SW, Washington, DC 20202; telephone: (202) 205-5451.

Office on the Americans with Disabilities Act, Civil Rights Division, U.S. Department of Justice, Post Office Box 66118, Washington, DC 20035-6118; telephone: (202) 514-0318.

Social Security Administration, U.S. Department of Health and Human Services, Post Office Box 17743, Baltimore, MD 21235; telephone: (800) 772-1214.

CLEARINGHOUSES AND INFORMATION AND REFERRAL RESOURCES

Clearinghouse on Adult Education and Literacy, U.S. Department of Education, 4090 MES, Office of Vocational and Adult Education, 400 Maryland Avenue, SW, Washington, DC 20202-7240; telephone: (202) 205-8270; e-mail: OVAE@inet.ed.gov; http://www.ed.gov/offices/OVAE. Provides referral services and disseminates publications of state and national significance and other reference materials on adult education and literacy-related activities.

HEATH Resource Center, American Council on Education, One Dupont Circle, NW, Suite 800, Washington, DC 20036-1193; voice/TTY: (800) 544-3284; (202) 939-9320; e-mail: heath@ace.nche.edu; http://www.heath-resource-center.org. A national clearinghouse on postsecondary education for individuals with disabilities, collects and disseminates information nationally about disability issues in postsecondary education. The clearinghouse provides information on educational support services, policies, procedures, adaptations, transition, and opportunities at American campuses, vocational training schools, adult education programs, independent living centers, and other training entities after high school for individuals with disabilities. Numerous publications are available upon request.

National Council on Independent Living (NCIL), 1916 Wilson Boulevard, Suite 209, Arlington, VA 22201; telephone: (703) 525-3406; TTY: (703) 525-4153; e-mail: ncil@ncil.org; http://www.ncil.org. A national membership association of local nonprofit corporations known as Centers for Independent Living. As the only cross-disability grassroots national organization run by and for people with disabilities, NCIL provides technical assistance, training, and leadership to independent living centers and information and referral services to adults with disabilities and their families.

National Respite Locator Service, 800 Eastowne Drive, Suite 105, Chapel Hill, NC 27514; telephone: (800) 773-5433; http://www.chtop.com/locator.htm.

II

Finding Meaningful Support

3

And Now What?

Parent Support Opportunities

"It is one of the beautiful compensations of this life that no one can sincerely try to help another without helping himself."

—Charles Dudley Warner

Perhaps you and your family have just learned your child has special needs, or perhaps you have known for some time. You may have shared the same emotions that the families in Chapter 1 experienced—denial, anger, sadness, anxiety, guilt, and fear. You may have juggled the same logistical realities described in Chapter 2—caregiving demands, learning to live with new professionals, understanding the myriad of acronyms, finding services and child care, and meeting the concerns of siblings. At one time in history, families were usually not spread out geographically and extended family members were available to help parents meet the challenges of family life. But today grandparents, aunts, and uncles often live far away. As a result, your family may be facing these challenges alone.

This chapter tells you about parent support opportunities that may help you meet your family's needs. Along with the professionals who provide medical, educational, and other related services to children with disabilities to ensure their optimal growth and development, there are parents who are willing to walk with newcomers to show them the way.

FAMILY STORIES: FINDING A GUIDE

Although there is progress that needs to be made in providing services to children with disabilities, families are benefiting from more information about disabilities, options for medical treatment, and available services. But because there is so much information, parents are being asked to learn a lot in a short time and to interpret and use this information to make important decisions. Families often mention how helpful it would be to have a *tour guide* to help them learn the new terminology, figure out how to manage the day-to-day responsibilities, understand the services that are available, and be supported as they consider their options.

In each of the stories presented in Chapters 1 and 2, the parents connected with helpful resources at different times after finding out about their child's disability. Some of the families were lucky—their connections came early. Catherine and W.C. met Jean while they were in the hospital following Karl's birth and diagnosis. Jean showed them a window to the future and offered them hope that their lives would go on in a meaningful way. She encouraged them to take their first steps to learn about and find services for Karl; she suggested strategies for recognizing, understanding, acknowledging, and meeting their own needs, and she answered questions about early intervention services and what they might expect as Karl got older. Cathryn and Richard connected with their tour guide 4 months after Gregory and Daniel were born. Cathryn was able to share her innermost thoughts and feelings about running away and abandoning her family without fear of being judged.

For Jane and Rodney, Zachary was almost 3 years old before the diagnosis became clear, and it was years later before Jane found support. Initially all that Jane had was a toll-free telephone number that her pediatrician had given her when he informed her that Zachary had autism. Information from the toll-free telephone number was minimal, and although it answered a few of Jane's questions, it didn't give her the support and encouragement she was looking for. Responding to an invitation to a seminar hosted by Parent to Parent of Pennsylvania opened the door to the support that helped her feel less alone.

For Maria and David, there were many weeks in the NICU and multiple surgeries that kept everyone's focus on Lucia's critical medical concerns. Finally, Lucia was stable enough to be discharged. Although the discharge nurse at the hospital provided the link to services in the community for Lucia, there was not a similar link to parent support for Maria and David. Through California Children's Services and United Cerebral Palsy, 3 years later they finally found support for themselves from professionals and parents who gave them hope about the future.

TYPES OF PARENT SUPPORT AND INFORMATION: CHOICES FOR PARENTS

As you can see in Figure 3.1, opportunities for sharing parent support and information can be directed and provided by professionals or by parents themselves. Parent support also can be provided either in a group setting or through a one-to-one connection. These different opportunities can be useful at different times and for different reasons. Each parent is unique and has his or her own preferences about support, and these preferences may vary over time. Sometimes one-to-one contact with another parent is needed; other times the support of a group of parents is helpful. When medical information is needed, then informational support from a professional may be preferred. It is crucial that parents find the information and support that suits them.

	Group setting	One-to-one setting
Professionally directed and delivered		
Parent-directed and delivered		

Figure 3.1. Opportunities for sharing parent support and information can be directed and provided by professionals or by parents themselves, either in a group setting or through a one-to-one connection.

Support and Information Provided by Professionals

There are professionals available to provide support and information to parents who have a child with a disability, including doctors, nurses, social workers, teachers, lawyers, counselors, therapists, and religious leaders. Sometimes these professionals provide their support to parents in a group setting. In other instances a professional may meet with a parent individually and provide support and information one to one.

Group Support Many agencies that provide services to children and adults with special needs offer families an opportunity to come together in a group setting with other families. Parent support groups are organized and facilitated by a professional staff member, and these group meetings provide parents with emotional and informational support.

Parents are encouraged to share their experiences in emotional support group meetings so that they can learn from and support each other. The chance to share feelings about their child's disability with other parents is reassuring and comforting for many parents.

The informational support group meetings may have a guest speaker sharing information about a specific topic (e.g., early intervention services, cystic fibrosis, challenging behaviors, feeding tips, sibling issues). These meetings may allow time for discussion and questions so that parents take away new information and strategies. The role of the professional is to plan with the parents the content that will be shared.

Parent support groups can give parents a chance to hear from other parents about their experiences so they feel less alone and can provide opportunities for parents to share the *tricks of the trade* that can make caring for a child with a disability easier. Sometimes parent support groups become social groups as well, with parents meeting socially outside of the regular parent support group meetings. If you are interested in becoming part of a parent support group, ask the staff members at the place where your child receives services whether they offer or can direct you to a parent support group.

One-to-One Support Parents may want to talk individually with a professional about a particular issue or need. They may make an appointment with a therapist to discuss the services that are being provided for their child, they may speak with a counselor or social worker about their own feelings about the disability experience, or they might seek legal counsel from their lawyer.

Support provided by professionals in a one-to-one setting can be either informational (a teacher shares ideas about activities that can happen at home to encourage a young child with a speech impairment to use sign language) or emotional (a social worker helps a parent talk about and deal with fears about his or her child's future). The one-to-one nature of this support can be tailored to the specific needs or concerns of the parent. If you have specific questions for a professional, the service providers who are a part of your child's life should be able to help contact the appropriate person for the individualized support you seek.

Support and Information Provided by Parents

When parents of young children with disabilities are asked who can best support them emotionally, their first choice is other parents who have had or are having the same or similar experience as they are having. Sharing experiences with others in similar circumstances is an important source of social support.

Opportunities for connecting with other parents occur naturally and spontaneously for families—over the backyard fence, in playgroups, and through community programs. But families of children with special needs tend to have fewer of these natural opportunities because their children with disabilities are not easily included in these settings. Finding a family with similar experiences can be more difficult than forging connections with other families in the neighborhood. Fortunately, there are parent-directed support opportunities that put parents in touch with other parents who are sharing their life experiences—either as a group or one to one.

Group Support Hundreds of parent support groups have been started by parents wishing to talk with other parents about similar disability issues. Parent support groups usually have a single disability focus (e.g., Down syndrome, cerebral palsy), but other types of groups also can be found. For example, parents whose children attend the same early intervention program may form their own support group even though their children may have different disabilities. Or, parents who have children with challenging behaviors (whose disabilities may be different) get together to share support and strategies for managing these behaviors. For all of these groups, the parents develop the group and run the meetings themselves, offering opportunities for informational and emotional sharing.

There is a philosophical difference between support groups that are directed by professionals and support groups that are led by parents in determining the focus and direction of the meetings. Some parents may prefer that the group be led by a professional, who takes responsibility for the logistics and focus of the group. Parents may have some input, but these parents appreciate professional guidance. Other parents want to participate in a group that is led and directed by parents, with one or more parents determining the content of the group's meetings and facilitating each session. They feel that the group *belongs to them* if they determine the focus and activities of the group. Sometimes this sense of parent ownership and commitment to the group makes the difference between a support group that continues over time and one that does not. Regardless of whether a support group is parent directed or professionally directed, the more involved parents are, the more likely the group is to last.

Parent-directed groups can be harder to find than those directed by professionals; perhaps it is not easy for parents to get the word out about their support groups. Professionals have the resources of their agencies, and they network with other professionals as a part of their regular responsibilities. They are likely to be more aware of group opportunities for parents that are being offered by other professionals than those offered by parents. If you are looking for a support and information group that is being offered by parents for parents, begin asking other parents you meet about parent-led support groups.

One-to-One Support The final aspect of parent support is one-to-one support. Parent to parent support is parent directed and delivered one to one. Since 1975, Parent to Parent programs have been providing a unique form of individualized support to families who have a member with a disability. Trained, supporting parents are matched with parents newly referred to the program. Because supporting parents know the challenges and special joys that come with parenting a son or daughter with a disability, they are able to offer informational and emotional support.

Parent to Parent matches are made quickly, ideally within 24 hours of the referral, and are based on similar disability and family issues. Often the referred parent has just been given his or her child's diagnosis or is just beginning a new era in the life of his or her child with a disability. Once parents are matched, each relationship develops based on the needs and preferences of the referred parent. For some parents, the match is short term and involves an exchange of information; for others, the match lasts for years or develops into a lifelong friendship. Because two parents who share common experiences are matched, parent to parent support is different from that provided by professionals. And because the relationship between the parents is one to one, the nature of the support is different from that found in parent support groups.

FINDING SUPPORT AND INFORMATION

Professional Support and Information

Each state has agencies that serve children with special needs in communities across the state. For example, each state has an education agency (usually called the Department of Education) that oversees the educational services provided by local school districts for children with special needs. A state health agency (usually called the Department of Health or the Department for Children with Special Health Care Needs) is responsible for local health agencies in communities around the state.

Every state also has a developmental disabilities council that receives federal funds to provide support services for people with developmental disabilities and their families. And each has a Department of Rehabilitation to help with adult issues such as job preparation and procurement. These agencies will be able to help you find services in your community for your child and your family.

You can find out how to reach these state agencies by looking in your telephone book under the listings for state offices. Service providers who are working with your child should be able to tell you about related services available in your community. You also can contact the National Information Clearinghouse for Children and Youth with Disabilities (NICHCY), which offers information about disabilities and related services, assists with referrals, produces resource sheets with contacts for disability-related services and programs in each state, and publishes a newsletter (contact information can be found in Appendix C). NICHCY maintains an updated directory of local and state agencies—be sure to ask them to send you the resource sheet from your state (or you can download it from the NICHCY web site at http://www.nichcy.org). State agencies will be able to put you in touch with their local counterparts in your area. Some of these state and local agencies may offer parent support activities for parents of children with disabilities who are receiving services within their agency.

Parent-Directed Support and Information: Parent to Parent

Local Parent to Parent Programs There are more than 600 local Parent to Parent programs that offer community-based information and support to parents of children with disabilities, ongoing medical conditions, or other special education and health care needs. As you will read in Chapter 10, many of these programs offer not only a one-to-one match but also other support opportunities for parents, children with disabilities, and other family members. Ask the professionals providing services to your child if they know of a Parent to Parent program in your area. Other parents who have children with special needs may be able to link you to a Parent to Parent program. The Beach Center on Families and Disability at The University of Kansas maintains a current listing of Parent to Parent programs (contact information can be found in Appendix C).

Statewide Parent to Parent Programs In 30 states there are not only local Parent to Parent programs but also statewide Parent to Parent networks. Statewide programs provide training and technical assistance to local programs in a variety of ways and make it possible for parents to be matched statewide when a local match isn't available. You will read more about statewide Parent to Parent programs in Chapter

14, and a list of statewide programs appears in Appendix C. If you are interested in finding a local program in your area so that you can be matched or if you want to talk with someone about starting a program in your own community, contact the statewide Parent to Parent program in your state. If there is not a statewide Parent to Parent program in your state to help you find a local program or to match you with someone who lives close to you, there are resources to help put you in touch with local Parent to Parent programs all across the country. These resources can be found in Appendix C.

National Parent to Parent Activities There are Parent to Parent efforts that help match and support parents who cannot find a parent connection or information at the local or statewide level. Usually these parents have children with rare disabilities, and there may be only a few families nationally whose children have the same disability. Finding this type of match requires a national or even international search.

One group that has access to national and international databases of information is Mothers United for Moral Support (MUMS). MUMS provides support to parents of a child with any disability or rare disorder in the form of a networking system that matches them with other parents whose children have the same or a similar condition. A national/international database of families enables MUMS to match parents who have not been able to find a match at the local or state level. Contact information for MUMS can be found in Appendix C.

Despite the fact that there are hundreds of local and statewide Parent to Parent programs and that MUMS exists to help parents find national matches, there is no national Parent to Parent organization that coordinates activities nationally and helps families to find national connections when local or statewide matches cannot be found. You will read in Chapter 15, however, about the efforts of some parent leaders to design a national infrastructure that will support local and statewide programs while serving as a coordinating hub for all Parent to Parent programs.

Parent-Directed Support and Information: Other Resources

In addition to Parent to Parent programs, there are numerous other parent-directed groups available to help families who have a child with a disability. Contact information for these organizations can be found in Appendix C.

Beach Center on Families and Disability The Beach Center on Families and Disability is a federally funded research and training center at The University of Kansas working to improve the quality of life for individuals with disabilities and their families through research, training, technical assistance, and dissemination activities. The Beach

Center houses research data on Parent to Parent programs and their effectiveness.

Family Voices Family Voices is a national grass roots organization directed by parents of children and adults with special health care needs and is comprised of families and professional friends who care for and about children with special health care needs. Family leaders organized Family Voices to ensure that children's health is addressed as public and private health care systems undergo change in communities, states, and the nation. Family Voices gathers and provides information about health care issues affecting children so that everyone can advocate for and obtain the health care that children deserve. Every state has a Family Voices coordinator who assists families at the local and state levels. The national Family Voices office can provide you with the name of the Family Voices coordinator in your state.

Grassroots Consortium on Disabilities The Grassroots Consortium on Disabilities is a national coalition of parent-directed, community-based parent support programs that provide support and information to traditionally underserved families who have children with disabilities. Serving culturally diverse families who may face issues such as poverty, English as a second language, and migrancy, in addition to disability-related issues, the Grassroots Consortium on Disabilities focuses on reaching and meeting the concerns of families in underserved communities through individualized supports and services presented in the native language of the family. A list of the programs of the Grassroots Consortium on Disabilities appears in Appendix C.

National Center on Parent-Directed Family Resource Centers The National Center for Parent-Directed Family Resource Centers at PHP, Inc. provides training and technical assistance to parents and professionals who are interested in developing a parent-directed family resource center (PDFRC). PDFRCs provide emotional support, information, and training to parents who have a child with special needs.

National Coalition for Family Leadership The National Coalition for Family Leadership is a group of parent leaders who have had many years of experience in the Parent to Parent movement. They meet annually to identify emerging trends, plan national responses, share recommended practices in family support, and nurture each other and new parent leaders.

National Fathers Network The National Fathers Network provides information, support, and resources to fathers of children with disabilities or an ongoing medical condition. Supporting the efforts of 83 fathers' programs in the United States, the National Fathers Network publishes a newsletter and a column in *Exceptional Parent* magazine and operates a web page.

National Organization for Rare Disorders The National Organization for Rare Disorders provides callers with information about rare disorders and brings families with similar disorders together for mutual support. Single printed copies of disability information sheets are available through a literature order form.

National Parent Network on Disabilities The National Parent Network on Disabilities is a consortium of parents and professionals, Parent Training and Information Centers (PTIs), parent support programs, service provider organizations, and university programs that are working together for legislative awareness and systems change on behalf of families who have a family member with special needs.

Parent Training and Information Centers PTIs are directed primarily by parents of children and adults with disabilities. The mission of PTIs is *to provide training and information to parents to enable them to participate more effectively with professionals in meeting the educational concerns of children with disabilities.* PTIs provide training and information to parents of infants, toddlers, children, and youth with disabilities and to the professionals who work with these parents. PTIs can help parents to 1) understand their children's specific concerns, 2) communicate more effectively with professionals, 3) participate in the educational planning process, and 4) obtain information about relevant programs, services, and resources. There is at least one PTI in every state, and a complete listing of the PTIs can be found at http://www.taalliance.org or at http://www.brookespublishing.com/ptop/.

Technical Assistance Alliance for Parent Centers The Technical Assistance Alliance for Parent Centers (the Alliance) coordinates the delivery of technical assistance to the PTIs through four regional PTI centers located in California, New Hampshire, Texas, and Ohio.

The Sibling Support Project The Sibling Support Project is a national program dedicated to the interests of brothers and sisters of people with special health and developmental concerns. The primary goal of The Sibling Support Project is to increase the availability of peer support and education programs (through interactive workshops for siblings, called *Sibshops*) for brothers and sisters of people with disabilities and special health care concerns.

Specific Disability Groups The number of specific disability information and support groups has grown since 1980 because parents find it helpful to connect with other parents who have children with similar disability issues. Many of these groups are directed by parents who believe in the value of mutual support and information sharing. These groups often offer support groups for parents, referrals to local resources, informational materials, advocacy efforts, networking opportunities, and a program newsletter. There are local, state, and national organizations for some of the groups, and the national office can usually provide the names of state and/or local chapters. Although there are too many specific disability groups to list in this book, there are directories that contain extensive listings. Two that you might find helpful are the annual *Resource Directory* produced by *Exceptional Parent* magazine (available from Exceptional Parent, 555 Kindercamack Road, Oradell, NJ 07649–1517; telephone: [201] 634-6550; http://www.eparent.com) and the *Self-Help Sourcebook: Finding and Forming Mutual Aid Self-Help Groups* (available from American Self-Help Clearinghouse, Northwest Covenant Medical Center, 25 Pocono Road, Denville, NJ 07834–2995; telephone: [973] 625-7101; http://www.selfhelpgroups.org).

SUMMARY

Parents' concerns for support and information will vary from week to week and from parent to parent. Fortunately, the options for support and information mean that parents can choose according to their own concerns and preferences. Unfortunately, sometimes it takes time for parents to find out about all of these options. Informed parents who have had experience in finding services for their children with special needs and support and information for themselves can serve as important resources for parents who are just beginning to find their way. Experienced parents know about professionally directed services as well as about parent-directed services, they know about local, state, and national resources, and they understand the importance of working alongside parents and helping them.

Parent to Parent programs help parents to connect with experienced and informed parents who can tell them about various support options and walk with them as they try them out. In the next several chapters, you will read more about parent to parent support—why it is unique, how it complements other services, and how you can bring the Parent to Parent experience to families in your community, whether you are a parent or a professional.

4

What Is Parent to Parent?

"Although the world is full of suffering,
it is full also of the overcoming of it."

—Helen Keller

Parents often find that a combination of support options helps them address their emotional, informational, and logistical concerns. Thousands of parents also are finding that the one-to-one support that they receive through a Parent to Parent program is especially helpful as they adjust to their child's disability. There are many examples of the kind of support that families receive from their Parent to Parent match.

Supporting parents are seen as reliable allies who immediately understand the situation because they have been through it themselves:

After our daughter was diagnosed with a major heart defect that would require open heart surgery, we were matched with a couple who had a 2-year-old with Down syndrome who had gone through the same surgery. They adopted us as their couple to support. Our daughter had been in hospitals constantly. Our support parents came down to see her in the hospital, called us, and sent letters. The dad even gave blood for our daughter's surgery. They took us out to dinner when our daughter was in intensive care. They came to our daughter's first birthday party. They have become our close friends.

The match provides support that is available 24 hours a day—not just Monday through Friday from 8 A.M. to 5 P.M.:

Without question, my match with my pilot parent was my single most valuable resource since my son was born. She and her husband listened daily to our questions about the immediate and the future and didn't give us too much information, just enough to help us cope at each stage. The value of talking to a parent who is 3–5 years down the road is immeasurable, and I wish that every parent could take advantage of this valuable resource, critical to raising a child with special needs.

Parents who have already learned about the service system can interpret the jargon and help the referred parent find his or her way through what sometimes feels like a maze of service providers, regulations, and forms:

Being directly involved with a supporting parent has given me a lot of information on how to best plan for my child's emotional and educational development and how to facilitate all facets (medical, educational, and emotional) of her development. Without this contact I would be lost in a muddle of misinformation.

Seeing another family with a child who has a disability and is older than their own child gives the referred parents a sense of hope for the future. Because their experiences are similar, parents in a match can be mutually supportive to each other—sharing information and support both ways—so the support is reciprocal:

Seeing another young couple with a happy, typical family and household that happened to include a child with a disability enabled us to see that we could go on with our lives and plans, that the world had not come to an end, and that things were not as bleak as we had feared. Our supporting parents made us feel like we were not horrible for having negative reactions in the beginning to our child's disability. They shared their own experience, and we saw that we were not alone. The whole experience helped us accept the situation, establish plans and goals, and get on with doing everything we could to help our son. Without this contact I am sure that our grieving process would have extended for longer than it actually did.

This chapter introduces you to Parent to Parent programs. Each program has its own story and its own unique characteristics. And yet each program has an underlying commitment to the importance of the match between a supporting parent and a parent who is looking for the emotional and informational support that only another parent can provide. This chapter includes stories from different programs to show you how Parent to Parent developed and how the programs offer one-to-one support to parents who have a family member with a disability. Once you have been introduced to these programs and their characteristics, you will find information in Chapters 5–13 about how to start a Parent to Parent program and develop different program components.

In the Beginning: Pilot Parents Program

A young couple living in Omaha, Nebraska, in the 1960s waited 2 years before their suspicions about their son Dana were confirmed—he did indeed have Down syndrome. They waited 2 more years before they met other parents of children with Down syndrome. Fran, Dana's mother, remembers the fears and frustrations of facing the unknown and the endless questions: Would Dana grow and develop? Would he ever go to school? Could he ever hold a job? And most of all, what was that mysterious label stuck to him—Down syndrome? Dana's family felt isolated because they were certain that no one could understand or empathize with their feelings of anguish and helplessness.

When Dana was 4, Fran met another parent of a child with Down syndrome during a chance meeting in a grocery store. Within minutes Fran realized how much she had been yearning to talk to someone who could understand the doubt, worry, and frustration that she and her husband had been experiencing. It was a new beginning for the family—there were services for Dana and for Fran and her husband. For the first time there was hope.

Fran and her husband joined the Greater Omaha Arc (a branch of The Arc of the United States) and learned all that they could about mental retardation. They met more parents, and over time Fran grew to appreciate how helpful these connections were. In 1970, after attending a series of training sessions given by a psychologist for parents of children with disabilities, Fran realized how much she had learned over the years, from professionals and from other parents who were sharing her journey. She wanted to connect and share her knowledge with parents who were starting out. She yearned to find a way to help parents connect with other parents so that information and emotional support could be easily shared.

At the same time, Shirley, a social worker at the Greater Omaha Arc, came to know Fran. Shirley realized that although she could be helpful to Fran and other parents in many ways, there was one way in which she could not. Because Shirley was not a parent of a child with a disability, she could not provide the kind of support to parents of children with disabilities that other parents could. Fran and Shirley knew that psychologist Wolf Wolfensberger, a leader in the field of services for individuals with mental retardation, shared their beliefs in the value of mutual support among those with similar experiences. An alliance formed around this vision, and the trio spent almost a year developing the Pilot Parents model and planning the first formal Parent to Parent program.

PILOT PARENTS MODEL

The heart of the Pilot Parents model is a one-to-one match between an experienced, trained mentor parent, called the *pilot parent,* and a parent seeking individualized support from another parent who has *been there.* The pilot parent (sometimes called a *supporting parent,* a *veteran parent,* a *resource parent,* or a *visiting parent*) helps to guide the new parents as they begin to deal with the realities of their child's disability. Pilot parents have children with disabilities and are familiar with disability issues. Pilot parents receive training to help them make use of their own experiences in ways that are helpful to referred parents. Pilot parents commit to the program for 1 year, agree to be available to be matched with a new parent, and attend monthly meetings designed to hone their skills as mentors.

Originally the Pilot Parents program served families who had children with mental retardation, but the cofounders realized that the mutual sharing of information and support was beneficial regardless of the disability—as long as the matches could be made based on similar disability and family experiences. By 1974, the Pilot Parents program was training parents whose children had a wide range of disabilities and special health care needs. Funding from the Developmental Disabilities Council of Nebraska allowed the Pilot Parents program to hire its first paid parent coordinator.

GROWTH OF PARENT TO PARENT SUPPORT

The Pilot Parents model was such a success in Nebraska that soon the program was matching hundreds of parents each year. Parents in neighboring states began to hear about the parent matching that was happening in Nebraska and were interested in creating this same opportunity in their communities. In 1975, the Pilot Parents program received a federal grant that allowed them to train parents and professionals who were interested in developing parent support programs in Nebraska, Missouri, Kansas, and Iowa. Within 3 years, 33 new Pilot Parents programs emerged within these four states. Parent to Parent programs based on this model began to spring up in every state in response to the needs of parents for support and information from other parents.

From the single Pilot Parents program in Omaha, the number of Parent to Parent programs has grown to more than 600 local and statewide programs, with at least one in every state. Although each has its own identity, all of these programs have the one-to-one match between a veteran parent and a parent seeking support.

Parent to Parent began serving families in the United States in the early 1970s, and some of the earliest programs (including the Pilot Parents program in Omaha) are still in existence today. Although many programs have been around since 1985 or earlier, more than half of the programs that responded to a national survey in 1995 were less than 6 years old (see Table 4.1 in Appendix A). In many communities Parent to Parent programs are new additions to the set of services available for families.

CHARACTERISTICS OF PARENT TO PARENT PROGRAMS

Parent to Parent programs range in size from very small programs that match a few supporting parents with a few referred parents, to larger programs that match hundreds of supporting and referred parents each year. Most Parent to Parent programs are small, and the greatest percentage provide services to 13–25 referred parents annually (see Table 4.1 in Appendix A).

WHO DOES PARENT TO PARENT SERVE?

Parent to Parent programs serve families who have children with a broad range of physical, intellectual, and emotional disabilities, ongoing medical conditions, and other special health care needs, including those acquired later in life. And although the severity of the disabilities of the children whose parents are participating in Parent to Parent programs varies significantly, more than half of the referred parents who responded to the survey reported their child's disability to be moderate or severe. Generally, the children of parents being matched by Parent to Parent programs have a developmental disability that is moderate or severe (see Tables 4.2 and 4.3 in Appendix A).

Parent to Parent programs also serve parents whose family members with disabilities are at different ages. Although most of the children of referred parents receiving services from a Parent to Parent program are between birth and 6 years old, as Parent to Parent programs and their supporting parents and their children age, more matches are being made for families who have adolescents or young adults with disabilities (see Table 4.4 in Appendix A).

PARENT TO PARENT'S IMPACT

A team of parents and researchers from around the United States conducted a 3-year national study to determine the effectiveness of parent to parent support. Several hundred parents in five states filled out a set of questionnaires at four times during the study (a brief summary about this research appears in Appendix A). Some of these parents were matched right away with a supporting parent who had received at least 8 hours of training. Other parents waited 8 weeks before being matched with a supporting parent. Parents answered questions about how they felt they were coping, how they felt about their situation, how empowered they felt, whether they felt they had social support and a reliable ally, and how much progress they had made in getting their child's needs met.

Simply put, an overwhelming majority of parents find parent to parent support helpful, and this kind of support cannot come from any other source. The more contacts a referred parent has with a supporting parent, the more helpful the match is. Parent to parent support increases parents' acceptance of their situations and their sense of being able to cope. It also helps parents make progress on resolving the need or problem that they or their child had when they first contacted a Parent to Parent program. Because parent to parent support offers a unique form of help to parents of family members with a disability, it needs to be an essential component of a comprehensive family support system. This system provides services to families to support not only the emotional needs described in Chapter 1 but also the logistical and informational needs described in Chapter 2.

ORGANIZATIONAL CHARACTERISTICS OF PARENT TO PARENT PROGRAMS

Parent to Parent programs are sometimes sponsored by another agency (e.g., The Arc, hospital, social services agency) that offers administrative and financial support to the program leaders. Sometimes a Parent to Parent program becomes incorporated as an autonomous not-for-profit agency, giving parent leaders the flexibility to develop the program in directions that they determine. There are advantages and disadvantages to each organizational structure, and you will read more about these in Chapter 7. (Table 4.5 in Appendix A provides information about the sponsorship status of and the types of agencies that sponsor Parent to Parent programs.)

Most programs are directed by parents—underscoring the importance of parent leadership in Parent to Parent. When a Parent to Parent program is independent, directed by a parent, and guided by a board of directors of whom the majority are parents, then ownership of the program belongs to the parents. Chapters 7 and 8 provide you with information for building a strong organizational foundation for your Parent to Parent program.

The level of support and technical assistance available to newly developing programs varies considerably. Some local Parent to Parent programs develop in states that have a statewide Parent to Parent program that provides technical assistance to new local programs. The statewide program may have a manual on program development to share, or parents from the statewide program may assist with the training of supporting parents. Some statewide programs offer annual training for coordinators of local programs. Although there is no doubt that the presence of a statewide Parent to Parent program can be beneficial to a new local program, there also may be program development and implementation guidelines that the statewide program will expect you to respect as you develop your program. In other states a statewide Parent to Parent program does not exist and local programs develop on their own. You will read in Chapter 14 about statewide Parent to Parent programs and the services they provide to families and to coordinators of local programs.

PROGRAM SERVICES

Most smaller and younger Parent to Parent programs concentrate their activities on recruiting and training supporting parents, establishing a referral system, and making and supporting one-to-one parent matches. These activities are the foundation of all Parent to Parent programs, and programs strive to have these activities in place before taking on any additional activities.

Although the majority of Parent to Parent programs offer training to supporting parents before they are matched with another parent, the length and content of this training varies from program to program. As you will read in Chapter 6, the training for parents wishing to be supporting parents provides them with a time to 1) reflect on their own journey and the adjustments they have made along the way, 2) learn specific communication and listening skills, 3) gather information about community resources, 4) consider the role of the supporting parent, and 5) practice using their own experiences and their new information and skills in ways that will be helpful to another parent. In many cases the program director trains the supporting parents, so the training sessions provide the program director with an opportunity to get to know the supporting parents in ways that will be useful when matches are being considered.

Once a pool of trained supporting parents exists, then Parent to Parent programs will work to provide a match for any parent referred to the program, but some may only match parents of infants, parents whose children are in the school district, or parents who have a child with a specific disability. Chapters 5 and 6 provide more information and strategies for bringing a group of trained supporting parents together and matching those supporting parents with other parents looking for support.

Once a foundation has been created for ensuring the availability of trained supporting parents, making parent matches, and supporting matches once they are made, the program leaders add other components based on the needs and preferences of the families participating in the program. Some programs add only one or two program activities (e.g., social events for families, a program newsletter). Other programs grow to be comprehensive family resource centers offering an array of services for all members of the family and for professionals. You will find tips for adding program components in Chapter 10.

PROGRAM STORIES

The following Parent to Parent program stories will help you to understand how and why Parent to Parent programs grow in the directions they do. They begin with a commitment to the importance of individualized and flexible emotional and informational support provided through the parent match. Then the programs work to develop activities that are responsive to the needs of the families served.

Special Care Parents

Special Care Parents is a hospital-based Parent to Parent program in California—a volunteer organization that connects parents who have similar experiences with a high-risk pregnancy or the delivery of a high-risk, medically fragile, or premature infant. Special Care Parents was launched in 1985 by parents whose son spent 11 months in the neonatal intensive care unit (NICU) because they could not find an organization in the Sacramento area in which they could discuss their experiences with other families. Because this period in their lives was one of emotional turmoil and their experiences were incomprehensible to family and friends, the founding parents worked to create a link among parents sharing the NICU experience. Special Care Parents is a nonprofit organization that is not sponsored by a hospital or any agency providing services to families. Its many activities are supported by fundraising efforts, contributions, and grants.

Special Care Parents provides support to families in four hospitals in the region that have NICUs. Babies born prematurely or with special health care needs may be transferred to these institutions from northeastern and central California and northwestern Nevada. Special Care Parents has provided support and information to thousands of families that have experienced their child's early days, weeks, and months in these hospitals.

Special Care Parents' mission is to assist families with the social, emotional, and informational concerns related to having an infant in a NICU. Parents share their experiences and offer support to one another through the Parent to Parent Telephone Network. A parent new to the NICU experience is matched with a trained graduate parent who experienced similar medical problems and concerns. Once a match is made, the number and frequency of contacts are determined by the concerns and preferences of the new parent. For new parents who would like to meet the graduate parent personally, Special Care Parents offers a Hospital Visitation Program that allows trained parent volunteers to talk with new parents at their infant's bedside. New parents also may connect with other parents at monthly support group meetings.

The coordinator of Special Care Parents provides graduate parents with 8 hours of training before they are matched with another parent. During the training the graduate parents recall their own NICU experiences and consider what was helpful and challenging to them. Training also includes communication and listening skill development and strategies for using personal experiences in supportive ways with another parent. Information about the NICU procedures and equipment and other community resources also is an important part of the training for graduate parents. The coordinator of Special Care Parents is available to assist with any aspect of the match once training is complete and the graduate parent is connected with a new parent.

Some of the other services provided by Special Care Parents include a monthly Crib Decoration Program in which the babies' isolettes are decorated with pictures and bows to make the hospital environment seem less sterile and institutional; monthly group meetings with speakers on various topics; a resource library of information on such topics as the NICU experience, prematurity, family support, and community resources; a quarterly newsletter; and information packets for parents and other family members to demystify the NICU, to acknowledge feelings, and to provide resource information. Because many of the parents do not speak English as their first language, Special Care Parents has translated the information packets into Cambodian, Chinese, Hmong, Korean, Lao, Russian, Spanish, and Vietnamese. The availability of multilingual NICU parent packets has meant that families whose first language is not English have a greater understanding of their situation and are better equipped to handle its realities.

Special Care Parents' High Risk Pregnancy Program provides similar supports to families who are experiencing high-risk pregnancy. During the pregnancy, the expectant parent(s) receives support through parent to parent telephone contacts or hospital visits from a graduate parent. Special Care Parents ensures that each family receives a countdown calendar and a packet of information on coping with high-risk pregnancy by distributing these resources through area hospitals and perinatologists.

Special Care Parents is an example of a hospital-based, but not hospital-sponsored, Parent to Parent program that provides informational and emotional support to parents with a high-risk pregnancy or an infant in a NICU. Through one-to-one matches between graduate parents and parents new to the high-risk pregnancy or the NICU experiences, Special Care Parents supports parent connections that otherwise might not occur and facilitates the sharing of perspectives that are unique to the parents' experiences.

Family Support Network of Eastern North Carolina

In 1987, a group of parents and professionals started Family Support Network of Eastern North Carolina to provide parent to parent support for families who have children with special needs or who have experienced the death of a child. Beginning with a grant from the United Way, a part-time coordinator, and a few volunteers, Family Support Network of Eastern North Carolina has evolved into a private, nonprofit agency that has a full-time director, a part-time secretary, 85 trained support parents, and an annual budget of $121,000. Remember, parents are not paid to be supporting parents. Family Support Network of Eastern North Carolina also has benefited from training and technical assistance provided by the statewide Parent to Parent program in North Carolina.

Family Support Network of Eastern North Carolina serves families and professionals in six counties in eastern North Carolina. The main office for the program is located in an evaluation clinic, whereas the second office is in a regional hospital that serves families in 29 eastern North Carolina counties. From these two locations, Family Support Network of Eastern North Carolina serves more than 1,000 families and professionals each year.

Using training materials provided by the statewide Parent to Parent program, the director of Family Support Network of Eastern North Carolina provides small groups of prospective support parents with 12 hours of training. The content of this training includes the history of Parent to Parent, the grieving process, active listening, communication and problem-solving skills, and the role of the support parent. The training sessions are held on Saturdays, and professionals are asked to share their expertise during the training sessions.

Referrals to Family Support Network of Eastern North Carolina come from a variety of sources, but many come from the two agencies where the network's offices are located. Sometimes referrals to Family Support Network of Eastern North Carolina come from the statewide Parent to Parent program. Matches are made for parents who have a child or young adult with any disability, and the staff at Family Support Network of Eastern North Carolina work hard to match a referred parent within 24 to 48 hours of the initial referral. When the disability of the child is rare and a match cannot be found locally or regionally, then the network's staff ask the statewide Parent to Parent program to search its statewide database of support parents to find an appropriate match.

Family Support Network of Eastern North Carolina offers activities and supports above and beyond the one-to-one match to parents and professionals. In response to requests from families and professionals for training in family-centered care (care provided by professionals that views the needs of the family as central and provides services that revolve around those needs), the network hosted the first parent–professional collaboration conference in eastern North Carolina. The network encourages parent and professional presentations at workshops; provides names of parents to speak to local organizations, community colleges, university students, and hospital and medical staff; and chairs an annual legislative breakfast to ensure that families attend and present their stories to the local, state, and federal legislatures.

Other program activities include groups for siblings of children with special needs to share their feelings and experiences and annual picnics and holiday parties to encourage families to develop a support system for themselves in the community. Parents appreciate that they are connected to other parents who can be there to say, "I have been where you are, I have felt those same feelings, I have experienced the same uncertainty, and I am here to walk with you."

Parent to Parent of Northeast Kansas

After several years of offering parent support groups to parents of children with special needs in northeast Kansas, a school social worker, Carrie, began to look for other support that she might offer to parents. Also a parent of an adolescent with a disability, Carrie knew firsthand about the challenges and joys that come with the disability experience and about the importance of flexible parent support. Because Kansas did not have a statewide Parent to Parent program that she could contact for technical assistance in developing a Parent to Parent program, Carrie contacted another local program in Kansas for advice. She recruited a group of parents to work with her to establish Parent to Parent of Northeast Kansas.

The group of parents presented their vision to the special education parent advisory council, school administrators, and members of the school board and then launched Parent to Parent of Northeast Kansas under the sponsorship of the special education cooperative. Carrie's office was home to the fledgling program, and she assumed the role of the program coordinator as a part of her paid position with the special education cooperative.

Parent to Parent of Northeast Kansas designed its training based on an informal needs assessment of the parents who were interested in becoming supporting parents. Sample training materials received from other local programs in Kansas helped to give the group ideas about the content that is included in the training. Six months after the establishment of the program, the first group of supporting parents received 8 hours of training.

Once a core group of supporting parents had been trained, Parent to Parent of Northeast Kansas focused its efforts on letting school district personnel know about the program and its readiness to take requests for matches. With the support of the special education cooperative as the program sponsor, the program leaders found it easy to develop a program brochure, post fliers, speak about the program at in-service training sessions, write articles for school newsletters, and send home announcements with students. A special education teacher made the first referral to the program—a single mother of a 7-year-old boy with cerebral palsy.

For the next 3 years, the program operated successfully out of Carrie's office under the sponsorship of the special education cooperative. Referrals and matches were made for children with a wide range of disabilities who were students in the school district. When a statewide Parent to Parent program was funded in Kansas and stipends became available to local coordinators, Parent to Parent of Northeast Kansas moved into the community and one of its supporting parents became the program coordinator. Once the program became community based, referrals and matches were no longer limited to students in the school district.

You have been introduced to four Parent to Parent programs—the original Pilot Parents program in Omaha and three newer programs. Each of these programs has its own unique characteristics, but each offers support that is one to one, personalized, flexible, community based, and available 24 hours a day. For some parents the match consists of a few contacts by telephone around a specific informational need. For others, the match evolves into a lifelong friendship with the parents (and often the entire family), becoming mutual emotional and informational resources for each other. You will read more about the matched experience in Chapter 5—how matches are made and supported and why the match is a meaningful form of support for the thousands of parents who are participating in Parent to Parent programs in the United States and around the world.

SUPPORTING PROFESSIONALS AND SERVICE PROVIDERS

Many professionals who refer parents to a Parent to Parent program discover how parent to parent support complements their own roles. Service providers have a lot of information that they can and do share with families, but they cannot (unless they also are parents of a family member with a disability) offer parents immediate support that is based on a shared reality and common understandings. Professionals find it comforting to refer a family to a Parent to Parent program. They know that the referred parent will receive emotional support from someone who has had firsthand experience with the same emotions—and they know that the information that families receive from the supporting parents will be shared and interpreted in ways that are not overwhelming. Because service providers usually have many appointments in a single day with little flexibility in their schedule, it is reassuring to know that the families they refer to a Parent to Parent program will receive responsive, flexible, accessible, and individualized support when they need it, rather than by appointment only. Professionals familiar with Parent to Parent programs know that parents will be supported regardless of what the family is facing and that the nature of the support will not be determined by agency guidelines. Here is an example of how Parents Helping Parents in Santa Clara, California, was able to support the efforts of another service provider agency:

Parents Helping Parents

The agency director who was calling me started out apologizing. "I feel terrible calling you. We are a multimillion dollar agency with numerous staff, and we're dealing with another agency in town. I know how small your group is; I'm not sure you can do anything." I interrupted her, pointing out that helping is the middle name of Parents Helping Parents. The director told me about a single mom who was threatening to leave her 13-year-old daughter (who had been diagnosed as having a developmental delay and an emotional disorder) on the doorstep of another service provider agency in town because she couldn't take it any longer. The caller went on to explain that her own agency, by law, could not intervene until the mom had actually taken an inappropriate action. The other agency where the mother was threatening to leave the girl had no placement for the child.

With permission from the mom, we were able to send over a supporting parent to listen to and support her. This support for the mom through our Parents Helping Parents program gave the two agencies the time that they needed to locate an out-of-home placement for the child. When a placement was found, the supporting parent rode with the mom and daughter to transfer the daughter there so that the mom would not have to drive back home alone. This mom needed Parents Helping Parents while she had her daughter with her, and she also needed it as she let go. The professionals involved in this situation needed a different kind of support than what either agency provided—the support that another parent can give. And, they needed another agency with flexibility enough to provide the parent some immediate help while they worked through their processes for providing services.
A Parent to Parent program worked ideally in this situation.

When service providers who work with individuals with disabilities and their families collaborate with a Parent to Parent program in their communities, they find that their own capacity to support families is enhanced. Parent to parent support expands the options that agencies can offer to parents. When parents come to agencies, they are seeking different kinds of services. When parents mention an interest in talking with another parent or when it seems that this opportunity might be helpful, providers are able to refer parents to a Parent to Parent program. A school administrator shared the following:

When the Parent to Parent program was established, we knew that it would be helpful for families, but we didn't realize until later that it would also be helpful to our staff. As professionals, we often feel inadequate because we cannot understand what families are going through because we haven't actually experienced what they have. Our staff became aware that the Parent to Parent program could fulfill a need for families that they could not. In this way the Parent to Parent program supports the professional as well as the family.

SUMMARY

Many parents and professionals live in a community that has a Parent to Parent program, and it provides support to parents and contributes to the overall quality of the professional services that are available to families. If you find that there is not a local Parent to Parent program in your area, you can make a difference by leading or joining an effort to start a local program. You will find the how-to information that you will need to develop a Parent to Parent program in the next several chapters. There are many resources available to help emerging Parent to Parent programs. Parent to Parent program directors are eager to share resources and their recommended practices with those who want to start a program. All that is needed is the leadership of at least one parent who has a family member with special needs and is committed to the success of the program. When there is a group of parents working together to develop the program and perhaps a service provider who believes in the importance of a parent-directed Parent to Parent program, then the effort will be even easier.

RESOURCES

Ainbinder, J., Blanchard, L., Singer, G.H.S., Sullivan, M., Powers, L., Marquis, J., & Santelli, B. (1998). How parents help one another: A qualitative study of Parent to Parent self-help. *Journal of Pediatric Psychology, 23,* 99–109.

Santelli, B., Singer, G.H.S., DiVenere, N., Ginsberg, C., & Powers, L. (1998). Participatory action research: Reflections on critical incidents in a PAR project. *Journal of The Association for Persons with Severe Handicaps, 23*(3), 211–222.

Santelli, B., Turnbull, A., & Higgins, C. (1996). Parent to Parent support and health care. *Pediatric Nursing, 23*(3), 303–306.

Santelli, B., Turnbull, A., Lerner, E., & Marquis, J. (1993). Parent to Parent programs: A unique form of mutual support to families of persons with disabilities. In G.H.S. Singer & L.E. Powers (Eds.), *Families, disability, and empowerment: Active coping skills and strategies for family interventions* (pp. 27–57). Baltimore: Paul H. Brookes Publishing Co.

Santelli, B., Turnbull, A., Marquis, J., & Lerner, E. (1993). Parent to Parent programs: Ongoing support for parents of young adults with special needs. *Journal of Vocational Rehabilitation, 3*(2), 25–37.

Santelli, B., Turnbull, A., Marquis, J., & Lerner, E. (1995). Parent to Parent programs: A unique form of mutual support. *Infants and Young Children, 8*(2), 48–57.

Santelli, B., Turnbull, A., Marquis, J., & Lerner, E. (1997). Parent to Parent programs: A resource for parents and professionals. *Journal of Early Intervention, 21*(1), 73–83.

Santelli, B., Turnbull, A., Marquis, J., & Lerner, E. (2000). Statewide Parent to Parent programs: Partners in early intervention. *Infants and Young Children, 13*(1), 74–88.

Santelli, B., Turnbull, A., Sergeant, J., Lerner, E., & Marquis, J. (1996). Parent to Parent programs: Parent preferences for support. *Infants and Young Children, 9*(1), 53–62.

Singer, G.H.S., Marquis, J., Powers, L., Blanchard, L., DiVenere, N., Santelli, B., & Sharp, M. (1999). A multi-site evaluation of Parent to Parent programs for parents of children with disabilities. *Journal of Early Intervention, 22*(3), 217–229.

III

Starting and Developing a Parent to Parent Program

5

Matching Parents

The Heart of Parent to Parent

"It is when we try to grapple with another man's intimate need that we perceive how incomprehensible, wavering, and misty are the beings that share with us the sight of the stars and the warmth of the sun."

—Joseph Conrad

Parent to parent support grew out of a need that parents of children with special needs have to connect with parents who have children with similar needs. We all sometimes feel this need to share experiences with and receive support from others who have had similar experiences to our own. People are comforted when they can connect with someone else who understands their situation. In Parent to Parent programs, the connections between parents are one-to-one, and the matches are made carefully so that the support is personalized.

What happens in a parent to parent match that makes it helpful? In this chapter, Catherine and W.C., who were introduced in Chapter 1, tell you more about their match with Jean. You will learn why the support they received from Jean was different from, but also complementary to, all the supports they received from professionals, family, and friends. This chapter introduces key strategies for making the best possible parent to parent matches and for following each match to be sure that the experience is comfortable and productive for both matched parents. There are resources available from Parent to Parent programs to help you establish your own referral and match activities and provide parent to parent support in your community. You will find information about some of these resources at the end of the chapter.

CONNECTING WITH ANOTHER PARENT

Some families are connected with another parent shortly after they learn of their child's disability or special needs. Catherine and W.C.'s match with Jean happened right after their son was born and provided them with emotional and informational support that was tailored to their needs.

Catherine and W.C. Meet Jean

When I held our beautiful boy in that hospital room after the neonatal specialist confirmed the diagnosis of Down syndrome, I felt lost and overwhelmed. We had no knowledge of whether he was physically healthy, and we had no previous experience with an infant with special needs. The nurse gave us a stack of literature in a folder. As we read, we began to wonder: How serious would our son's delays be? Would he be excluded by other people? Would he feel left out? Would people think he was capable of less than he actually was? Would his friends, his teachers, and others accept him with a clean slate? All these thoughts, emotions, and questions flooded our minds.

We had friends come by with words of encouragement and hugs and kisses. It was the strangest sensation that even though we were feeling lost, none of these kind visitors could give us a road map with directions for navigating through this. What we really needed was a personal guide—someone who once was as lost as we were now feeling. And that is what Jean was to us.

How did we connect with Jean? A neonatal specialist who knew about The Family Connection of South Carolina asked us if he could contact them on our behalf. Because the neonatal specialist had met with The Family Connection staff and heard stories about families who had been matched, he had an understanding of parent to parent support and believed in its importance. He also knew what to do to make a referral on our behalf—first obtain our permission and then call The Family Connection. Not knowing what to expect of this referral but at the same time looking for anything we thought might make our lives easier, we gave our approval. The Family Connection found a match for us that day.

Although we didn't realize it at the time, the process that The Family Connection used to match us with Jean was a careful one. When the neonatal specialist called The Family Connection, he spoke with the referral coordinator and shared general information about our family—Karl was our first child, he had Down syndrome but there were no other medical issues, W.C. and I were in our thirties and had careers, and we both wanted to talk to another parent who had a child with Down syndrome. The referral coordinator used this information to check the Family Connection database of trained supporting parents to find the best match for us. Jean called our hospital room later that day. She introduced herself to us as a support parent and told us that she had a son who had Down syndrome. She asked if she could stop by. Although it was the end of a long day and we weren't sure that we wanted to meet her, we knew that she had experienced a day like ours when her son was born. That made her different from the others who had come to visit, and that made the difference.

When she came I remember acting cool toward her—after all I didn't know this woman. Could she help us? She looked normal, but how could she be? Yet I know on that day I had more in common with this woman than with any of our other visitors. She remembered the confusion, the fear, the loneliness, and the sense of being lost. And yet she knew her way around.

Jean briefly told us about her son, who was 7 years old. We asked about his birth, his life, and his future. She described him as quick, active, and a lover of T-ball. She showed us pictures, and everyone looked happy. For the first time we had hope that our family could go on and do things that typical families do.

When Jean left she promised to give us a call in a day or two to see if there was anything she could do. She left us her telephone number in case we wanted to call her. She called us several times to see how we were doing. It seemed as though she would call at the right time—like the day we got Karl's official diagnosis from the geneticist. She listened and understood. That was what we needed.

Over the next several months, our appreciation of Jean and her family grew. Jean continued to encourage us through her telephone calls and visits, and she helped us connect with the organizations that could provide Karl with the early intervention services that he needed. Over the course of the last several years, we have had at least 30 contacts with Jean. Now that Karl is 5, we don't connect with her as much. But we know that she is a telephone call away.

WHY MATCHES WORK

Catherine and W.C. were part of a parent to parent match that worked for them. They, like many parents who are matched with a supporting parent, feel that the success of the matched experience depends on how much the supporting parent feels like a *reliable ally*—someone they can count on no matter what. Whether the supporting parent is seen as a reliable ally depends on three components:

- Similarities, or a sense of sameness, between the parents and their children with special needs and their situations
- Around-the-clock availability of support
- Support that flows both ways

Sense of Sameness

A sense of sameness is the basic principle of self-help support, and in Parent to Parent this sense of sameness is established because the support parent has experienced the same challenges as the referred parent. Referred parents consider this sense of sameness to be the most important and distinguishing feature in a match. Shared experiences facilitate a fuller understanding and a greater acceptance of thoughts and actions without judgment. When the referred parent discovers that the supporting parent *has been in his or her shoes,* a unique connection is established.

You realize that you're not alone dealing with problems. You have someone there who has similar experiences and understands. The common thread is your child and the problems that he or she has and how you cope with them.

Parents also find that the act of comparing their situation with another person's similar situation is helpful. Parents are relieved to find someone with whom they can compare their lives—someone whose similar experiences prove that there is nothing abnormal about their own situation. When the supporting parent's child has more challenges than the referred parent's child, the referred parent may gain a new perspective on his or her own child's disability.

Another benefit for parents comparing their own situations is feeling hopeful about the future. When the supporting parent's child is older than the referred parent's child, the supporting parent is a window to the future and helps the referred parent anticipate future events and feel optimistic about them.

It's reassuring, you know. My son doesn't walk yet but my supporting parent helps me see that there is light at the end of the tunnel.

Hearing family stories and experiences of a supporting parent also helps referred parents learn about practical parenting tips, links with other support services, and information about their child's disability. For parents, gaining ideas and information from a supporting parent leads to better management of day-to-day challenges.

I take my child to behavior specialists . . . and it's good to talk to them, but they don't have to deal with my child and her problems every day. A parent going through similar circumstances can tell you how they handled something. You aren't going to get that from a doctor.

Availability of Support

Having a supporting parent who is easily accessible adds to the effectiveness of parent to parent matches. Although only a few contacts may actually occur, referred parents have an ongoing sense that the supporting parent can be called on if needed. This sense of availability gives referred parents a feeling of control and security. One parent shared her relief.

That really lightened the load for me. If I didn't feel confident in going to someone else, I knew that I could always pick up the telephone and call my support parent.

Mutuality of Support

Parent to Parent programs promote equal relationships between supporting parents and referred parents. Unlike the relationship between a parent and a professional, the parents in a parent to parent match share a similar background. Both parents have learned through life experiences and are experts in their child's care. There often is reciprocity in the support that occurs in a match. Parents say that giving support is as important and helpful to them as receiving support.

She just tries to help me out. . . . If she's having a bad day, I'll try to help her out. . . . She'll call me one week, or I might call her one week. We just take turns calling each other and checking up on the kids and the family. . . . It makes me feel so good to help people because that's the way it should be in life—people helping people.

Once a match has been made, the relationship offers parents a range of emotional and informational supports. Most important, matches offer the presence of a reliable ally—someone to listen and understand.

The light at the end of our tunnel came in the form of Nancy, our supporting parent. She had encountered all that we were facing, and she listened with a sensitive ear. Her own experiences meant that she understood every-

thing I was feeling, and when I needed to vent, she was a patient sounding board. She always answered my never-ending questions, and when I needed someone to cry with, Nancy was there.

Supporting parents also provide information to referred parents through the match, such as information about the disability, community resources, caring for a family member with a disability, insurance issues, eligibility requirements for services and financial assistance, and finding a baby sitter. Often information is shared as the supporting parent helps the referred parent think through the steps that need to be taken on behalf of the child with special needs.

When I was first learning about early intervention services for my daughter and was asked to decide what we wanted for her, I realized that I had no frame of reference at all for making these decisions. I didn't know what questions I should be asking. Fortunately, my supporting parent did, and without recommending specific service providers or programs, she helped me understand what to look for and what to consider as we made our decisions.

A high percentage of parents found that a match with a veteran parent provided them with someone to listen and understand; someone to give them information about their child's disability, community resources, and caring for a child with a disability; someone to help them with referrals to other agencies; and someone to provide problem-solving support (see Table 5.1 in Appendix A).

MAKING PARENT MATCHES

How do parents get matched so that they can begin to benefit? Catherine and W.C. were lucky. The neonatal specialist at the hospital where Karl was born knew that The Family Connection could offer a parent to parent match and mentioned this opportunity to Catherine and W.C. The call from the neonatal specialist to The Family Connection launched the matching process. Parents find parent to parent support in different ways. Some see a flier in a waiting room and contact the program on their own, others hear about Parent to Parent from another parent or a friend. If the child's diagnosis is made when the child is in school, perhaps the referral comes from a teacher. Ensuring that all potential referral sources know about the program and how to make a referral is critical.

Fostering Referrals

An essential step in the match process that needs to occur before referrals are made is ensuring that those most likely to make the referrals know about the program. Parent to Parent programs receive the greatest percentage of referrals from medical personnel (e.g., doctors, nurses) and early intervention services providers. As programs consider referral sources to whom they will target awareness efforts, they should keep these percentages in mind. Your own experiences with parents and providers in your community also will help you to know which individuals and agencies are likely to refer parents to your program. You will want to be sure that these community contacts have the information that they need about your program so that they can tell parents about it and refer parents to it.

Once you have identified likely referral sources, you will need to consider how you will get the word out to these sources, particularly to parents. A program brochure placed in settings where parents who have children with disabilities visit (e.g., clinics, early intervention programs, schools, community recreation programs) will make it easier for parents to refer themselves. Share information about the program and publicize the telephone number for your program widely in your promotional literature. Be sure to list contact information in the telephone book as well. Parent to Parent programs have developed strategies and resources for getting the word out about their programs, and you will find more ideas for promoting a Parent to Parent program in Chapter 11.

Getting professionals to refer parents to a Parent to Parent program is a challenge, even with an aggressive public relations effort. Some professionals don't understand the unique support that one parent can provide to another, and they may hang on to fears that parents are going to do or say something wrong. They may feel that a supporting parent should not be trying to offer support without training to do so, not realizing that supporting parents are trained and as parents themselves are uniquely qualified.

Other challenges have more to do with professional realities than with professional attitudes. High staff turnover in the helping professions means that even when a Parent to Parent program has established a strong referral link with an agency, this connection may evaporate if the key staff person leaves that agency. Then the Parent to Parent program must build that link all over again with a different contact. Moreover, some professionals worry that they will be breaking some kind of client–professional privilege or confidentiality if they refer a parent to a Parent to Parent program. This concern is unfounded because Parent to Parent programs do not accept referrals without the permission of the parent who is being referred.

Once you have informed the potential referral sources about your program and services, be sure that you have a system for responding to those who contact your program to request a match. Because first contacts with a Parent to Parent program are usually via telephone, you will want to lay the groundwork so that this first contact feels comfortable, friendly, and supportive. Sometimes parents call a Parent to Parent program themselves, so it is important to have a parent respond to incoming calls. The contact may be the first one that a self-referring parent has with another parent who also has a child with a disability. For these parents, parent to parent support begins with this first telephone call. Reaching out to a Parent to Parent program to request a match may not be easy to do, and having a parent answer the telephone will increase the comfort level of parents who contact your program.

Although Parent to Parent program coordinators may prefer not to have an answering machine or a voice mail respond to telephone inquiries, these devices are better than having a call go unanswered. With a messaging service, callers will at least have an opportunity to leave their name and telephone number. Be sure that your program has the resources to be responsive to incoming calls and to return calls in a timely manner. The impressions that first-time callers form about your program at the initial contact may determine whether they participate.

MAKING THE BEST MATCH

Matching a referred parent with a supporting parent is the heart of Parent to Parent programs, and the success of the match determines the quality of support the referred parent receives from the Parent to Parent program.

Considering Family Characteristics

Because matches tend to be more successful when there are common family characteristics between the supporting parent and the referred parent, programs gather and consider the following information from a parent seeking a match:

- Age and sex of the child with a disability
- Nature and severity of the child's disability
- Members of the family as defined by the parent—the parent(s), siblings, and extended family members and their ages
- The structure of the family (e.g., biological parents, single parent, foster parents, adoptive parents)
- Geographic location—where the family lives and in which school district
- Primary language spoken
- Issues of greatest concern (e.g., impending surgery, the transition to preschool, Medicaid waiver, behavioral issues)

Parent to Parent programs use as many of these factors as possible to determine an appropriate match between a referred parent and a supporting parent. The factor that most influences the match is a similarity in the disability of the child—simply because most parents want to be matched with a veteran parent whose child has the same disability as their own child.

Considering Personal Characteristics

Whenever possible, Parent to Parent programs strive to match parents around similar personal characteristics as well. Interviews with referred parents suggest that aside from disability and family characteristics, the quality of the parent match is enhanced if their supporting parents have similar personal characteristics. These individual and personal characteristics and styles may be more difficult for Parent to Parent program staff to be aware of than other factors, such as disability of the child, but they are important to consider when making parent matches.

Similar Personality

Parents who are outgoing and extroverted will appreciate being matched with a supporting parent who is more social. As their match evolves they may find it easier to spend time together in social settings or community activities because of their similar personalities. A parent who is quiet and reflective will probably feel more comfortable with a supporting parent who is also more introverted. They can begin to get to know each other around shared preferences. Some Parent to Parent programs gather information about personal interests or hobbies from supporting parents and referred parents so that these factors can be taken into account when matches are made.

Similar Philosophy About Parenting

Parents have their own style of parenting and their own beliefs about their role in the lives of their children. A parent's philosophy about parenting comes from a variety of sources—parenting styles of family and friends, books about parenting, classes on parenting skills, or cultural influences. There is no one correct philosophy about parenting, and parents feel strongly about raising their children according to their own beliefs and values. Some parents value a structured approach to parenting—one based on routine and well-defined consequences. Others may be more laid back and less structured. When a supporting parent and a referred parent have a similar philosophy about parenting, the emotional and informational support around child-rearing issues is more compatible.

Similar Communication Style

In the same way people have different personality characteristics, everyone has his or her own style of communication. Although there are communication skills that can be learned (see Chapter 6), everyone's communication style is unique. Some people are naturally talkative and can keep a conversation going with little input from others. They find it easy to talk to anyone in any setting. Others have a quieter communication style, perhaps preferring to listen and respond rather than initiate a conversation. Although referred parents express a preference for being matched with a supporting parent whose communication style is similar to their own, a naturally talkative supporting parent who is matched with a conversational referred parent will need to recognize their similar styles and be able to take on the role of the reflective listener. A quiet supporting parent who is matched with a referred parent whose communication style is reactive may have to make more of an effort to lead the conversation and create a comfortable environment for the referred parent to talk.

Similar Attitudes About Disability and Expectations for Their Child

Most people are not aware of their own attitudes about disability until they have an opportunity to interact with individuals with disabilities—either as a parent, family member, friend, or service provider. Most people have had little or no experience with children or adults with a disability, so they have no frame of reference on which to base their attitudes and expectations. One of the reasons that parents feel scared and confused when they find out that their child has a disability is that they don't know what to expect or they may be basing their expectations on their worst fears. Supporting parents have an opportunity to educate a new parent and model a positive attitude about disability. A new parent who is matched with a supporting parent who sees the child first and the disability as secondary may gain a new perspective on disability.

Supporting parents offer a new parent courage to have hope for the future. For example, in the area of *self-determination,* a movement that strives to include individuals with disabilities in the planning of their lives (e.g., education, housing, employment, social activities) in the same way that individuals without disabilities are included in these plans, supporting parents can help other parents feel comfortable with the concept. Parents may have different attitudes about self-determination that are based on their own interpretations of disability, their expectations for their child with special needs, and cultural views on independence and autonomy. Program coordinators will be able to make compatible matches when they have an awareness of the supporting and referred parents' expectations and their attitudes about disability.

Generally, the more the veteran parent and the referred parent have in common, the easier it is for them to relate to each other. This seems true not only for obvious factors, such as the disability of the child, but also for less obvious factors, such as personality. In order to ensure a compatible match, Parent to Parent coordinators take time during the referral process to get to know the referred parent. Maryellen Sullivan, Director of Parent to Parent of New Hampshire, stated,

There are no hard and fast rules for making matches. When I am getting a referral or speaking with a parent calling for him- or herself, I listen for clues and for hard facts. The clues help me know a little about the parent's personality and expectations—those qualities that are difficult to match. The hard facts help me match the disability and age of the child as well as the issues that the family is dealing with right now. Sometimes initial telephone calls with a referred parent end up being long, particularly when I am talking to parents who have not had a chance to share their story with another parent. I appreciate the longer calls because they give me a better opportunity to get to know the parent. Sometimes a possible match will pop into my mind as we are talking. Some supporting parents I know well; others I have spoken with briefly. The better I know the referred parent and the supporting parent I am considering for the match, the more confident I am that the match will be a success.

Issue-Based Factors

Parent to Parent programs also match parents around similar issues that have been or will need to be addressed. For example, parents may have questions about their child's impending heart surgery and can be matched with a supporting parent whose child has undergone the same procedure. Another parent may be about to request a due process hearing about the educational programming for his or her child, and the opportunity to be matched with another parent who has had this same experience will be supportive and informative. Maryellen continued:

One of our matches involved a parent whose 18-month-old was temporarily disabled with a broken femur [upper leg bone]. The parent asked where she could borrow or rent a car seat that would accommodate the child and his cast. Then she asked if there was anyone she could speak with about caring for the cast, keeping it clean, and keeping her toddler clean because the cast nearly reached his lower ribs. No one came to mind as I was speaking with her, and I knew there was no one in the network whose toddler had had a broken leg. But I did know someone whose child had been in a similar cast and who had dealt with the hygiene of the cast and body for weeks. It turned out to be a great match.

Parent to Parent programs honor the preferences of parents about the factors they hope will be considered in their matches. The top factors considered when making a parent match are similarity in the child's disability and in family issues. Additional factors that should be considered but were rated as less important by programs and parents are 24-hour availability of the supporting parent, similarity in age of children, proximity of referred and supporting parents, and similarity in family structure, cultural background, parents' age, education, and income levels. See Table 5.2 in Appendix A that describes the factors that are used by Parent to Parent programs to match referred parents, the percentage of programs that use each factor in making parent matches, and the factors that parents prefer to have considered in their match. Because the preferences of referred parents vary, talk with the referred parent (or the person making the referral on behalf of the parent) about the parent's personal preferences to ensure a good match.

DOCUMENTING INFORMATION FOR MAKING MATCHES

Similar information also is available on parents who have been trained and are available to be matched as supporting parents, so matching around several factors is possible. Some of the larger statewide Parent to Parent programs are using computers to store information about referred parents and supporting parents, and many of these programs have developed their own software that allows them to make matches by computer. (A list of statewide programs can be found in Appendix C.)

It is not necessary, of course, to use technology if your program does not have a computer. You can keep track of this information through traditional paper-and-pencil methods. This information can be organized by using a notebook or note card system. Pages can be included in a notebook (or index cards in a shoebox) in alphabetical order according to a specific issue (e.g., educational assessment, Medicaid waiver), a specific disability (e.g., autism, learning disability), or a specific concern a family might have (e.g., upcoming individualized education program [IEP] meeting). Listed below the topic are the names, telephone numbers, and addresses of supporting parents who are experienced in that topic. Under the name of each supporting parent is a line to record the name of a referred parent he or she is supporting to ensure that a supporting parent is not involved in multiple matches. Most programs have developed systems and forms to record information for referred parents and supporting parents. These forms include demographic and descriptive information, such as parent(s) name, address, and telephone number; the child's name, date of birth, and disability;

siblings and ages; ethnic background; primary language spoken at home; family structure (including extended family members involved in the child's care); and family issues for which support is requested (see Figures 5.1 and 5.2).

AVAILABILITY OF THE SUPPORTING PARENT

Once a supporting parent is identified, the referral coordinator calls the prospective supporting parent about the opportunity to participate in a match. The referral coordinator shares all of the available information about the referred parent. It is important for supporting parents to have a feel for the nature of the match before accepting. Because participating in a match with a referred parent is a gift of time, the referral coordinator asks the supporting parent whether the timing of the potential match is suitable for his or her own family life. Supporting parents are encouraged to be mindful of their own needs and not to take on a match if there are activities in their own lives that need attention first.

Because Parent to Parent programs strive to make matches within 24 to 48 hours of the referral, the supporting parent also is asked to consider whether they will be able to contact the referred parent within the next few days. Supporting parents are reassured that turning down a match opportunity is acceptable for any reason. If the feel of the match and the timing of the match are comfortable for the supporting parent, then the match is made.

LAUNCHING THE MATCH

Once a supporting parent agrees to participate in the match, every effort is made to contact the referred parent within 24 to 48 hours of the referral. Parent to Parent programs are committed to the idea that timely responsiveness to a parent who is seeking support is essential. More than half of local Parent to Parent programs nationally reported that the first contact occurs within 24 to 48 hours of referral to the program; the vast majority of programs indicated that the first contact happens within a week of the initial referral (see Tables 5.3 and 5.4 in Appendix A).

Generally, the initial contact between a supporting parent and a referred parent is by telephone, but sometimes the two parents actually meet during this first contact. Some hospital-based Parent to Parent programs encourage supporting parents to stop by the hospital room for the initial visit. In other instances, the referred parent may have spoken with the referral coordinator and given permission for a supporting parent to come visit right away.

Referred Family Information Form

Referred by ______________________ Date ______________________

Matched to ______________________ Date ______________________

Family information

Name ____

Address ____

Telephone (home) (___) ______________ (work) (___) ______________

Occupation/employer ____

Interests/hobbies ____

Language(s) spoken other than English ______________________________

Relation to child ____

Partner's name ____

Address ____

Telephone (home) (___) ______________ (work) (___) ______________

Occupation/employer ____

Interests/hobbies ____

Language(s) spoken other than English ______________________________

Relation to child ____

Marital status ☐ single ☐ married ☐ separated ☐ divorced ☐ widowed

Names of children	Date of birth	Sex

Figure 5.1. Referred parent form. (Courtesy of Parent to Parent of Virginia.)

Figure 5.1. *(continued)*

Child with disability

Name ________________________________

Nature of disability ________________________________

Age of child at time of diagnosis ________________________________

Special concerns

____

____

____

Other information related to match

____

____

____

Release of information

Parent to Parent has my permission to release my name and telephone number to another parent for a parent match.

________________________	____________
signature	date

Parent to Parent has my permission to release the information on this form to the following Parent to Parent networks (please check all that apply)

- ☐ Parent to Parent local network
- ☐ Parent to Parent statewide network
- ☐ Parent to Parent nationwide network
- ☐ Other

________________________	____________
signature	date

Notes/Remarks

Date	
________	________________________
________	________________________
________	________________________
________	________________________
________	________________________

Supporting Parent Information Form

Referred by ______________________ Date ______________________

Matched to ______________________ Date ______________________

Family Information

Name ____

Address ____

Telephone (home) (___) ______________ (work) (___) ______________

Occupation/employer ____

Interests/hobbies ____

Language(s) spoken other than English ______________________________

Relation to child ____

Partner's name ____

Address ____

Telephone (home) (___) ______________ (work) (___) ______________

Occupation/employer ____

Interests/hobbies ____

Language(s) spoken other than English ______________________________

Relation to child ____

Marital status ☐ single ☐ married ☐ separated ☐ divorced ☐ widowed

Names of children	**Date of birth**	**Sex**

Figure 5.2. Supporting parent form. (Courtesy of Parent to Parent of Virginia.)

Figure 5.2. *(continued)*

Child with disability

Name ______________________________

Nature of disability ______________________________

Age of child at time of diagnosis ______________________________

Special issues/expertise (use space below and/or attached checklist)

____

____

____

Other information to consider in a match

____

____

____

Release of information

Parent to Parent has my permission to release my name and telephone number to another parent for a parent match.

______________________________ ______________

signature date

Parent to Parent has my permission to release the information on this form to the following Parent to Parent networks (please check all that apply)

☐ Parent to Parent local network

☐ Parent to Parent statewide network

☐ Parent to Parent nationwide network

☐ Other

______________________________ ______________

signature date

Notes/Remarks

Date

__________ ______________________________

__________ ______________________________

__________ ______________________________

__________ ______________________________

__________ ______________________________

Figure 5.2. *(continued)*

The following is a checklist that will help us make the best match possible. Please check all items that best describe your child, including past and present.

Degree of Disability:

Mild O Severe O

Moderate O Unknown O

Mobility:	PRESENT	PAST
Delayed	O	O
Normal for Age	O	O
Walks Independently	O	O
Crawls, Scoots	O	O
Wheelchair Self-Operated	O	O
Wheelchair with Assistance	O	O
Walks with Supportive Devices	O	O

Speech:		
Delayed	O	O
Clear & Understandable	O	O
Difficult to Understand	O	O
Not Understandable	O	O
Nonverbal Communication	O	O
Augmentative Communication	O	O
Does Not Communicate	O	O
Sign Language	O	O

Vision:		
Normal Vision	O	O
Corrective Lenses	O	O
Partial Loss	O	O
No Vision	O	O

Diet/Eating Skills:	PRESENT	PAST
Regular Diet	O	O
Special Diet	O	O
No Help Needed	O	O
Some Help Needed	O	O
Fed by Others	O	O
Feeding Tube	O	O
Gastrostomy Tube	O	O
Feeding Problems	O	O

Behavior:		
Typical for Age	O	O
Overactive	O	O
Underactive	O	O
Aggressive	O	O

Treatments:		
Physical Therapy	O	O
Occupational Therapy	O	O
Speech Therapy	O	O
Chemotherapy	O	O
Radiation Therapy	O	O
Lovaas Therapy	O	O
Auditory Training	O	O
Patterning	O	O
Vision Therapy	O	O
ECMO	O	O

Other (list): ______________________

____

Figure 5.2. *(continued)*

Hearing:

Normal Hearing	O	O
Hearing Aid	O	O
Partial Loss	O	O
No Hearing	O	O
Cochlear Implant	O	O

Toilet Skills:

Normal for Age	O	O
Some Help Needed	O	O
Not Trained	O	O
Catheterization	O	O

Special Conditions/Equipment:

Apnea Monitor	O	O
Colostomy	O	O
Computer	O	O
Heart Monitor	O	O
IV	O	O
Oxygen	O	O
Shunt	O	O
Suction	O	O
Tracheostomy	O	O
Ventilator	O	O

Other (list): ______________________

____

Type of School/Program (circle):

Not Attending	Regular Child Care
Special Child Care	Early Intervention
Regular Preschool	Special Ed Preschool
Regular Class	Self-Contained Class
Resource Room	Psychoeducational Class
Public School	Private School
Home School	

Special Education Classification:

____

____

____

Special Schools/Programs Attended (list):

____

____

____

Hospitalization/Surgery:

Surgery/Procedure	Hospital
______________	______________
______________	______________

Medication (list):

____

____

____

Doctors Used:

Name	Specialty	City
______________	______________	______________
______________	______________	______________
______________	______________	______________

Knowledge/Expertise in the Following:

Inclusion O Adoption O Insurance O ADA O

Breast Feeding O Genetics O School Advocacy O

O Others ______________________________________

Follow-up contacts occur based on the needs and preferences of the referred parent and the schedules of the veteran parent and the referred parent. These contacts may be made by telephone or in person, and as more parents have access to home computers, contacts between referred parents and supporting parents also are happening via e-mail.

Some Parent to Parent matches are short term and consist of a few contacts over a few weeks, whereas others evolve into lifelong relationships. Although programs reported that 41% of matches last between 1 and 6 months, each match follows its own path, with the timing of the contacts and length of the match being determined by what best meets the needs of the referred parent. The beauty of parent to parent matches is that each is different and uniquely responsive to the needs of the referred parent (see Tables 5.5 and 5.6 in Appendix A).

Generally, the more contacts a referred parent receives from a supporting parent, the more satisfied the referred parent is with the match. Supporting parents should try to arrange a minimum of four contacts during the first 8 weeks of the match. It is important, however, for supporting parents to recognize that each match will be unique and that the number of contacts preferred by one parent may be different from that preferred by another parent. As you will read in Chapter 6, the training sessions for parents who wish to be supporting parents recommend that supporting parents talk with referred parents about the nature, timing, and frequency of contacts that will be most helpful.

FOLLOW-UP SUPPORT FOR THE MATCH

Once the program coordinator has made the match between a referred parent and a supporting parent, the evolution of the match (including the frequency and number of contacts) is left up to the parents. The program coordinator, however, remains an important resource. Ideally, the referred and supporting parents know that if there is a need for assistance (e.g., information, a referral for additional support, an additional match, a rematch), the program coordinator can be called on for help. Because research suggests that referred parent satisfaction with the matched experience depends on the family, personal factors on which the match is made, and on the number of contacts the referred parent receives, many Parent to Parent programs are building in follow-up activities to ensure that the match is going well.

Initial Follow-Up Activities

One follow-up activity involves the program coordinator calling the referred parent and the supporting parent several times to offer any information or support that may be needed. Such follow-up calls to the support parent and the new parent are important to be sure that the match actually took place and that contacts are occurring. These follow-up calls are sometimes known as *HAT calls* because they are social calls to ask, "**H**ow **a**re **t**hings?" HAT calls give the program coordinator a chance to evaluate how things are going in the match and to determine whether a new or different match is needed. Often HAT calls are made about 2 weeks after a match is made and again at 6 weeks and 3 months from the start of the match. Program coordinators also use HAT calls to share new resources or information with either parent and to answer any questions that come up. Maryellen Sullivan, Director of Parent to Parent of New Hampshire, stated,

I used to think that I was muddying the waters by calling back each parent. I worried that these follow-up calls might be intrusive and that the supporting parents would feel that I was checking up on them. I also was concerned that referred parents would be confused by my calls and begin to consider me their supporting parent. But every now and then I would learn that for some reason contacts had not been happening even though I thought the match had been launched. Perhaps the supporting parent misplaced the referred parent's telephone number or was dealing with an unexpected family need. Whatever the reason, it was important for me to know and to do whatever was necessary to facilitate those contacts. These follow-up calls give me the information that I need to know—that the match has occurred. Now I find that both the supporting parent and the referred parent appreciate hearing from me, and they like knowing that I care.

Ongoing Follow-Up Activities

Some programs use a set of reminder and follow-up postcards to facilitate contacts, particularly early in the match. A reminder postcard sent to a matched supporting parent encourages a first contact if one has not been made. Reminder postcards also may be used to encourage successive contacts. In some programs, supporting parents receive follow-up postcards to use to let the program coordinator know about contacts as they are made and the outcome of those contacts. Some programs provide logs that supporting parents can use to keep track of their contacts and any follow-up activities that need to occur (see Figures 5.3 and 5.4).

Follow-Up with Referral Source Activities

It also is important to follow up with the person who helped connect the referred parent to your Parent to Parent program—to thank them for their referral and to let them know the outcome of their effort on behalf of the family. This contact can be by telephone, postcard, or letter,

Telephone Log for Supporting Parents

Name of parent seeking support ______________________________

Address ______________________________

Telephone (home) (___) ______________ (work) (___) ______________

E-mail ______________________________

Name of child ______________________________

Age ______________________________

Siblings ______________________________

____

Situation/reason for contact (remember to share your experiences, be positive, but realistic, ask how he or she is doing, and LISTEN):

Information requested (remember your resource guide):

Notes/remarks (Before you hang up, promise to call again. Below is space to record the date you called and comments about that call. Remember to send a postcard to your Parent to Parent coordinator after each call!):

Date

__________ ______________________________

__________ ______________________________

__________ ______________________________

__________ ______________________________

Figure 5.3. Sample log form for supporting parents. (Courtesy of New Jersey Statewide Parent to Parent.)

1st I have contacted my referred parent. Date ____________ Signed ____________	2nd It has been 2 weeks, and I have contacted my referred parent. Date ____________ Signed ____________
3rd It has been 1 month and, yes, I have talked/visited with my referred parent. Date ____________ Signed ____________	4th Within this second month, I have contacted my referred parent again. Date ____________ Signed ____________

Figure 5.4. Sample reminder postcards for supporting parents. (Courtesy of Parent to Parent of Vermont.)

and it need not be lengthy. You will find that the time you spend thanking your referral sources generates good will for you and your program and encourages future referrals as well.

RECOMMENDED PRACTICES AND RESOURCES FOR MATCHING

Parent to Parent programs connect parents with other parents who share similar family and disability experiences. The presence of another parent as a reliable ally is a source of emotional and informational support. Because the quality of the match determines how helpful parent to parent support will be, the following tips are important to remember as you establish the matching component of your program.

Gather Relevant Information Before the Match

Learn as much as possible about the referred parent in the initial conversation. Information about the child and the disability are important, but also gather information about the parent's own situation, needs, and specific challenges; the reasons for seeking support; hopes for a supporting parent; and any preferences related to the match (e.g., a parent prefers mail or e-mail to telephone contacts). Take time to establish a relationship with a referred parent. This time will lead to an understanding of the referred parent's personality and preferences and may help to make a more meaningful match.

Follow-Up After the Match

After the match is made, follow-up activities can help ensure the success of the match. Checking in with each parent a few days after the match has been made may encourage the initial contact. Regular and ongoing check-in calls with the referred parent and the supporting parent provide an opportunity to resolve the logistical problems that may arise in the match (e.g., replacing lost telephone numbers). Although check-in calls may sound invasive, most parents prefer an intensive and systematic follow-up on the part of the program.

Check on the Match from Time to Time

Timely check-ins with the referred parent and the supporting parent will help find out when a match is not working. After talking with the parents, the coordinator may offer them the opportunity to try a new match. Reassure the parents that not all matches are comfortable, and make rematches as necessary. Referred parents and supporting parents need to understand that parent to parent support is an ongoing resource that can be tried out several times until a successful match is established.

Encourage More Contacts

Supporting parents should be encouraged to make regular and consistent contacts with the referred parent, even if these contacts are brief. Many programs encourage supporting parents to contact the referred parent at least once a week during the first few weeks of the match so that they can get to know each other more quickly. Recognizing how full family calendars are, some supporting parents find it helpful to plan the next contact or visit before the current one ends. Another strategy that is used when parents meet in person is for the supporting parent to bring along a personal copy of a helpful book or adaptive equipment to loan to the referred parent. A follow-up contact is guaranteed to retrieve the shared item.

Although in many parent to parent matches contact is initiated by both of the parents, some referred parents are not comfortable calling the supporting parent. Yet referred parents welcome a contact that is initiated by the supporting parent. Parents need to hear in their support parent training how important it is for them to take the initiative in making contacts on a regular and frequent basis. These early contacts will help the referred parent feel sure that the supporting parent is a reliable ally who will be there for him or her.

RESOURCES WHEN A MATCH IS HARD TO FIND

In some instances it may not be possible for a local program to achieve a close match (e.g., child has a rare disability, parents live in rural area). When a local effort is not successful, check with the statewide program in your state to see if a statewide database exists for connecting parents (see Appendix C).

If you do not live in a state that has a statewide Parent to Parent program or if a statewide match cannot be found, there are options at the national and international levels. In Chapter 3 you learned about several organizations that maintain national and international databases of parents who are seeking a match or who are available to be matched around rare disabilities. One of these resources may be able to find a match for you with a parent whose disability and family experiences are similar to your own.

Suppose you can't find a match at the national and international levels. Parents report that even though a veteran parent may not have a child with the same disability, that parent can still be helpful by listening and giving guidance and emotional support. Sometimes the shared disability experience is enough to ensure a good connection between parents. Although matches need to be made whenever possible according to the child's disability and age, family issues, family size and structure, geographical location, and language spoken at home, lack of a perfect match should not stop you from making a match. It is more important that parents seeking support be in touch with other parents than not in touch at all.

SUMMARY

The parent match is the vehicle for support to parents who have a child or adult family member with a disability, and the care with which Parent to Parent programs make and support their matches is one reason for the success of thousands of matches that are made every year. Another reason for the success of matches is the supporting parents who volunteer their time to be matched. In the next chapter you will read more about supporting parents and how they are prepared for their role.

Many well-established Parent to Parent programs have program development manuals available for purchase that provide information about handling referrals and making parent matches. These manuals often contain sample record-keeping forms and descriptions of how the program manages referrals and makes and follows parent matches. A list of some of these program development manuals and contact information for purchasing them follows.

RESOURCES

Local Coordinator Training Manual: Kansas Parent to Parent, Families Together, Inc., 501 Jackson, Suite 400, Topeka, KS 66603; telephone: (785) 233-4777; fax: (785) 233-4787

Mentor Visiting Parent Training Manual: Parents Helping Parents, 3041 Olcott Street, Santa Clara, CA 95054-3222; telephone: (408) 727-5775; fax: (408) 727-0182

Parent to Parent Program Manual: Washington Parent to Parent Programs, State Office, The Arc of King County, 10550 Lake City Way NE, Suite A, Seattle, WA 98125-7752; telephone: (206) 364-3814; fax: (206) 364-8140

Parent to Parent Support in North Carolina: The Manual for Program Development and Support Parent Training: Family Support Network of North Carolina, CB# 7340, Chase Hall, University of North Carolina, Chapel Hill, NC 27599-7340; telephone: (919) 966-2841; fax: (919) 966-2916

Parents Encouraging Parents (PEP) Program Manual, PEP Resource Parent Manual Tennessee Department of Health, and *PEP Staff Training Manual:* Cordell Hull Building, Fifth Floor, 425 Fifth Avenue N., Nashville, TN 37247-4750; telephone: (615) 741-0353; fax: (615) 741-1063

Regional Coordinator Manual: Parent to Parent of Pennsylvania, Gateway Corporate Center, 6340 Flank Drive, #200, Harrisburg, PA 17112; telephone: (717) 540-4722; fax: (717) 657-5983

Steps to Starting a Self-Help Group: Parents Helping Parents, 3041 Olcott Street, Santa Clara, CA 95054-3222; telephone: (408) 727-5775; fax: (408) 727-0182

When You Reach Out to Others, You Are Not Alone: Parent to Parent of New Hampshire, 12 Flynn Street, Lebanon, NH 03766; telephone: (603) 448-6393; fax: (603) 448-6311

6

Finding and Preparing Supporting Parents

The Strength of Parent to Parent

"You know more of a road by having traveled it than by all the conjectures and descriptions in the world."

—William Hazlitt

In Chapter 5 you learned how matches are made between a trained supporting parent and a referred parent. Integral to the success of this match is the availability of trained supporting parents who are ready and willing to share their experiences and wisdom with other parents. Consequently, once you have made the decision to launch a Parent to Parent program and have established a mechanism for taking in referrals and making matches, you need to be sure that the program has a core group of supporting parents who are ready to be matched. There are four phases to building and sustaining a core group of supporting parents:

1. Recruiting potential supporting parents
2. Screening parents who wish to become supporting parents
3. Training new supporting parents
4. Nurturing and celebrating veteran supporting parents

This chapter describes specific strategies for recruiting, screening, training, and nurturing supporting parents. Also, you will learn how and why programs occasionally match untrained supporting parents.

SUPPORTING PARENT STORIES

Catherine and W.C.—Giving Back

By the time Karl was 2 years old and Franklin had joined our family, we had learned and benefited so much from Jean that we wanted to share those same gifts with other parents. We were at a stable place in our own lives, despite our busy schedules, and we knew that we had a lot to offer. We decided to take the training to serve as supporting parents. We called The Family Connection of South Carolina because we had been working with them on a respite program and knew that they needed supporting parents.

At the beginning of the training, we had a chance to share our own story and celebrate with other parents how far we had come and appreciate how much we had to give. As we each told our story, we supported each other—we were practicing being supporting parents as we were training for the role. We heard about the experience from supporting parents who were already matched. One of the messages I took away from the training was that a supporting parent doesn't solve problems for other parents but provides parents with information about options. A supporting parent encourages parents to think about each option and decide what is best for their family.

The training also included speakers who talked with us about issues in families with children who have disabilities and the adjustment process that parents go through. There was a terrific speaker who was a supporting parent who spoke on nurturing ourselves as caregivers and reminded us that we can help others only when our own needs are met.

We also spent time learning about and practicing communication strategies and active listening skills. Although everyone has his or her own personal style of communication, there are helpful strategies for starting a conversation and keeping it comfortable. As we practiced, I was amazed at how effective these communication and listening skills were and how good I felt at knowing that I had skills I could use.

A very important part of the training for us was the explanation by The Family Connection staff about their role as supporters for us. They assured us that once we were matched, they would check in with us regularly to see how our match was going and to answer any questions we might have.

RECRUITING AND SCREENING SUPPORTING PARENTS

Qualifications

The first step in recruiting supporting parents is to decide on important qualifications. The first criterion is that supporting parents be parents of children with special needs so that they will have the voice of personal experience. What about other caregivers who are serving in the parent role? Many Parent to Parent programs match around foster and adopted child issues. Foster and adoptive parents can be supporting parents in these situations because they know the disability issues and are familiar with aspects of the foster or adoptive parent experience. When grandparents are raising their grandchildren, a grandparent to grandparent match can be made. The program development team will need to consider the kinds of matches the program will make and then recruit supporting parents accordingly.

There are other qualifications that Parent to Parent programs consider as they recruit supporting parents. Programs look for supporting parents who

- Have a genuine interest in reaching out to help other parents. Ninety percent of supporting parents get involved because they want to provide support to other parents.
- Are at a stable place within their own families. Although the emotional reactions to having a child with a disability never completely disappear, supporting parents should have come to a certain level of comfort about their situation.
- Have natural empathy and strong communication skills. One of the roles of a supporting parent is to listen and understand. Many referred parents rank having another parent to listen as the most important part of the support for them.
- Are nonjudgmental and have an appreciation of diversity. An open, nonjudgmental attitude is critical to the success of the match. Everyone has his or her own style, and it is this diversity that makes each

match different. To be effective, supporting parents need to recognize and respect these diversities.
- Are committed to the Parent to Parent philosophy.

Most supporting parents and Parent to Parent program directors have a philosophy about the rights of individuals with disabilities and their families that includes the following: 1) Individuals with disabilities are people first and are more similar to people without disabilities than dissimilar; 2) individuals with disabilities contribute in positive ways to families and to society and need to be afforded the same rights and respect as people without disabilities; 3) families know best about their own needs, strengths, and preferences and should be included in planning and decision making that occurs on behalf of their family member with a disability; 4) supporting parents are qualified to provide a special kind of support to referred parents that complements and enhances the support provided by professionals; and 5) confidentiality is essential and nothing is shared without the permission of parents. Supporting parents introduce and model this philosophy in their conversations with referred parents.

Expectations

Parents who are considering becoming supporting parents need to know about expectations so that they will understand their obligations. You will want to be sure that parents have answers to the following questions:

- *What will be the time commitment to the program?* Many programs ask for a 1-year commitment from supporting parents, with an opportunity at the end of the year to recommit. Flexible availability to a supporting parent sets parent to parent support apart from professional and group support; therefore, parents interested in becoming supporting parents must have time to give to the match. Prospective supporting parents need to consider their other obligations and the amount of time they can give. In some Parent to Parent programs, supporting parents understand that they can shift from active status to inactive status if their family circumstances make it difficult for them to support another parent. In all Parent to Parent programs, supporting parents know that they never have to accept a match if the timing is not right for them and the needs of their families.
- *What type of training is involved before a match is made?* The majority of programs match trained supporting parents and use untrained parents only when necessary. Training usually takes 6–10 hours

and includes sharing family stories, informing parents about the adjustment process, teaching communication and listening skills, talking about community resources, and explaining the role of the supporting parent and the matching coordinator. You will read more about the training for supporting parents later in this chapter, and can find research-based information about the content and format of training in Tables 6.1 and 6.2 in Appendix A. Once supporting parents complete the initial training, many programs offer additional opportunities for training and support.

- *What documentation do supporting parents need to keep about their matches?* Most programs have forms for supporting parents to log and document their contacts with referred parents. Supporting parents use these forms to make notes about the issues that the referred parent is dealing with and any follow-up activities needed. Program directors find the forms helpful in documenting the number and nature of contacts between supporting parents and referred parents.

Recruiting Supporting Parents

The program's next step is to find the right supporting parents. In the early stages it is understandable that a Parent to Parent program may want to build a base of trained supporting parents as quickly as possible; however, experienced program directors recommend starting with a small number of supporting parents. Beginning slowly will ensure that quality training and support are available to each supporting parent and that the program has the capacity to give each match the follow-up support it may need. Starting small and gradually increasing the number of active supporting parents will enable the program to maintain quality.

Mature Parent to Parent programs find that many parents who wish to be supporting parents entered the program as referred parents. Their training begins as they receive support and experience how they are helped by their supporting parent. The support they received was so helpful that they want to give back to the program and to other parents.

Until programs have a base of referred parents to which they can turn to recruit supporting parents, they will need other ways of gaining access to potential supporting parents. Recruiting requires knowing where to find prospective supporting parents and how to reach them. It is important to use a variety of recruitment activities. Supporting parents can be recruited by the same efforts you will be using to promote your program to referral sources and to parents themselves (see Chapter 11).

Consider where potential supporting parents can be reached, and target your recruitment efforts in a variety of places. If the program has a sponsoring agency, it may be able to assist in the location of prospective supporting parents. Other community agencies that provide services to children with special needs and their families will know parents. Confidentiality usually prohibits these agencies from releasing parents' names, but agency personnel can forward information about a Parent to Parent program activity to parents. Your program would need to supply the agency personnel with information that they could include in their newsletter. In addition, you could prepare a mailing and request that the agency attach address labels of the families to the envelopes. Be sure to include information that tells the parents how to request additional information or contact you about their interest in becoming a supporting parent. Many programs have developed letters and fliers that they use in recruiting supporting parents (see Figures 6.1 and 6.2). Once interested parents contact the program and share their name and address, you can begin to communicate with them and no longer need the assistance of another agency.

Be sure that you build a core group of supporting parents that has as much diversity as possible—parents from all social, economic, educational, and racial backgrounds; from different family structures; from different disability experiences; and from different geographic locations.

Screening Supporting Parents

Some Parent to Parent programs have a screening process to ensure that supporting parents are ready to take on the role. Generally, the process involves a parent interview during which the program coordinator shares information about Parent to Parent, its philosophy, and the role of and expectations for being a supporting parent. This conversation can happen in person or over the telephone, and sometimes the program coordinator will use a screening questionnaire. The coordinator also talks with the prospective supporting parents about their own families and disability experiences and usually asks why they would like to be supporting parents.

Other Parent to Parent programs hold an introductory meeting to explain the program. Either way, it is important for parents to have a chance to learn more about the role of the supporting parent, the training, and the match before they decide whether to participate. Similarly, it is important for the program coordinator to meet prospective supporting parents and learn about why they are interested in becoming supporting parents and where they are in their family lives. Occasionally parents will express interest in becoming supporting parents when their personal situations suggest that they might not be ready. By meet-

Date ______________________________

Dear ______________________________,

As you know, parents of children with disabilities and health problems provide invaluable support to each other by sharing experiences, frustrations, knowledge, and joys. There is a common bond between parents of children with disabilities. Yet, many times parents are not able to discover this bond because they don't know where to turn to find other parents facing similar situations.

Parent to Parent is a network of volunteer parents of children with a wide range of disabilities and illnesses who are available for telephone contact with parents facing a new diagnosis.

You have been recommended as a parent who might be willing to volunteer to become a support parent. We would like to invite you to join us at a training workshop. Our training workshops focus on communication skills, listening skills, the process of grieving, confidentiality, and local resources. We will also discuss different disabilities and illnesses, how the network functions, and our public awareness activities.

Our next workshop will be held on _____________ at __________________. Please think about this. If you are interested in participating, please call us at ________________ to register. The registration deadline is ________________.

We believe that this service—which only parents can provide—will enable other parents to view, in a positive manner, their child's ability to grow, learn, and develop to his or her fullest potential. We hope you agree.

We look forward to hearing from you.

Sincerely,

____

Figure 6.1. Sample letter for recruiting supporting parents. (Courtesy of Parent to Parent of Virginia.)

Our goal at

Parent to Parent

is to give families

the skills and support

they need to help

their children with special needs

reach their full potential.

Our hope

is for families

to feel less isolated and more confident

about themselves.

All information is kept confidential.

Postage

New Jersey Statewide
Parent to Parent
35 Halsey St., 4th Floor
Newark, NJ 07102

Parents Supporting Parents

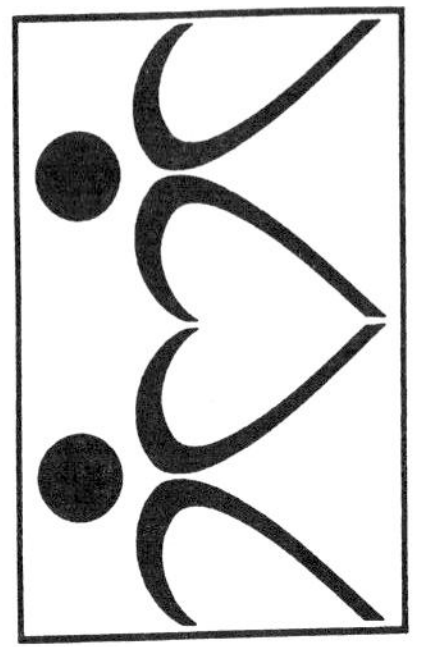

New Jersey Statewide
Parent to Parent

Parents Supporting Parents

1-800-FSC-NJ10
(1-800-372-6510)

Figure 6.2. Sample flier. (Courtesy of New Jersey Statewide Parent to Parent.)

Figure 6.2. (*continued*)

New Jersey Statewide Parent to Parent

Parent to Parent is a statewide network of parents supporting families of children with developmental delays, disabilities, or other special health needs.

As trained *supporting parents*, we offer emotional support and information, and act as a valuable resource to families. We offer assistance in learning the necessary skills to help parents face the challenges of raising their child.

We are not counselors or therapists. We are parents who have experienced the feelings and emotions that come after learning that our children have a developmental delay, disability, or other special health needs. We offer moral support and encourage parents to feel comfortable and optimistic about the future.

Parent to Parent is dedicated to supporting families at their most challenging times and to celebrating each new victory. Parents helping parents ... it's a simple concept that works.

What Parent to Parent Offers

- One-to-one matches of families who have similar needs and experiences.
- Emotional support for parents when they learn their child has a developmental delay, disability, or special health needs.
- Current information on a variety of disabilities and health issues.
- Training for parents who would like to become a *supporting parent.*
- Information on local, state, and national resources for the child and family.
- List of informative books on issues related to children with special needs.

All information is kept confidential.

If you would like to be matched with a supporting parent or would like to become a supporting parent, please complete and mail the form at right or call us at:

1-800-FSC-NJ10

(1-800-372-6510)

OUT OF STATE CALL 732-974-1144

New Jersey Statewide Parent to Parent

If you would like more information, please call us at 1-800-FSC-NJ10 or complete this form and mail it to:

Parent to Parent
c/o Statewide Parent Advocacy Network
35 Halsey St., 4th Floor
Newark, NJ 07102

Name ______________________

Address ______________________
Street

____
City *State* *Zip*

____
County

Telephone ( ) ______________________
Area Code *Phone Number*

Please check all that apply:

- ☐ I would like to be matched with another parent.
- ☐ I am interested in becoming a supporting parent.
- ☐ I would like to receive more information on **Parent to Parent**.

Parent to Parent is funded by
The NJ Department of Health and Senior Services
in cooperation with:

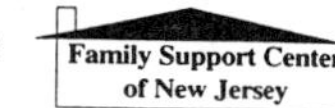

and

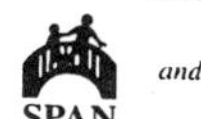

ing with prospective supporting parents, the program coordinator is better able to determine their readiness levels (see Figure 6.3).

Whether through a group meeting, through an individual conversation, or as part of the supporting parent training, many Parent to Parent programs screen prospective veteran parents in terms of the following:

- Acceptance of their child and adjustment to their family situation
- Ability to reach out and provide support to other parents
- Ability to cope with other people's problems and tolerance of values and feelings that may be different from their own
- Willingness to share their family story with others
- Communication skills
- Maturity and empathy
- Time availability

Most programs also ask prospective supporting parents to complete an application form that includes contact information and a demographic description of the family—information that will be considered in making parent matches (see Figure 6.4).

Most screening occurs before interested parents take part in the training, but there are many opportunities during the training session(s) to determine a parent's readiness. The training sessions give parents a chance to reflect on their experiences and how far they have come and to become more familiar with the role of the supporting parent. Occasionally program coordinators encounter a parent who wishes to be a supporting parent but who is not ready. Depending on the circumstances, the program coordinator may talk with the parent and suggest that the parent be matched with an experienced supporting parent before serving in that role. Another option is not to match a trained supporting parent who may not be ready for that experience, even if a possible match could be made. Sometimes extra time is all that is needed. Even parents who are ready to be matched as supporting parents may wait several weeks or months until the right family presents itself for a match. Fortunately, there are many ways for parents to be involved in a Parent to Parent program. Parents can take part in program activities and volunteer to support the work of the program (see Chapter 10). A third possibility is to make a double match between a parent who is not quite ready to be a supporting parent and an active supporting parent. They connect with a referred parent, and the mentor supporting parent models effective supporting parent strategies.

Parent to Parent Screening Guide

The following list is an informal guide to determining whether volunteers would make effective helping parents. As you interview prospective helping parents, keep these questions in mind. Do not ask parents these questions directly. Record your impressions of your conversation. Remember that these are sensitive questions and each person may react differently. The most important question is: What message would this prospective helping parent give to a referred parent?

Acceptance of the child:

- Do they view the child as a valuable person?
- Do they accept the child's strengths and weaknesses and have expectations that seem realistic?
- Do they believe their child can learn? Do they feel learning opportunities are important?
- Do they participate in services provided to their child? Do they advocate for change when necessary? Do they monitor services?
- Have they successfully worked through most of their anger and fear surrounding the birth of a child with a disability?

Ability to provide support to other parents:

- Are they willing to share their own experiences?
- Are they concerned about others?
- Are they nonjudgmental?
- Do they view their role as prospective helping parents as a supporting role rather than a decision-making one?
- Are relationships within their family relatively stable?
- Are they coping well with emotional issues?
- Do they have an ability to identify the needs and feeling of others?

Ability to cope with other people's problems:

- Are they willing to become personally involved with other people?
- Can they cope with the problems of others without being hurt themselves?
- Can they handle confidential information without the need to discuss it with other people?

Ability to communicate:

- Do they express themselves well?
- Are they good listeners?
- Do they know when to be quiet?

Maturity:

- Are they able to accept rejection by others without being personally offended?
- Can they work without a lot of praise or recognition?
- Are they willing to give to others without the expectation of returns?

Time:

- Do they have the time to be involved in Parent to Parent?

Final things to consider when recommending a parent as a helping parent:

- Do they convey a sense of calm reassurance?
- Do you think that they are ready to share their knowledge and experiences effectively with another parent?

Figure 6.3. Sample screening guide. (Courtesy of Parent to Parent of Washington.)

Parent to Parent Volunteer Application

Name ______________________________ Date ______________

Street address ____

City ______________________________ Zip ______________

Telephone (home) (   ) __________________ (work) (   ) __________________

Occupation ____

Place of employment ____

Language(s) spoken other than English ______________________________

Names of children	Birthdate	Sex	Disability

(Please use the back if you need more room.)

1. Please describe the adjustments you and your family have made.

2. What have been the most rewarding events, or the easiest years, for you in your role as the parent of a child with a disability?

3. What has been the most difficult for you in your role as a parent?

Figure 6.4. Supporting parent application. (Courtesy of Parent to Parent of Washington.)

Figure 6.4. *(continued)*

4. Please indicate those characteristics that most closely describe your parenting style. The purpose of this checklist is to gain an idea of your parenting style. This may be useful in matching you with another parent.

Please check the appropriate boxes.

Characteristics	Usually 1	2	3	4	Rarely 5
Patient					
Flexible					
Strict					
Energetic					
Physically affectionate					
Emotionally expressive					
Able to admit mistakes					
Accepting					
Frustrated					
Supportive					
Perfectionistic					
Able to make decisions					
Outgoing					
Organized					
Objective					
Passive					
Trusting					
Optimistic					
Easygoing					
Impulsive					
Open to new ideas					
Accepting of change					
Protective					
Self-confident					
Lenient					
Consistent					
Logical					
Content					

Figure 6.4. (*continued*)

5. Please explain which of these characteristics have been the most helpful to you in parenting your child.

6. Please explain which of these characteristics have been the least helpful to you in parenting your child.

7. If given the opportunity, what would you do differently in your role as the parent of a child with a disability?

8. Please describe briefly how and from what source you received the most support in adjusting to your child's disability.

9. Would parent to parent support have been helpful to you? If so, at what point and why?

10. What do you expect to gain from the experience of being a supporting parent?

11. What would you describe as your goal as a supporting parent in a relationship with a newly referred parent?

12. What characteristics on the list would you describe as being a help to a supporting parent in his or her role? What characteristics would you consider harmful?

Please feel free to make any further comments:

TRAINING NEW SUPPORTING PARENTS

Training supporting parents before they are matched is one of the foundations of Parent to Parent, and three fourths of all local Parent to Parent programs have a formal training component for supporting parents. Additional training sometimes also occurs as part of the ongoing support that is offered to supporting parents as they participate in parent matches.

Initial Training for Parents

The training that parents receive before they are matched with a referred parent is one of the features that sets Parent to Parent apart from many other parent support programs. During the training, parents who wish to be supporting parents are given time to reflect on their own experiences as parents of children with special needs and to develop communication and listening skills that will help them to use and to share their experiences in effective ways.

Content

As your program considers the content areas of the training for supporting parents, remember that more than half of local Parent to Parent programs have developed training materials themselves and are willing to share with others. You can get ideas about the content and format of training from existing training manuals. In many instances, these training guides provide all of the content, suggested resources, audiovisual materials, sample handouts, and suggested group and individual training activities for the total sequence of training sessions. (A partial listing of Parent to Parent programs and their training materials appears in the resources at the end of this chapter. The data from the national survey of Parent to Parent programs that appear in Table 6.1 in Appendix A can give you an idea of what is included in supporting parent training.)

A typical training program gives supporting parents a solid foundation of information about disabilities, available community resources, and skills in communication and empathetic listening. A comprehensive training program also gives supporting parents opportunities for self-evaluation and a time to look at their own values, beliefs, and actions. Strong communication skills, a knowledge base about disabilities and community resources, and a firm sense of self and respect for others are essential qualities for supporting parents, and the training is designed to prepare supporting parents in these areas. Although many content areas are common to most supporting parent training components, each program's training is unique. Nancy DiVenere, Director, Parent to Parent of Vermont, stated,

Our supporting parent training offers families an opportunity to reflect on their experience as parents and to begin to consider what was helpful to them when they first learned about their child's disability. It asks experienced parents to think about how they feel today and to think about some of the things that they can do today that they might not have been able to do earlier. Many families tell us they are better able to solve problems, find resources for their child in their communities, talk to health care providers, and plan for their future. They tell us they're able to see what their child can do, instead of what he or she cannot do. This activity is just one component of our training for parents who wish to volunteer as supporting parents. Our training is also designed to enhance supporting parents' communication and listening skills. Training gives parents confidence to share their stories, their expertise, and their wisdom through experience. It gives them tools for careful listening and for communicating with referred parents in ways that make it easy and comfortable for conversations to continue.

Amount and Format of Training

The majority of supporting parents receive at least 4 hours of training before they are matched, and some programs offer up to 18–20 hours of training (see Table 6.3 in Appendix A). The amount of training that your program provides depends on the decisions you make about the content and format of the training, as well as on the preferences of parents and program staff.

As the training component of your program grows, you will need to consider the format of your training. Will training meetings be scheduled as one longer session or several shorter time periods? Will training occur on the weekend or in the evening during the week? Will there be a small or large group of parents? Will there be alternative training formats for parents who cannot come to a group training? If so, what might these alternatives be? Answers to these questions may be based on an informal needs assessment that the program conducts with parents to learn more about their preferences. You may decide to provide a certain number of hours of training before parents are matched and then offer ongoing training opportunities once parents are matched. You also may decide to offer training on a one-to-one basis if interested parents cannot attend a group training session.

Supporting parent training generally consists of group training for 6–10 hours. Most programs choose to use a full-day training format (9 A.M. to 5 P.M.). Typically, supporting parent training sessions occur on Saturdays, and refreshments and lunch are provided. But in some programs the parents prefer to attend supporting parent training in the evenings rather than on the weekends. These programs typically offer two to four evening sessions (perhaps from 6:30 P.M. to 9:30 P.M.) over a 2- to 3-week period. Some programs may start earlier and provide a light dinner.

The vast majority of Parent to Parent programs limit the number of parents participating in the training to 8–12 parents. A group of this size is large enough for the parents to appreciate the diversity of the experiences within the group and participate in a lively exchange of ideas, but it is small enough for the parents to feel comfortable (and have enough time for) sharing their own family stories, participating in role-play activities, and bonding with one another. If factors mean that a larger number of parents will be trained together, consider subdividing the group into smaller working groups for most of the training activities.

Sharing Family Stories

Often training begins with an opportunity for each of the parents to introduce him- or herself and to share his or her family story. There are several reasons for beginning supporting parent training in this way:

- A supporting parent's relationship with a referred parent is likely to begin with a sharing of family stories. Supporting parents need to share just enough of their story to establish common ground with the referred parents and to help the referred parents feel comfortable telling their own family story. As referred parents share their stories, supporting parents have an opportunity to learn more about the issues that are of greatest concern to the referred parents. Beginning the training with this opportunity provides a simulation for supporting parents' early interactions with referred parents.
- Supporting parents can reconnect with their early feelings on learning about the diagnosis by sharing their family story. By re-experiencing their feelings, supporting parents are better able to empathize with the referred parent and recognize where the referred parent is in the adjustment cycle.
- As indicated in the previous real-life stories, as the family stories are shared, the other parents in the training group respond in comforting ways—just as they will do in their match. The activity allows them a chance to practice their supportive responses and to recognize how many of the supporting parent skills they already have as a result of their experiences.

You need to allow plenty of time for this story sharing, but you also may have to limit it. You might suggest that each person take about 10 minutes so that everyone will have ample time. If you know one of the parents, you may want to talk to him or her ahead of time and ask him or her to go first and model a 10-minute family story sharing. The trainer's role is to move on from one parent to the next and to acknowledge strong emotions and affirm the support efforts of the group. Beginning with family stories provides the trainer with relevant content from which to draw examples during the rest of the training. Referring back to individual family stories adds greater relevance to other training activities.

Adjustment Process

The transition to a discussion about common emotional reactions is natural (see Chapter 1). Although emphasizing that each family story is unique, trainers might suggest that there are some common stages of adjustment that parents experience in individual ways. The group can discuss any common emotional reactions they heard in the family stories.

By sharing family stories and discussing the adjustment process, supporting parents can get in touch with where they are in this experience and learn to recognize where referred parents may be in the adjustment process (sample handouts that are used to support this discussion appear at the end of this chapter). The group needs to recognize that there is no set way in which these reactions are experienced—some parents feel each of these stages intensely and for long periods; others may know only some of these stages. Some parents cycle through the stages in one sequence, whereas other parents may move in and out of stages in a different sequence, and stages are reexperienced as the child reaches various developmental milestones and makes transitions within the service system.

Role of the Supporting Parent

The role of the supporting parent is to recognize and understand where referred parents are in the adjustment process and help them know that their feelings are normal. The sharing of family stories and the identification of the stages in the adjustment process help supporting parents to remember what their own early experiences were like and to anticipate what their role as a supporting parent will be like.

Being a supporting parent can be hard work, given the emotions that are involved. It is helpful for supporting parents to take some time during the training to consider their role and define what they will be doing, as well as identify what may be outside the scope of being a supporting parent. Listing the roles of a supporting parent in small groups is a good way to build on the initial training activities and add a different style of learning into the training. After talking as a large group, the parents may be ready for a different, more informal venue. Brainstorming in small groups is a good way to collect a lot of ideas in a short time period.

Divide the group into smaller groups of three or four parents. Ask half of the groups to talk about what they think the role of the supporting parent includes (e.g., listener, provider of information, role model, window on the future, source of encouragement, friend). Ask the other groups to identify roles that they think are not appropriate for a supporting parent (e.g., medical specialist, counselor, lawyer, social worker). Bring the small groups back together after 10 minutes, and ask them to share their discussions with the larger group. Stress that an essential aspect of their role as supporting parents is confidentiality and that every interaction with their matched parents must guarantee privacy.

Communication and Listening

Training parents about communication and listening can be interactive, giving them a chance to identify and practice new skills and hone old ones. One way to encourage parents to think about the importance of communication and listening is to ask them to remember a positive and productive conversation that they had with someone. Ask them to identify specific actions that made the conversation successful. As the discussion unfolds, write all of the ideas on two large pieces of paper. Although these sheets are not labeled, the trainer can write down examples of verbal communication on one page and examples of nonverbal communication on the other page. As the pages fill up, it is easy for the parents to identify the differences between the two, reinforcing the idea that communication happens both verbally and nonverbally.

The trainer can introduce the idea that most communication is nonverbal and that supporting parents will need to be aware of how much is communicated without a spoken word. Try the following simulation activity. Ask each parent to find a partner and to have a 2- to 3-minute conversation. As the pairs are talking, notice which ones are demonstrating nonverbal communication strategies, such as eye contact, body posture, facial expressions, and gestures. Ask one or more of these pairs to freeze their positions so that the other parents can observe nonverbal communication in action.

To introduce verbal communication, consider inviting a supporting parent to join you in a role play. Ask the parent to begin talking to you about any issue. As the parent talks, model verbal responses (e.g., open-ended questions, paraphrasing, summarizing, reflecting back feelings) to keep the conversation going. Think about the verbal communication strategies that will be discussed in the next segment of the training so that you can be sure to model these during the role play. Ask the observing parents to write down all of the verbal communication strategies that they hear the trainer using. Adding an element of competition to the role-play observation (a small prize for the parent who contributes the greatest number of verbal communication strategies) motivates full participation and makes it more fun. Then it becomes easy to go over the handouts on communication skills because the parents have seen and described them (sample handouts on verbal communication strategies appear at the end of this chapter).

To introduce the section on listening, you might start with an activity in which parents are asked to practice listening to a story (a sample story appears at the end of this chapter). Using a story with a twist ending and specific bits of information emphasizes the importance of two kinds of listening: absolute listening (listening to the whole story for facts) and selective listening (listening to parts of the story for feelings and hidden meaning). Parents may use different nonverbal and verbal communication responses depending on the kind of listening they are doing and the reason for the listening.

Allow plenty of time (1–3 hours) for parents to practice all of these skills. Then as a summary activity, try breaking the group into sets of three. One parent is the speaker, the second is the listener, and the third is the observer. The speaker begins a conversation with the listener. The listener practices using all of the communication and listening skills to keep the conversation comfortable and productive. The observer reflects back to both parents the communication and listening skills that were a part of the conversation. The parents can repeat this sequence so that each parent gets to try each role. This offers an active way for parents to practice these skills in a comfortable environment. And because this activity allows parents to talk about their own experiences, it may be easier than a role-play activity in which parents are asked to take on a new role.

Referral Process and Tips for the First Contact

End the training session with a discussion about how the referral and matching process works, and summarize what supporting parents can expect to happen now that they have taken the training. There are important points to emphasize:

- It may take a while to get the first match.
- A supporting parent can refuse a match at any time.
- Rematches are fine—not all matches are comfortable for both parents.
- Anxiety about the first contact is typical.
- Plenty of time is needed when making the first contact.
- Supporting parents should take the initiative for making early contacts and should strive for at least four contacts during the first 2 months of the match.

- Supporting parents can't and shouldn't try to respond to all of the referred parent's needs. Offer to help the referred parent with a referral to a professional when he or she needs more support than another parent should give.
- The program coordinator is available to supporting parents and referred parents for assistance and/or additional information at any time.

Simulation Activities

Because the timing for various training activities varies depending on the needs and characteristics of the group, consider preparing several supporting parent simulations on index cards that can be used in small groups just in case you finish early (samples appear at the end of this chapter). Even if you don't use them during the initial training, they can be used in ongoing training or other support activities for supporting parents.

Additional Training Content Areas

There are training content areas beyond those described here that are often included in supporting parent training. Many programs offer training on community resources and specific disabilities. You may want to develop your supporting parent training by considering which training content areas are being used by the greatest percentage of Parent to Parent programs and by listening to the needs and preferences of parents who are interested in becoming supporting parents (see Figure 6.5).

General Training Tips

Regardless of the format of supporting parent training, most Parent to Parent programs strive to ensure that child care and transportation realities are not barriers to parents' participation. Parent to Parent programs can support the child care needs of parents who are attending the training sessions by providing child care on site or by reimbursing parents for child care expenses. If a parent needs assistance with transportation to attend the training, most programs will help the parent find a ride with another parent who also is attending or will provide reimbursement to the parent for the travel expenses incurred through the use of public transportation.

Just as children with disabilities have different strengths and learning preferences, adults bring with them different learning styles. You may find that varying the learning activities to meet the different learning styles of the group is helpful. Some parents learn better by listening, some by doing, and some by talking. Large groups are better for some,

Arrival and Get Acquainted Time Informal Interaction	15 minutes
Welcome, Introductions, Overview	15 minutes
Sharing Family Stories Large-Group Sharing	75 minutes
Break and Stretch	15 minutes
Common Stages of Adjustment Large-Group Discussion of Handouts	30 minutes
Role of the Supporting Parent Small-Group Brainstorming/Large-Group Sharing	45 minutes
Lunch	60 minutes
Communication Skills Large-Group Brainstorming Simulations Large-Group Discussion	75 minutes
Listening Skills Large-Group Response to Story Practice Activity in Small Groups Self-Assessment	30 minutes
Break and Stretch	15 minutes
The Referral and Matching Process Large-Group Discussion of Handout	30 minutes
What Ifs, Simulations, Other Questions, Wrap-Up Small-Group Discussions Large-Group Summary Large-Group Question and Answer	30 minutes

Figure 6.5. Sample supporting parent training outline.

whereas others prefer small groups. At the end of the training, acknowledge the importance of becoming a supporting parent, and present each parent with a certificate. Parents who participate in the training together have shared a special experience and may appreciate getting a roster of the parents in their group so that they can keep in touch and become informal supports for each other as they experience their matches.

Who Conducts the Training?

Once decisions about the format and content of the training have been made, your program will need to find a trainer who will lead the training sessions. Will it be a parent in your local program? Will professionals be involved? Most programs have a parent leading the training but also use professionals (e.g., social workers, nurses, physicians) for various aspects of the training. Because most Parent to Parent programs are parent directed, they don't exclusively use professionals for training supporting parents.

If a program is new, then the coordinator of another Parent to Parent program in the same state may offer to do the first round of training and serve as a mentor trainer. If a new program emerges in a state that has a statewide Parent to Parent program (see Chapter 14), staff from the statewide program can assist with the training. Because there is no national Parent to Parent organization that ensures that all new trainers receive the support they need and because there is no standard training curriculum, the best resource for a new program is a veteran trainer from another Parent to Parent program.

Ongoing Training and Supports

Local and statewide Parent to Parent programs provide other training and supports for their supporting parents (see Table 6.4 in Appendix A). Programs not only provide training for prospective supporting parents but also may have a manual for supporting parents to use as a resource. This manual contains handouts related to the content of the training, a summary of the forms that the veteran parent uses to document the progress and outcome of each parent match, as well as information about community and state resources that are available to families.

After supporting parents complete the initial training, programs continue to offer supports to them as they participate in their matches. Most programs offer one-to-one consultation to supporting parents to answer any questions that arise during the match.

Most of the larger programs offer supporting parents the opportunity to participate in ongoing training sessions with other trained supporting parents. The agendas of these training opportunities vary depending on the needs and requests of the supporting parents, but they include time for supporting parents to brainstorm together about common issues (e.g., being available without being intrusive, knowing when to refer, supporting a couple when each parent's needs are different) related to their matches and time to share tips with each other. Statewide programs sometimes provide a statewide conference or retreat for supporting parents—settings in which supporting parents have a chance to participate in further training and network with one another.

Some statewide Parent to Parent programs recognize that there are expenses related to serving as a supporting parent, and program coordinators try to minimize these extra expenses for supporting parents. Some larger statewide programs reimburse supporting parents for long-distance telephone calls to their match family. More than half of the statewide programs reimburse for postage expenses, and close to half of these programs cover supporting parents' travel expenses related to their match.

Of all of the supports offered to supporting parents, training is the most requested by parents; a manual and reimbursement for expenses also are highly requested. As you consider ongoing training and other opportunities for supporting parents, keep in mind that the activities presented in Table 6.4 in Appendix A are being implemented by large, well-established statewide Parent to Parent programs. These programs represent a vision of what is possible as small, local Parent to Parent programs grow and mature in their capacity to offer services to parents.

NURTURING AND CELEBRATING VETERAN SUPPORTING PARENTS

Just as Parent to Parent programs recognize the importance of preparing supporting parents for their matched experience, they also work to acknowledge and celebrate the voluntary contributions of supporting parents. Some programs hold regular celebration or education meetings for supporting parents and honor outstanding supporting parents annually. Other programs may hold an annual special retreat for supporting parents, offering them a chance to spend a day or weekend in a relaxed setting with other supporting parents. Sharing information that may be useful in matches, celebrating each other, and having fun together to reenergize are common retreat activities and serve as the program's way of thanking the parents.

MATCHING UNTRAINED SUPPORTING PARENTS

Occasionally some programs will ask an untrained parent to participate in a match with a referred parent. Parent to Parent programs typically have fewer untrained parents than trained supporting parents available to participate in one-to-one matches, and untrained parents are used only when a trained supporting parent cannot be found or when the needs of the referred parent are unique. Generally, untrained parents are parents known to a program who have not been able to participate in supporting parent training. When using these parents for matches, programs usually provide them with an abridged version of the content that is included in the supporting training sessions. This information is provided through written materials or a one-to-one conversation between the program coordinator and the untrained parent.

SUMMARY

Training for supporting parents before they are matched is one of the key components of a Parent to Parent program, and this orientation, along with the match, sets Parent to Parent apart from other programs that connect parents. Although supporting parents do not need training in how to be a parent of a child with a disability, there is no question that the training they receive from their Parent to Parent program helps them to be more effective in helping other parents. Use any of the training strategies presented in this chapter as well as existing training materials described in the resources that follow to develop the training activities for your program.

Many Parent to Parent programs that have been training and matching supporting parents for years have developed training manuals for those leading the training and for the supporting parents participating in the training. These manuals include tips for developing and carrying out the training for supporting parents. They also include copies of all of the handouts and a list of other resources that might be used. Existing program directors share these training manuals with those developing a new Parent to Parent program, and they make their manuals available to others at nominal cost. A list of training manuals, along with contact information for obtaining the manuals, follows.

REFERENCES

Perske, R. (1977). *Improving the quality of life: A symposium on normalization and integration.* Arlington, TX: Association for Retarded Citizens National Headquarters.

Perske, R. (1978). *A coordinated effort to take the risk out of "at risk:" The report to the President, mental retardation the leading edge—service programs that work.* Washington DC: President's Committee on Mental Retardation.

Perske, R. (1981). *Hope for the families.* Nashville: Abingdon Press.

RESOURCES

Basic Parent Partner Training Manual, Advance Parent Partner Training Manual: Parent to Parent of Virginia, c/o The Arc of Virginia, 6 North Sixth Street, #403-A, Richmond, VA 23219; telephone: (804) 222-1945; fax: (804) 222-3402

Family TIES Training Manual: Family TIES, Massachusetts Department of Public Health, 109 Rhode Island Road, Lakeville, MA 02347; telephone: (617) 727-1440; fax: (617) 727-9296

Family to Family Volunteer Training: RAISING Special Kids, 4750 North Black Canyon Highway, Suite 101, Phoenix, AZ 85017; telephone: (602) 242-4366; fax: (602) 242-4306

Parent to Parent of Florida Support Training Manual: Family Network on Disabilities of Florida, 2735 Whitney Road, Clearwater, FL 34520; telephone: (727) 523-1130; fax: (727) 523-8687

Parent to Parent Training Manual: Parents Reaching Out, 1000 Main Street, Los Lunas, NM 87031; telephone: (505) 865-3700; fax: (505) 865-3737

Support Parent Training Manual: The Family Connection of South Carolina, 2712 Middleburg Drive, Suite 103B, Columbia, SC 29204; telephone: (803) 252-0914; fax: (803) 799-8017

Supporting Parent Training Manual: Kansas Parent to Parent, Families Together, Inc., 501 Jackson, Suite 4000, Topeka, KS 66603; telephone: (785) 233-4777; fax: (785) 233-4787

Supporting Parent Training Manual: Parent to Parent of New Hampshire, 12 Flynn Street, Lebanon, NH 03766; telephone: (603) 448-6393; fax: (603) 448-6311

Supporting Parent Training Manual: Parent to Parent of Vermont, 1 Main Street, 69 Champlain Mill, Winooski, VT 05404; telephone: (802) 655-5290; fax: (802) 655-3507

Visiting Parents: A Training Manual: Parents Helping Parents, 3041 Olcott Street, Santa Clara, CA 95054-3222; telephone: (408) 727-5775; fax: (408) 727-0182

Appendix

Sample Adjustment Process Handout

You will have bewildering, weird times, all right. You may wonder if you are losing your mind. Probably not. But strange times will come, and getting through them takes energy and grit.

Some experts have described in detail the stages you are expected to face. The only trouble is that parents who are adjusting to children with disabilities do not follow a set course. Each parent reacts differently.

Here are a few oversimplified descriptions of stages you may—or may not—experience. And many parents could add to this list.

The Drags: It is as if your spring had run down. You feel so tired you can hardly drag yourself around. The sun may be shining, but to you the day seems cloudy. You may feel a lump in your throat or a knot in your stomach. It is hard to breath, and every once in a while you may hear yourself sighing. You may even wonder if you have the flu. When these times come, you wish you could find a warm, cozy hole, crawl into it, and close a lid after you.

This may be your mind's way of telling you that "out there," there is too much to take. So you slow down, withdraw, move within yourself, interact less with the world around you, and take some time out. This is okay, providing you do not stay out too long.

The Speeds: When this stage approaches, you feel as though somebody has wound your spring too tightly. You move around at a frenzied pace . . .

- So much to think about
- So much to do
- So much ground to cover
- So many places to go
- So many people to see

It is as if a combination of the Ten Commandments and St. Vitus' Dance energizes your movements. Many new ideas and concepts which need to be acted upon come to your mind. It is your personality's way to "get at it," even if some motions are wasted.

This material is reprinted by permission from Perske, R. (1981). *Hope for the families.* Nashville: Abingdon Press.

The Blocks: Tough news came from the doctors. But somehow your ears refused to hear what they told you, and your eyes remained blind to the evidence they presented. The knowledge that your child possesses a disability is hard to take. You may even talk to others as if your child has no disability. That is okay for a while. Parents' minds need time to change from believing their child's a superbaby to seeing that child as he or she really is. It is all right to make this shift slowly. But it is unhealthy if it is never made.

The Hurts: No professional can describe all the types of anguish and pain parents feel after learning their child has a disability. Nevertheless, all of them hurt; they hurt badly! Such pain can force you to become edgy and nervous; to walk floors or lie awake all night, tossing and turning; or to break down and cry—fathers included.

Bear in mind that when you do feel such pain, it may be your body and mind saying to you that you are strong enough to bear the hurt you must feel. It is my hunch that you will never suffer pain beyond what you can endure. There are many mechanisms within you to dull the sense when things become overwhelming. Some people can become stronger from enduring pain.

If you happen to be hurting while reading these sentences, you may feel anger toward the author of these words. That is okay, too. This book is not intended to bring you comfort. Its purpose is to help you grow and adjust so that you can accept, love, and act creatively on behalf of your child. You cannot do this without experiencing some hurts, enduring them, and working your way through them.

The Guilts: At times you may feel you have committed some horrible sin against God and man. You may even look deeply into your past, searching for that single horrid act that caused it all. But I am willing to wager that no matter how hard you search, you probably will never find such a cause.

Nevertheless, on some days you feel sure that you must be the worst human specimen on the face of the earth. Somewhere, somehow, you committed an unpardonable sin, and now you are paying for it.

Such guilt is phony. It is not the same kind of guilt you feel when you are caught with your hand in the cookie jar—or when you commit other real transgressions of greater magnitude. Therefore, you need not drag out all the black [bad] things in your life, examining them one by one. This exercise only gets in the way of adjusting to your child's handicap.

The Greats: While a few days earlier you may have felt that you were the world's worst mom or dad, now it may come to you that you are one of the greatest. You secretly may feel that God has chosen you to bear this extra burden because you are more special than other human beings.

Of course, it is more pleasant to fantasize yourself as being great. It is better than feeling you are the world's worst. So enjoy it while you can. But be careful. Sooner or later somebody will say or do something to send you crashing off your pedestal. When that happens, it is to be hoped you will not fall into the guilt trap again. Instead, you may achieve a fresh stability from knowing you are not a superparent. But you aren't a superdemon either. You have your weaknesses and strengths, like everyone else.

The Hates: After hurting for a time, you may search irrationally for chances to blame others and hurt them. Almost anybody you can think of may become a target:

- Your spouse
- Your neighbor
- Your doctor
- Your minister
- Your children
- Your parents
- Your in-laws

So you watch and wait. Sooner or later, someone—being human—will say or do something to "justify" unleashing your anger at them. Fortunately, your gracious friends and relatives often remain unruffled when you blow your stack at times like these.

It is all right to feel such anger and hatred, even though it is irrational. Acting on that anger, however, can be precarious. It could make others hurt . . . then you hurt because you caused them pain . . . and the vicious circle starts over again.

The Escapes: Sometimes when you awaken at 2:00 A.M., you may wish you could close your eyes and never open them again. These wishes usually will remain secret because you will be ashamed of them. Nevertheless, many parents of children with disabilities openly confess to going through stages when they felt such an urge to escape. In spite of such in-the-wee-hours-of-the-morning urges, grit your teeth and hang on. By the time the sun rises, the situation often looks brighter.

OPTIONS TO CONSIDER

- If you feel like ending it all . . . wait. In time you will realize that such escapes are stupid. They create more problems than they solve.
- Do not divorce your mate this week. Better to wait, even though you harbor fears that your spouse has rotten genes . . . or that it is

all his or her fault. (Your marriage partner may be secretly harboring the same fears about you.) It is better to contain such fears for the present and try to work together as a team.

- Shout epithets if you must. But let it come as no surprise that your curses lack the power to shake the foundations of God, nor do they wither the earth. It may be wiser, however, to utter them under your breath, in order to save wear and tear on your throat.
- Do not blame your doctor. The news that your child has a disability will hurt no matter how he or she breaks the news to you. However, if your physician, in relating to you and your child, develops irrational blocks, guilts, and greats because of the disability . . . get yourself another doctor.
- If you find yourself in the drags, enjoy the misery only for a limited time. Move those muscles! Work! Scrub that sink or mow that lawn. Do it even though you do not want to.
- When the speeds come on, stop. Sit down for a moment. Then talk slowly, walk slowly. Pick only 1 of the 241,000 things you feel you should do that day, and do it.
- Learn to admit to yourself that no matter how real these feelings may seem, they are strange and irrational. They will pass.
- Know that time is your best friend. In time, beautiful sanity can grow out of the terrible chaos.
- Look around and choose genuine support persons—key professionals, advocates, relatives, friends—who are capable of entering your struggle in a helpful way. More are available than ever before, so do not try to "go it alone." In an international symposium on people with disabilities, the participants asserted that although the initial pain in parents (upon learning their child has a disability) remains high, their ability to move through those bewildering stages became easier because of the outside support they received (Perske, 1977). Also, in a report to the President it was learned that child abuse in one program was nonexistent because of the many helpful family supports from the outside (Perske, 1978).
- Try to keep the "unbearables" you experience from overflowing onto your child with the disability. After all, the barriers he or she must overcome or live with are almost unbearable, too. It does not help to heap more burdens on these children when it is all they can do to carry their own.

So, there will be bewildering times in your lives. But as you hang on and move through each one, you will find precious opportunities to be strong and tender at the same time—with yourself, with your child, and with those around you.

Appendix
Sample Verbal Communication Handout

BASIC COMMUNICATION SKILLS

When you talk with a new parent, the initial task is to allow the parent to express the situation as he or she sees it. Most useful in determining this is the technique of providing limited structure through the use of an open invitation to talk.

An open invitation to talk may be best understood when compared with a closed approach. For example:

- OPEN: Tell me about your child? How are things going?
- CLOSED: How old is your child? What is his or her disability?

Open comments provide room for the parent to express his- or herself without imposed categories. An open comment allows the parent an opportunity to explore him- or herself with the support of the pilot parent. A closed invitation often emphasizes the factual content as opposed to feelings and sometimes demonstrates a lack of interest in what the parent has to say. Closed questions can usually be answered in a few words or with a *yes* or *no*.

Although the pilot parent does ask questions, the questions are centered around the concerns of the new parent. Questions should be designed to help the parent clarify his or her own concerns or feelings, rather than provide information for the pilot parent. If the pilot parent relies on closed questions, he or she often is forced to concentrate so hard on thinking up the next question that he or she fails to listen to and attend to the parent.

ACTIVE LISTENING RESPONSES

Active listening responses include door openers, noncommittal responses, paraphrasing, focusing on feelings instead of facts, pointing out nonverbal behaviors, and silence.

Examples of some of the responses to use include

- Door openers: "Would you like to share more about that?"
  "I'm interested in what you are saying."
  "That sounds important to you."

"Do you want to talk about it?"

- Noncommittal: "Uh-huh," "Yeah," "Really," "I see," nodding your head
- Paraphrasing: "What I hear you saying is . . ."
  "In other words . . ."
  "Let me make sure I'm hearing this correctly; you are saying . . ."

The caution in paraphrasing: Do not interpret what the person has said. When you are paraphrasing, you are only repeating back in fewer words what the person has said. Be careful not to let your own feelings or opinions slip in.

- Focusing on feeling: "You sound . . ."
  "You seem . . ."
  "You look . . ."

These are to help the person focus on the feelings behind the words. Many times the person gets so caught up in the words that they lose sight of exactly what they are feeling. Silence: "Silence is golden." Try not to feel uncomfortable when there is silence. Many times the speaker is refocusing and he should not be interrupted. Sometimes this silence is very productive, so don't feel that you should constantly be talking in order for anything to be happening.

WORDS NOT TO USE

1. "If I were you . . ."—because you are not them.
2. "Should" or "shouldn't" phrases—"You should be happy" or "Your husband shouldn't be so negative" imply advice giving and judgments on the family. Could and couldn't phrases work better in any situation. They imply that the family has options.
3. "Don't" phrases—"Don't worry" or "Don't feel guilty" are judgments on your part.
4. "Be realistic" and "Face the reality"—your opinion is not what they need. Remember to support them where they are in their grieving.
5. "It's going to be okay" and "Everything will be okay" are phrases that imply you think that they are not normal in feeling the way they do.
6. "I know how you feel"—you don't know how they feel, only how you felt. You might say, "I remember how I felt when they told me" or "If they told you that, no wonder you are feeling so bad."

7. "Oh, you don't mean that"—they may very well mean exactly that. All of us have had terrible feelings at one time or another. It is all a part of grieving and should be respected.
8. "Because you have worked so hard, the baby has come so far"—this makes the parent feel that he or she will have to work harder and can't take a rest, for fear the baby will lose ground.
9. "Special"—most days we are all doing the best we can with what we have, and we don't necessarily feel anyone is special.
10. "You're so strong"—don't put that kind of burden on a parent. Other people do enough of that. We are all just doing the best we can, no better or worse than any other parent.

Appendix

Sample Story for Listening

PUPPIES FOR SALE

A man was putting up a sign that read, *Puppies for Sale,* and before he had driven in the last nail, there was a small boy at his side. That kind of sign seems to attract small boys.

The youngster wanted to know how much the puppies cost. The man told him they were very good dogs and that he did not expect to let any of them go for less than $35 or $40. There was a look of disappointment and then a lot of questions: "I've got $2.37. Could I look at them?"

The man whistled and called *Lady,* and out of the kennel and down the runway came Lady, followed by five little balls of fur, with one lagging considerably behind. The boy spotted the lagging puppy and pointing asked, "What's wrong with him?" The reply was that the vet had said there was no hip socket in the right hip and that the dog would always be lame.

The boy's immediate reply was, "That's the dog I want to buy. I'll give you $2.37 and 50 cents a month until I get him paid for."

The man smiled and shook his head. "That's not the dog you want. That dog will never be able to run and jump and play with you."

The boy very matter-of-factly pulled up his little trouser leg and revealed a leg brace running down both sides of his badly twisted right leg and under the foot, with a leather cap over the knee. "I don't run so well myself," he said. "And he'll need somebody who understands him."

QUESTIONS

- How much were the puppies?
- How much money did the little boy have?
- What was the mother's dog's name?
- How many puppies were there?
- What was the little boy's proposed deal to buy the puppy he wanted?
- Why did the boy want that particular puppy?
- When did you know that?

Appendix
Simulations and Role Plays

You can use the following simulations and role plays with a small group of three to four parents toward the end of the supporting parent training. Give each group one of the simulations and ask the members to discuss how they would respond to each situation as supporting parents. Allow 10–15 minutes for the discussion and then have each small group report back to the larger group so that all participants benefit from the ideas generated by each small group.

Mr. and Mrs. E. have recently had their first child, a little girl named Sara, who has severe birth defects. They waited a long time to have this child and are feeling very overwhelmed and sad. They cry during most of the first visit.

Mr. and Mrs. C. have just been given a vague diagnosis of mental retardation for their son, Matt, from their pediatrician. He has evaluated their child developmentally and gave them a poor prognosis for Matt's future and was very negative about what he would be able to do.

Mrs. B. is a single parent with a daughter, Susan, who has cerebral palsy. She spends almost every waking minute with her, ignoring household tasks, her other child, and herself. She feels that she may have caused the disability because she needed to take large doses of medication during the first months of her pregnancy. Now she feels totally responsible for her daughter's disability and that she must somehow compensate for it.

Mr. and Mrs. H. have a 2-month-old daughter who has hydrocephalus. They were told by the doctor that their daughter had a high probability of having developmental disabilities. The shunt surgery was successfully performed when she was 3 days old. They wonder if they should get a second opinion or if they should change doctors altogether because this one doesn't seem to be very understanding of their feelings. He told them the baby may develop seizures, and they are very scared. They also are worried that the shunt will stop working.

This material is reprinted by permission from the New Hampshire Office of Community & Public Health, Special Medical Services Bureau.

Mr. and Mrs. A. have been home for 2 weeks with their son, Jamie, who has Down syndrome. Mr. A. is very accepting of the child, wants to plan for the future, and seems very positive in his expectations for his son. Mrs. A., however, is focused on the physical needs that Jamie has and says little that is positive about him. She is very quiet during the first meeting and makes little eye contact.

Mr. and Mrs. F. were referred to Parent to Parent by their local pediatrician. She thought that they might learn more about community resources and gain access to some services for their child, who is now 4 years old and has severe developmental delays. The parents moved to the community 5 months ago and are very lonely. They have no family nearby.

Mr. and Mrs. D. have an infant son, David, who has spina bifida. They are involved with birth-to-3 services. However,

- Former friends have stopped coming by and calling. They seem to be uneasy around the couple, especially when David is present.
- The older children (ages 3 and 6) in the family seem to be placing extra demands for attention on their parents. They seem to be acting out and seeking attention in inappropriate ways. Mr. and Mrs. D. have cut back on other family activities in order to address David's needs.

7

Organizing Your Program

The Nuts and Bolts

"If a man will begin with certainties, he shall end in doubts; but if he will be content to begin with doubts, he shall end in certainties."

—Francis Bacon

In Chapters 5 and 6, you learned about how Parent to Parent programs find and train supporting parents and then carefully match them with parents who are referred to the program. Although these activities certainly can happen under the direction of a small group of parents, they are strengthened when they have a strong organizational base behind them.

This chapter describes how parents of children with special needs have successfully organized their Parent to Parent programs to serve children and families and the lessons they learned along the way. Within these stories you will find recommended practices and research-based data that will help you start a Parent to Parent program.

You also will learn how to 1) develop a leadership team and define its roles and responsibilities, 2) plan and facilitate organizational meetings using a written agenda, and 3) decide whether your program should develop a relationship with a sponsoring agency or a fiscal agency or stay an autonomous entity.

Some people may tell you that starting this kind of program cannot be done, at least not easily. You may have personal doubts about whether you can manage such a project. You may lack experience, training, or a formal higher education, and you may question your ability to organize and operate a program. You may wonder: Where will the money come from to do this? Will parents find the program? Will professionals refer families to the program? Will we find enough parents to volunteer as supporting parents? You are not alone with your concerns. This chapter answers your questions and gives you information to move ahead.

EARLY DEVELOPMENT PROGRAM STORIES

Hundreds of Parent to Parent programs have been started by parents across the country and around the world in the same manner and under similar circumstances. The following program story is just one of many.

The Beginning of Parents Helping Parents

In 1976, while attending a presentation on children with special needs, I mentioned to the social worker at my son Dean's early intervention program that I felt strongly about the need for a Parent to Parent program but did not have time to start one. She knew of two other parents who had been talking about starting a program and told me that they were planning to hold their first meeting within the next month. "Great!" I thought. "Now I won't have to start a program; I can just give them a hand."

Gita and Elayne were the catalysts for starting Parents Helping Parents (PHP). Gita's physician had called her and asked if she would go to the hospital to talk to a new mom who had just given birth to a child with a disability. After that visit Gita shared the experience and her ideas for a Parent to Parent program with Elayne and a few other parents. These parents became the program development team. They envisioned a program that would match experienced and new parents for support and information. After meeting informally for 2 months, they planned their first public gathering. Making arrangements for the gathering involved getting free use of a room at an agency, inviting a professional to speak free of charge, and distributing fliers about the event. I was excited to join the effort.

The first meeting was billed as a gathering because it was not a meeting to discuss strategies for organizing the program. And yet, the 40–50 parents who came to hear the speaker left as newly recruited supporting parents for the Parent to Parent program. At the next gathering we recruited more sup-

porting parents, and soon we had enough supporting parents to begin making parent matches.

Making parent matches was the reason we started, and initially this was the only service we envisioned. We believed that parents would be all right and could get their emotional and informational needs met if we would make sure they were matched with a supporting parent.

We called our supporting or veteran parents visiting parents, *and later* mentor visiting parents (MVPs). *After they were matched, MVPs would visit a new family in their home or in the hospital, invite the new family to their home, or maintain a relationship via the telephone. The MVPs always respected the preferences of the referred parents.*

After several planning meetings around our kitchen tables, we developed a PHP brochure. Several hundred copies were produced on a weird orange paper donated by a print shop. We took what we could get! We sent brochures to hospitals to increase referrals that were coming in by word of mouth. We developed two information forms: one to gather information about the new or referred family and the other to document information about the veteran supporting parent. Both parent forms provided the same information, except the section on special experiences for the supporting parent was replaced with the referred parent's areas of concern on the referred parent form.

The few dollars that we needed to run the program those first years came out of our own pockets. PHP's main expenses were related to producing and mailing fliers and brochures or purchasing refreshments for monthly parent support group meetings. I added a cardboard filing cabinet to my bedroom closet (our office in my home) and set up two boxes to hold information for the families. We collected information about diagnoses and resources from local, state, and national agencies such as Easter Seals and the National Information Center for Children and Youth with Disabilities. We used nearby print shops for reproducing documents and materials until a remade copier was purchased and housed at another parent leader's home. The minister of a church near my home gave us permission to use the church's fireside room for our gatherings.

The telephone was ringing overtime. We attached a remote control device to the answering machine so that our parent team could rotate the responsibilities of handling calls and matching parents by passing along the remote device.

In the beginning, matching parents was not easy because the number of supporting parents was small. Initially, we provided no formal training to supporting parents, but we added this important component as soon as we could. We matched about 20–30 parents the first year, 50 the second year, and continued to have about 40–50 people turn out for our speakers. The monthly parent support group sessions had an average of 12–16 parents in attendance.

As we reflected on our first year, we were proud of our successes. We had set up a system that would serve families and the community well into the future.

OVERVIEW OF STARTING A PROGRAM

Parent to Parent programs are organized in various ways. Early Parent to Parent program development teams did what they could to accomplish their mission, and Parent to Parent programs flourished because opportunities for parents to be matched with supporting parents were nonexistent.

In the PHP program story, a small group of parents came together as a team, without money and without elaborate plans, and decided to develop a program to help parents connect with other parents. They put referred parents in touch with mentor parents, and their parent matching services were started even before the program was formally organized. They used their homes as the program office from which to launch their services. They borrowed space from other agencies (churches, schools, and community centers) for larger gatherings.

Although every program development story is unique, generally parents involved in developing a new program spend the first year establishing a foundation by

- Defining the program and its mission
- Identifying the leadership team and deciding on individual responsibilities
- Creating a logo and developing a brochure
- Locating sources for free printing
- Finding free materials and information for families
- Adding names to the list of prospective supporting parents
- Thinking of ways to advertise the program

A Story from Parent to Parent of New Hampshire

It was 1979, and we were a group of 10 parents of children with special needs who met in Gerri's living room for a social evening once a month. Sometimes we had a guest speaker, and other times we would just talk with one another. Gerri's home was welcoming to all of us, but it was becoming inundated by calls from people who had heard about our group. We grew from 10 people to 110 people in 10 months and decided that we needed to have an office. The medical director of the Child Development and Genetics Department at Dartmouth's Hitchcock Hospital embraced the idea of a peer network and gave us a desk and a telephone in the developmental clinic.

Support groups come and go, and we learned that groups are not for everyone. It takes courage to walk into a group of strangers. And if the group has been together longer than a year or two, a newcomer can feel like an outsider as the intimacy of the original group changes. Sometimes one-to-one support is more enriching and fulfilling, and for us, it was the most easily arranged.

We all were familiar with writing grants, and even though we were developing our parent matching activities, we wrote our first grant to the local United Way to establish a respite care program. We had identified a need for respite as the biggest issue compromising our lives—the inability to go out to dinner, to the movies, or to friends' homes for a few hours. We identified respite care providers who were our friends and sought community volunteers whom we had recruited, and soon we had a teaming program for 30 families. We also responded to a request for proposal for a 3-year program to develop a peer networking program in our area.

In the beginning, Parent to Parent of New Hampshire called on untrained friends of the network to support referred parents. Some of these parents were veteran parents who were involved in earlier support groups that had been formed in the community. Encouragement, support, and follow-up were offered to untrained supporting parents just as it is offered to those who are trained, and both trained and untrained supporting parents offered new families support and information.

There were no set rules for making matches. We listened for clues as well as facts when getting a referral or when speaking with a parent who contacted our program. When we got off the telephone, we looked through the database for someone who would be a good match. If a match was not made around a specific disability, it was made around a specific issue, such as school, transportation, or moving to a new location.

LEARNING FROM EXPERIENCE

Your own innovation and creativity mean that your Parent to Parent programs will be unique. Taking a look at what successful programs have done and what research suggests as you go about planning your program is useful. Learning from the experience of other programs enhances the quality of new ones and saves time and energy while preventing problems.

CREATING A LEADERSHIP TEAM

A leadership team must have at least one or two people who are interested in helping others and willing to put time and energy into starting a program. If they are parents of children with special needs, they will use the knowledge and organizational skills that they have gained from their own experiences, their natural abilities, and their education. Parent leaders should keep in mind that they do not have to know how to do everything themselves. People in the community, in their state, and across the nation can supply answers and resources. The program organizers in the Family Support Network of Eastern North Carolina story in Chapter 4 used their statewide Parent to Parent program to boost their efforts. Professionals can and often do work as partners with parents to start a program. But because parents often prefer to be led by other parents, a parent should be found as quickly as possible to lead the program.

There is no magic in the number of members on a leadership team. The team can be 2, 10, 12, or 20. The leadership's active participation and commitment to the project will determine whether and how a Parent to Parent program is developed. Creating a team to share the work load is important, and the team members must take care of their physical, mental, spiritual, and emotional needs, as well as those of their nuclear or extended families, before they will be able to meet the needs of those involved in a Parent to Parent program.

Many programs begin with little or no money. Without money, early program leaders often recruit volunteers with specific skills to handle unfamiliar jobs and to help with some of the administrative tasks. For example, the members of a program development team that may not know financial systems for tracking might find a volunteer bookkeeper, accountant, or controller. The team that does not know how to write proposals or is unfamiliar with fundraising techniques might find a volunteer fund developer. Parents are often more interested in carrying out the service side of the program (matching parents) than the business side of running a program (financial management).

Program development teams may comprise, but are not necessarily limited to, parents of children who have a need for special services. Professionals from the educational, social, counseling, and health care arenas often volunteer to help. Later these same professionals may become part of an advisory board for your program (see Chapter 8).

Influential community leaders can provide knowledge and contacts as a program begins to organize, and they are invaluable networking connections who can help the program grow quickly and stabilize as it matures. Community members to consider for your organizing team (and perhaps later as members of future directing boards and collaborative partnerships) are

- Local political leaders (e.g., mayor, city council members, school board members)
- Corporate business leaders (e.g., company presidents, vice presidents, directors of human resources, personnel directors, directors of finance and administration)
- Members of service groups (e.g., Rotary Club, Kiwanis, Knights of Columbus)
- Staff of other nonprofit organizations (e.g., United Cerebral Palsy Association, Easter Seals, American Heart Association, American Cancer Society)
- People from technical assistance organizations (e.g., nonprofit development centers, Retired Senior Volunteer Program, Retired Executive Volunteers)
- Religious and spiritual leaders

Working together does not mean doing everything together. A well-functioning team learns to function independently as members while supporting each other as they share responsibilities. Supporting each other and keeping each other informed is a part of the team spirit and method. Being a team means coming together to decide what the issues are, what is to be done, and who can accomplish it. Parent to Parent of New Hampshire's team decided that providing respite was a priority for them. Parents Helping Parents decided that making parent matches and training physicians and nurses to work with families were top priorities. Mathematically speaking, good collaboration means coming together to add your expertise, divide the work, subtract your differences, and multiply your results.

Many leadership teams can start a program, but usually the one person committed to the mission sustains the program and sees it through to completion and stability. Usually this person is a parent and the commitment to the Parent to Parent program comes because the parent realizes the value of it from personal experience.

If you are excited about helping to develop a Parent to Parent program but are not interested in being the leader or being on the leadership team, be sure to make your desires known. Be open and honest about what roles and responsibilities you feel comfortable accepting. Program development teams need leaders, but they also need people who can help them get the job done.

FINDING MEMBERS FOR THE TEAM

Although often a program development team often begins with just a few people, there are creative ways to find more members for the leadership team, and it is important to do so. If you keep the team limited to a few, the team members are likely to experience burnout and the program may suffer. Here are some recruitment strategies:

- Make personal telephone calls to parents and professionals with whom you have been in contact—your child's pediatrician or teacher, your best friend who organizes events at church, or the parents you've met or heard at parent gatherings.
- Put a notice in the local newspaper about starting a Parent to Parent program. Ask interested parties to call you. Most newspapers have a free section for publicizing community activities.
- Put notices in magazines or newsletters of agencies and organizations that have an interest in children and families. Write letters to the editor to get your voice out to the public.
- Contact religious organizations, special schools, or organizations serving individuals with special needs such as the March of Dimes and United Cerebral Palsy.
- Give a copy of a letter about your intent to organize a program to other agencies so that they can add it to mailings to the families they serve. Put a telephone number, fax number, e-mail address, and mailing address on the letter so that families can get back to you. Create a tear-off section at the bottom of the letter so that they can fill in basic information (e.g., name, address, telephone number) and return it to you.

Sometimes organizing groups don't advertise their planning meetings and events because they are afraid too many people will respond. However, if you indicate in your publicity that you are in the process of developing a program, then you probably will attract only those who are ready to work. If, however, too many people attend, apologize for the cramped quarters, and get their names, addresses, and telephone numbers on a sign-in sheet. Don't lose any contacts who might make great future partners, supporting parents, committee members, or program volunteers.

PLANNING THE MEETINGS

Selecting a Place

Plan a meeting for those who respond to your advertising by picking a place that is easy to find and has convenient parking. First meetings often are held in someone's home, but they can be held at a school, a house of worship, a senior citizen center, a bank, a library, a community center, a hospital, a social services agency, a United Way office, or a hotel.

Because those who might allow you to use a meeting space sometimes worry about special accommodations and may be uncomfortable with individuals who have special needs, it may be easier to secure a place for your meetings if you leave the word *disability* out of your request. You could simply say that you are looking for a place for parents and professionals to hold a meeting.

Providing Refreshments

Have someone take responsibility for refreshments. Provide simple snacks, such as coffee, tea, juice, water, cookies, or fruit. People seem to socialize and relax more easily when food is a part of the activity. As the group grows, be creative and mindful of providing ethnically diverse treats.

Assembling Materials

Assign someone to gather materials, such as handouts, audiovisual aids, flip charts, marking pens, name tags, sign-in sheets, and overhead and videotape projectors. Create signs that will guide those attending the meeting to your location. In addition, find a dependable person to type information recorded or produced at meetings.

Arranging the Room

Avoid arranging the meeting space in classroom style, as this arrangement might suggest that the people seated in front have all the answers. When people are sitting in rows they can't see or interact with each other very well, and they have a harder time hearing what is being said. Arrange the seats in a circle, semicircle, or a U or T formation for the best interaction among people.

Creating an Agenda

Having a written agenda will help you avoid unproductive meetings, and when you hand out your agenda, those attending will know that you have prepared for the meeting (see Figure 7.1).

- Use odd but memorable times to start and stop the meeting (6:27 P.M. as opposed to 6:30 P.M.). These times may actually be easier for people to remember.
- Make sure the day of the week is included with the date. The word *Tuesday* or *Thursday* will help people determine their own availability for the meeting and will help them remember when to be there.

- Put the day and date on fliers, special event notices, and announcements.
- Decide who will open the meeting. The written agenda tells participants who will be the leader and also may indicate that multiple facilitators are sharing roles and working together.

CONDUCTING THE FIRST MEETING

Concentrate on four goals at this first meeting, and list them on your agenda. Introduce all four of these goals at the start of the meeting so that the team can see where the organization is heading.

Goal 1: Getting Acquainted with Each Other

Provide name tags to help people remember names, and invite participants to use a sign-in sheet with columns to indicate their name, address, telephone number, profession, and child's age and special need. To help people get acquainted, invite each person to stand and introduce him- or herself, giving his or her full name and area of expertise and a brief statement about his or her reason for coming. As participants share their reasons for coming, you will learn more about their children's ages and diagnoses. One of the team leaders can speak first to model the length of time and type of information to be shared in the introduction.

Various ice breaker games also can be used to encourage people to talk and interact with each other. For example, attach a piece of paper bearing the name of a famous person to each participant's back as they sign in. Everyone must circulate about the room asking others yes-or-no questions to guess which famous person he or she is. In doing so, they also get to know each other.

Goal 2: Creating Your Program's Mission, Goals, and Objectives

Before creating a mission statement, goals, and objectives for your program, begin with a brainstorming session to gather and record information about the needs of parents (e.g., problems, concerns, issues) and the philosophies (e.g., beliefs) and values that are connected to these needs. Understanding the needs of parents and a common philosophy about meeting those needs will make future proposal writing, long-range planning, and evaluation of your program easier.

Be sure that all information is recorded. Have two people take meeting notes so that recording can be done quickly and accurately. A second person can start writing the next idea while the first person con-

Agenda

Thursday, September 20, 2001

6:27 P.M. Call to order—Mary Jones, Facilitator

Logistical data (locate exits, restrooms, and refreshments)

Why we've called the meeting

6:45 P.M. Introductions—John Smith, RN, Co-facilitator

7:00 P.M. Brainstorm issues, concerns, and needs—Mary Jones and volunteers from the group

7:30 P.M. Facilitate the sharing of philosophy, values, and vision—John Smith

8:15 P.M. Begin to create a written mission statement, goals, and objectives—Mary Jones

9:17 P.M. Set next meeting date and adjourn—Mary Jones and John Smith

Respectfully submitted,

Mary Jones, parent

John Smith, RN

Friendly reminder: Leave in pairs or groups for safety.

Figure 7.1. Sample agenda for a first formal planning meeting.

centrates on writing down the current idea completely and correctly. The recorders should write large enough for the participants in the back of the room to be able to read what is written on the flip charts. Ask participants to read the documentation of their ideas for accuracy and to speak up if the recorder does not document it correctly. Using a flip chart keeps the group from repeating what already has been suggested, and keeps the group more focused on the idea being presented. Recording ideas also sends the message that each idea is important and will be used in the future. You may also notice that the group is more focused on the idea being presented.

Have someone else record the flip chart information onto paper to provide a duplicate copy. Try to keep recorded proceedings in binders in at least two different places. These notes provide a document that you can use as you continue to complete your mission, goals, objectives, and assigning roles and responsibilities. You will find that these records become invaluable time-saving tools for updating newcomers to the program.

At the end of the brainstorming session, the leaders can start formulating a vision by discussing how they would like to see the program develop. Participants add to this vision, and the group can work to achieve consensus about the future of the program. Clarity at the beginning helps the leaders explain their program succinctly, precisely, and easily to others later.

When the needs, beliefs, values, and vision are recorded, then proceed with the creation of a mission statement, based on those needs and beliefs (see Chapter 9). The process of outlining the future of your program will serve you well as you engage in long-range strategic planning later on (see Chapter 8).

Creating a written record of mission, goals, and objectives takes time, so start this process early so that your program proceeds in a focused manner. The program leadership should review the mission statement at least every other year. It can and should be revised as necessary to reflect the current program. Display your mission statement on your office walls, put it in brochures and newsletters, and use it in proposals. Consult the mission statement when you decide whether to add new program components (see Chapter 10).

Goal 3: Assigning Leadership Roles and Responsibilities

Assigning roles and responsibilities may not happen during the first few meetings. People often arrive at meetings with mixed emotions and unanswered questions, so you may need to allow time for parents to acknowledge and share their concerns. Being heard and acknowledged is therapeutic, and program development team members will be better prepared to move forward in a positive, more focused manner. If any of the parent leaders on the development team re-experience some painful emotions, they should be given support and time off so that they can return to the project refreshed and ready to work.

Distributing work seems easy when there are few people on the team. Each person tackles tasks according to his or her skills. Distribution of work can be done in the same manner in larger groups as well. Although a balanced load across the team is ideal, there are other ways to get things completed. One person may decide to take on 50%–75% of the work while 5–10 other people share the remaining responsibilities. Talking about roles and responsibilities will ensure that the work loads are acceptable to everyone on the team.

When assigning roles and responsibilities, you will need to be sure that two major program development areas are covered. The first centers around organizing the efforts of the team, and it includes the responsibilities of planning for the next meeting, finding a place to meet, preparing refreshments, arranging the room, creating the next agenda, and finding funds to pay for telephone, postage, and printing fees. The second area centers on providing the Parent to Parent program services even as the program development activities continue. This involves finding veteran parents who want to take on supporting or mentoring responsibilities; acquiring a telephone and answering machine for the program; advertising to the professional community; assigning someone to take responsibility for receiving referrals; assigning someone to make parent matches and document data; and training veteran parents as the program matures. Positions, roles, and titles can be clarified as the program matures and the number of people available to do the work increases. Be creative, and remember that there is no one right way to do things.

The only assignment after the first meeting may be that the leaders will take home all of the recorded information, type it up, and have it ready for the next meeting. Do not delegate a job this big so early, unless you have some assurance of dependability. The main responsibility of the participants at this point is to show up for the next meeting. Roles that can be assigned later include director, assistant director, chair, vice chair, secretary, treasurer, parliamentarian, or other positions the group may choose. If the leadership team does not yet have program objectives to which roles and responsibilities can be attached, then a list can be used to designate jobs to different people in the group.

As the program matures, detailed action plans should be created for each objective. Action plans include the objective (e.g., what is to be accomplished); the activities (e.g., how it is to happen); the person (e.g., who is responsible); the date of completion; and the list of targeted milestones and date for accomplishment. Action plan worksheets allow you to assign roles and responsibilities as your program grows.

Goal 4: Setting Dates for Meetings

During the beginning stages of a program, don't allow too much time between meetings; however, provide enough time for people to accomplish their tasks. Try to wait at least 2 weeks but not more than 1 month for the next meeting. Schedule monthly meetings 6 months at a time, and continue to plan business or organizing meetings.

IDEAS FOR SUCCESSFUL MEETINGS

Encourage people to stand when they talk so that they can be heard more easily. Standing tends to shorten the time a person keeps the floor—important when you have limited time.

Ask participants to volunteer to help during the meeting. This is your first opportunity to get people more involved in the organizing process. Call for two volunteers to perform each job to ease any anxiety the volunteers may feel. Invite active involvement if people don't step forward and volunteer. Ask them directly if they are willing to do a job, or have someone nominate a candidate for a position.

Set the next meeting date while everyone is present. This encourages people to return, is efficient because you don't have to call everyone about the next date, and indicates serious intentions.

Encourage participants and leaders to leave in groups when the meeting is over for safety and to give them another opportunity to talk and get to know each other better. Some of the best ideas come when walking to the car, and leaving together for protection models concern and care for others.

SEEKING A SPONSORING AGENCY

Another early decision that has to be made is whether to seek a sponsoring agency to assume responsibility for the program. A Parent to Parent program may be 1) established as a volunteer organization, 2) autonomously organized with paid staff, or 3) sponsored by any number of organizations. Many Parent to Parent programs are totally volunteer efforts with parents volunteering their time to the program. There are no paid staff and the program does not have a legal organizational status. Other programs choose to establish their own legal status as a not-for-profit organization autonomous from any other organization. Still, other programs decide to develop as a part of and sponsored by another existing organization.

There are advantages and disadvantages to being sponsored by another agency. Advantages include increased visibility and credibility for the program, financial and in-kind support, availability and access to professionals and resources, use of an existing program's nonprofit status for grant writing and fund raising, office space, and telephone lines. One disadvantage of sponsorship is some loss of autonomy to move the program in directions of your choice. Also, decisions about program philosophy, components, growth, and development may be determined by the sponsor rather than by the parents. The fact that there are both advantages and disadvantages in having a program sponsored is reflected in the fact that the survey of Parent to Parent programs reported that 52% of Parent to Parent programs were sponsored and 48% were nonsponsored.

If you decide to seek a relationship with a sponsoring agency, keep in mind that there are different kinds of programs that may be willing to sponsor a Parent to Parent program. The survey data indicate that sponsoring agencies for Parent to Parent programs tend to be disability and social services agencies, hospitals, school districts, and in some cases, the statewide Parent to Parent program itself (see Table 4.5 in Appendix A). If you get involved with a sponsoring agency, you may find it easier to maintain your program autonomy if the sponsoring agency also is not involved in providing direct services to children with special needs. You may find that a church, community center, or senior citizen center may be a more neutral sponsor than a school or hospital.

Because for most sponsoring agencies it is beneficial to have a Parent to Parent program as one of its program activities, a sponsoring agency may not be eager for the Parent to Parent program to leave and become its own entity in the future. So, if you elect to build a relationship with a sponsoring agency to help your program get started, it also is important that you begin planning for your program's independence and eventual separation from the sponsoring agency as well. Create a written Memorandum of Understanding that allows your program to depart from the sponsoring agency in the future so that there will be no misunderstanding when and if the time comes for your program to establish its independence.

FISCAL SPONSORSHIP

Until a program receives its nonprofit, tax-exempt status, it may consider using another nonprofit agency as its fiscal sponsor or fiscal agency. Having a fiscal agency before you acquire tax-exempt status means that people can give money to your program and get tax deductions for their contributions. Also, your program can receive funds from foundations and others who require funded programs to have a nonprofit, tax-exempt status.

A fiscal sponsor may charge you a percentage (usually from 8% to 25%) of the funds that they are holding for your program, and for this fee they will dispense and monitor your program funds for you. Sometimes a program uses a fiscal agency even though it has its own tax-exempt status because its funder insists that the funding it is supplying must be under another agency's fiscal sponsorship. Some funding sources may insist that a Parent to Parent program have a fiscal agency because they are not aware of the capacity of parent-directed groups to be a fiscal agency themselves.

COLLABORATION AND COOPERATION

A successful Parent to Parent program recognizes that collaborating with schools, hospitals, universities, and other organizations to produce workshops and various components of its program is a positive step toward growth. Collaborating is different from being sponsored because a program can seek assistance from other agencies while still remaining independent and autonomous itself. For example, PHP rented space at the Family Education Center for a small fee and had access to the center's copier at 10 cents per copy. The center's staff also were eager and willing to mentor PHP regarding insurance, proposal writing, long-range planning, and other nonprofit management and survival skills. They also allowed PHP to use their facility for meetings and workshops without cost. You will read more about collaborative partnerships in Chapter 12.

SUMMARY

Parent to Parent programs have been established successfully in many places, for many years, by many people, and you have every chance to be just as successful in creating your own Parent to Parent program.

Although there is no one right way to organize a program, several steps can help your program become successful. Learn from other programs, and use recommended practices. Parent to Parent programs are vulnerable for failure early on if one or two people lead it and do not seek help from others. Remember that it is best if parents are the leaders of Parent to Parent programs—self-help programs work best when run by people who have been there. Professional input also is valuable. Although now there are many experienced parent leaders who can mentor and train new parent leaders to create or operate programs so that program developers do not have to depend on professional help as they did in the past, having professionals who support your program's development can be very useful.

Directing a Parent to Parent program is an empowering experience for parents. Parents leading the program and those receiving services see that families can and do use their family and disability experiences in helpful and productive ways.

RESOURCES

Bradley, V.J. (1992). Overview of the family support movement. In V.J. Bradley, J. Knoll, & J.M. Agosta (Eds.), *Emerging issues in family support* (pp. 1–8). Washington DC: American Association on Mental Retardation.

Bradley, V.J. (1994). Introduction. In V.J. Bradley, J.W. Ashbaugh, & B.C. Blaney (Eds.), *Creating individual supports for people with developmental disabilities: A mandate for change at many levels* (pp. 3–9). Baltimore: Paul H. Brookes Publishing Co.

Carter, R. (1994). *Helping yourself help others.* New York: Random House.

Colvin, G.L. (1993). *Fiscal sponsorship—6 ways to do it right.* San Francisco: Study Center Press.

Hornsby, G. (1988). Launching parent to parent schemes. *British Journal of Special Education, 15*(2), 77–88.

Lutzker, J., Campbell, R.V., Newman, M., & Harrold, M. (1989). Ecobehavioral interventions for abusive, neglectful, and high-risk families. In G.H.S. Singer & L.K. Irvin (Eds.), *Support for caregiving families: Enabling positive adaptation to disability* (pp. 313–326). Baltimore: Paul H. Brookes Publishing Co.

Powell, T.J. (1990). *Working with self-help.* Washington, DC: NASW Press.

Poyadue, F.S. (1993). *Steps to starting a family resource center or self help group* (Rev. ed.). Santa Clara, CA: Parents Helping Parents, Inc.

Poyadue, F.S. (1998). *A unitary resource file.* Santa Clara, CA: Parents Helping Parents, Inc.

Poyadue, F.S. (1998). *In a nutshell* (a series of 17 booklets on Parent to Parent program services). Santa Clara, CA: Parents Helping Parents, Inc.

Santelli, B., Turnbull, A., Marquis, J., & Lerner, E. (1993). Parent to parent programs: Ongoing support for parents of young adults with special needs. *Journal of Vocational Rehabilitation, 3*(2), 25–37.

8

Institutionalizing Your Program

Parent-Directed Family Resource Centers

> "The problems of the world cannot possibly be solved by skeptics or cynics whose horizons are limited by the obvious realities. We need men who can dream of things that never were."
>
> —John F. Kennedy

Chapter 7 described the early development of a Parent to Parent program and step-by-step ideas for organizing a successful program. This chapter focuses on the mature development of a program that can best be accomplished through institutionalization. *Institutionalizing* your program means establishing a legal form of business that exists independent of its creators, owners, or developers; that has a place for carrying on its work; and that has perpetual existence with limited liability. Not all parent programs reach for or want this level of development, and institutionalization is not essential for maintaining a high-functioning program that offers parent to parent matches. But Parent to Parent programs that have grown to this level recommend it for the stability it brings.

This chapter introduces you to four key activities for institutionalizing your program: 1) becoming incorporated as a not for profit agency, 2) building a board of directors, 3) developing staff, and 4) undertaking long-range strategic planning.

GENERAL STRATEGIES FOR INSTITUTIONALIZING YOUR PROGRAM

Use experienced mentors as you build your program. Find someone who has experience directing a nonprofit agency or who is operating a parent-directed family resource center (PDFRC), and ask him or her whether he or she has time to be your mentor. Ask him or her specific questions, and share your thoughts and feelings about your concerns or plans. Use the mentor as a sounding board for new ideas. Your mentor may or may not be a parent of a child with special needs.

Use consultants who have very specific skills as well. Seek help from people who are successful at what they do and remember that getting help from others is a sign of wisdom, not weakness.

Ask other successful agencies to share their experience and copies of their documents, policies, and procedures with you; then adapt them to fit your own program. Collect three different samples of items that you want to develop—one from an agency about your size in scope and budget, one from a smaller agency, and one from a larger agency.

Build a cadre of grass roots volunteers to help you accomplish the agency's strategic goals and objectives to meet your funding needs.

Learn and implement five major fundraising techniques—proposal writing, direct mail campaigns, donor solicitation, special events, and planned giving (see Chapter 9). Many nonprofit organizations wait too long before hiring a director of fund development, so make sure that you hire someone as soon as possible.

Set up a formal manual or computerized financial system for checking and receipting. There are pegboard manual checking and receipting systems that are simple, effective, and efficient. If you use a manual system, maintain it while you make the transition to a computerized system. Once you are using computers, keep back-up copies on a disk and safely store them away from the office.

Use your auditor and your auditing team throughout the year to create, monitor, and maintain a financial system without loopholes and with good checks and balances. Keep a paper trail of invoices, bills, requests for funding, and receipts of all transactions. An internal audit is done by the agency's staff and board; an external audit, done at least annually, is performed by an auditing firm that is not connected to the agency. The cost of the audit will vary with the size of the agency and from firm to firm.

Create a procedure manual and a personnel handbook. Get acquainted with local, state, and federal laws governing nonprofit organizations and small business employers (e.g., payroll taxes, wages and benefits, rights, safety). Governments will provide copies of this information, and there are companies that put together packets of these materials that can and should be displayed in a conspicuous place at your business for employees to see. In addition, you will need to learn management skills, fiscal and administrative language and methods, and operation of a facility. You can learn at workshops sponsored by the United Way and Nonprofit Development Centers.

Although not everyone will be able to attend all of the organizational meetings, encourage them to come as often as they can. Some who cannot attend the full leadership or board of directors meeting may have done a lot of work during their committee meetings.

Start meetings on time, and don't keep those in attendance waiting. One of the marks of a good leader is keeping the process moving along and the program moving forward.

Implement public awareness programs by creating a marketing plan (see Chapter 11). Marketing and program evaluation are the most neglected areas of nonprofit organizational development, and this neglect often is cause for program failure.

Because the executive director will provide much of the vision for the agency and make the final decisions on the day-to-day operations, do all that you can to ensure that the executive director is a parent of a child with special needs. The board should be composed of at least 51% parents, and staff providing services to families should be parents as well. It is *not* essential that staff performing administrative duties and fund development be parents. You will learn as you grow by using your board of directors and your advisory board to guide you.

Perhaps two to four people from your program can attend Parents Helping Parents' (PHP) national symposium called "The Keys to Creating, Managing, and Maintaining a Parent-Directed Family Resource Center (PDFRC)." They will leave with common knowledge about next steps, recommended practices, and a shared team spirit for moving forward. Private foundations may be willing to provide funding for your leadership team to attend such a technical assistance symposium. To receive these funds you probably will be asked to submit a proposal seeking a *capacity building grant.* Foundations and corporations love to have you leverage their funds into greater assets, which is what capacity building accomplishes as it enhances your infrastructure.

By attending to these strategies and the steps outlined in the following PHP story, you can institutionalize your program in your community. These tasks are not hard, but they do take time to complete. The biggest decision about institutionalizing your program is deciding to take the necessary first steps. Once you start everything will come together.

PHP Program Story: Mature Development

PHP's success was overwhelming! In just 2–3 years, we were sending PHP's newsletter to more than 200 families. Information sheets had grown into information packets, and the special needs library had grown out of its box. Training for physicians was ahead of its time and well received. Nurses who were taking our 6-hour class on working with families who have children with special needs enjoyed it and earned continuing education credits. Workshops were provided to teachers and school psychologists as well. Veteran parents were trained in a 9-hour training program. Brothers and sisters were enjoying sibling therapeutic fun. A support group for single moms and a dad's night out were popular. And hundreds of parent to parent matches were being made each year.

But the years of volunteering had taken its toll on our leadership team. We could not continue to maintain our families, hold jobs, and volunteer for PHP. We needed to institutionalize PHP and make it our job. Could that be done? It seemed the only way that we and the program could survive. Here are the key activities our leadership team performed as we began to institutionalize PHP.

We separated the leadership team into a board of directors and staff. The staff were still unpaid, the chair of the board and the executive director were no longer the same person, and the executive director became part of the staff. Building a dynamic board to help guide and fund the program became our first priority.

We had already reserved the PHP name with the State of California by placing a telephone call to the Secretary of State's office. We incorporated as a 501(c)3 nonprofit agency and filed applications to gain state and federal tax-exempt status. We had to apply to the state to become a business entity that was either for profit or not for profit. When our not-for-profit corporation status was granted, we were eligible to seek funds and do business without paying state or federal taxes.

Two of us took proposal writing courses and learned to create PHP's first mission statement. Two board members and three staff members invested personal time and money in a 5-day fund-raising course.

We consulted the Retired Executive Volunteers (REV) for guidance on the next steps to take to stabilize PHP and move it forward. REV is a group of retired business executives who volunteer to share their knowledge, experience, and acumen with nonprofit organizations without charging a fee.

We held a long-range strategic planning retreat (facilitated by the REV). We then wrote and implemented a 5-year long-range strategic plan to build our program's infrastructure and enhance our program's services. PHP's strategic plan included goals for board development, diversified budgets with reserve funds, office space, fund development, public awareness and marketing, checking and receipting systems, program services, and the hiring of a paid staff. The first plan was about three pages in length, but it captured PHP's vision for the future and focused our growth and directed our activities.

As a result of these actions and over time, PHP completed the following accomplishments to further institutionalize the program. We rented a small office, then leased 2,000 square feet of office space, then leased 6,000 square feet of space before moving to our current 14,500 square foot building.

We set up a pegboard checking and receipting system and precise policies and procedures for tracking money in and out of PHP. We had already maintained checking and savings accounts for PHP that were separate from our personal accounts. We only needed to set up a money market account for reserve funds.

We developed written policies, procedures, and paid staff. We hired an auditing firm to do annual audits. We wrote and received ongoing federal grants to be a California regional Parent Training and Information Center and wrote proposals and received county, corporate, and foundation funding.

We conducted a feasibility study to gather information on how much support we had and our position in the systems of service in our community so that we could plan for the future. We became funded by the United Way, which provided part of our budget and enhanced our credibility with the community and other funding sources. Our local United Way had provided the necessary application forms and guidelines to help us through the required process of writing a grant proposal.

We continued to consult with the REVs as needed. As PHP became a well-known and respected institution locally, statewide, and nationally, we broadened our programs and partnerships with other agencies, as well as strengthened our infrastructure and stabilized our financial base.

Our successful efforts to institutionalize PHP led to many benefits. PHP became funded by the State of California as Santa Clara County's Early Intervention Family Resource Center and was selected as one of

California's five state technical assistance agencies for family resource centers by the State Department of Social Services. We also established and filled a parent liaison position in the State Department of Health, Children with Special Health Care Needs Division.

LEARNING FROM EXPERTS AND RECOMMENDED PRACTICES

Teams developing programs now can utilize recommended practices and direction from experts—parent and professional leaders who have spent 20–30 years learning by trial and error to create excellent programs. Contemporary program organizers also have the benefit of parent to parent research conducted by the Beach Center on Families and Disability at The University of Kansas (see Appendix A).

What are the steps to take to further organize or institutionalize a program that has mushroomed into other components? As described in the PHP story, in addition to ongoing fund-raising, there are several activities that program leaders need to perform as their attention is refocused on this transition to maturity.

BECOMING INCORPORATED

The leadership team needs to transform itself into or acquire other individuals to form the board of directors. For incorporation purposes, this board need only consist of a few people—a chairperson, a secretary, and a treasurer. These are the officers of the board. It is fine to have other board members and other officers, such as a vice chair, an assistant secretary, or a parliamentarian. This board of directors assumes responsibility for the corporation.

The board creates the by-laws and articles of incorporation as they prepare to apply for nonprofit status. By-laws and articles can be as simple as 2–4 pages or as elaborate as 20 or more (see samples of by-laws and articles of incorporation at the end of this chapter). You can get a book on nonprofit development (see resources section at the end of this chapter), or ask an organization similar to yours to share a copy of these items with you.

An organization can be incorporated as a for-profit business, a partnership, or a nonprofit business. Parent to Parent programs usually choose to become incorporated as a 501(c)3 public benefit, nonmembership charitable organizations. You will need to file three applications if your organization wishes to gain this status—one for incorporating, one for state tax-exempt status, and one for federal tax-exempt status. Benefits of being incorporated as a 501(c)3 nonprofit organization include cost savings (e.g., exemption from paying federal, state, and local taxes); lower mailing rates; better ability to attract money; a requirement for many grants (including United Way funding); limited liability for the organization; an increase in your standing in the community; better ability to receive tax-deductible donations; and the label of a legitimate business entity.

State and Federal Requirements for Nonprofit Corporations

Several requirements for nonprofit corporations are mandated by state and federal governments:

- Filing required annual information returns and payroll reports such as 990, Schedule A (IRS), CT2 (Registrar of Charitable Trusts), and 199 (Franchise Tax Board)
- Withholding and paying payroll taxes on time (e.g., federal income tax, Social Security tax, state income tax, state disability insurance)
- Filing federal payroll reports (e.g., W2 and W3 annually, 941 quarterly)
- Filing state payroll reports (e.g., DE43 and W2 annually, DE3 quarterly)
- Filing substantial limits on lobbying activities and prohibition against political activities statement
- Complying with additional standards (e.g., standards of conduct established by the state corporation code, by-laws and articles of incorporation, written personnel policies, accounting procedures)

The remainder of this chapter focuses on three other parts of mature program development—building a dynamic board of directors, developing staff, and embracing long-range strategic planning. There is a relationship between the accomplishment of the institutionalizing steps just outlined and these three subjects.

BUILDING A BOARD OF DIRECTORS

What Is a Board of Directors?

A board is the mechanism by which nonprofit organizations function, legally conduct their business, govern, and monitor themselves. Your by-laws and articles of incorporation require a board to take the lead in raising funds, creating policies, and guiding the organization. To approve grant requests, funding sources expect a board to be in place.

Tradition shows that a board works well by assisting the executive director with the tasks facing nonprofit organizations. Boards provide credibility and take on fiduciary responsibilities in the community. Basically, the community not only supports but also in a sense owns a nonprofit organization by allowing it not to pay taxes and by giving charitable donations. To ensure long-term success, having a strong and active board committed to the program's mission is a step in the right direction.

As the program grows, the *differentiation* of roles and responsibilities between the board (governing body) and the staff (volunteer and/or paid workers who provide the program services) is recommended. Funding sources want to see a separation of board and staff and prefer to fund agencies that have a board comprised solely of volunteers. Having your paid staff serve as board members provides a loophole for checks and balances and is a conflict of interest because the board is the staff's boss. Of course, having paid staff as board members is not *illegal* but is definitely frowned on in the nonprofit world.

Board Functions and Board Meetings

From the beginning it should be made clear to the board of directors that their roles and responsibilities lie in evaluating the organization's effectiveness and administering the corporation, including fund-raising and budgeting; long-range strategic planning; policy approval; and hiring, supporting, and evaluating the executive director, sometimes called the *chief executive officer (CEO).* It also is the board's job to oversee the proper use of the program's funds. The board becomes the community connection and the legal owners of the corporation when the group decides to incorporate as a 501(c)3 nonprofit charity organization. The board is legally responsible for the program and its welfare, and it defines the purpose of the corporation.

The board's duties, roles, responsibilities, and powers should be outlined and defined in the program's by-laws. The program, staff, and board are governed by the by-laws and policies. The board is concerned with the *business* of the program. The board members do not interact with the staff except through the executive director. The executive director is responsible for the staff and the day-to-day management and operation of the program. It is not the board's job to micromanage the services.

The executive director must keep the board informed of the state of the infrastructure, budget, and program services of the organization.

He or she hires, fires, and evaluates the rest of the staff. It is critical that the board not intrude on the day-to-day activities of the program.

Follow *Robert's Rules of Order* in your board meetings. Some members may request a less formal and less structured process, but this lack of formal parliamentary procedure can invite problems, waste time, lose community support, and lead to attrition of corporate leaders who join your board. For example, in order for a topic to be discussed during a meeting, it must be put in the form of a motion. That motion must be seconded. There is a specific agenda order or business to be followed, regulating powers of the chairperson and more.

Maintain at least 50% plus one member board attendance at meetings (a quorum) so that business can be conducted legally. The meeting can proceed, is recorded, and is counted as a meeting, but no final votes may be taken without a quorum of members present. If votes are taken, they are not legally binding. If a board member records all meetings, those absent can keep up by reading minutes of meetings and by reviewing committees' progress reports on their action plans. Develop the habit of treating recorded minutes of meetings seriously, and be sure all board members receive a copy. The recorded board minutes become important legal documents and are a crucial part of your annual audit.

Use committees to get more work done, to get more people involved, and to limit the time board members spend at meetings. Leadership meetings and board meetings are appropriate times for committee chairs to present summary reports of their progress and activities to the full group. The group either accepts, rejects, or sends back to the committee any area of the report that required a lot of discussion. Detailed discussion and major changes in the committe's projects should take place in committee, not at the leadership or board meeting.

Roles and Responsibilities of Officers

The board chairperson, who also can be called the *president,* is the presiding officer who facilitates board meetings and is responsible for the board's function as it accomplishes its tasks. He or she also chairs the executive committee and with the executive director creates meeting agendas.

The vice chair assumes the chairperson's duties in his or her absence, assists the chairperson in carrying out his or her role, and chairs other board committees, such as the marketing committee.

The secretary records the meeting minutes, provides a copy to each member, and maintains an official binder of the board's minutes (i.e., a legal document). He or she assists with typing, sending mail, and other secretarial duties. The assistant secretary performs functions of the secretary in his or her absence, assists the secretary with his or her duties and responsibilities, and can chair board committees.

The treasurer establishes and monitors a checking and receipting financial tracking system for the program. In addition, he or she creates written financial statements and gives reports on the status of the program's finances at board meetings. The treasurer works closely with executive committee members and creates with the CEO an annual budget for the board's review and approval. He or she also chairs an audit committee and ensures that an annual audit is performed.

Boards often choose one of their members to function as parliamentarian. This person maintains proper meeting protocol and adherence to Robert's Rules of Order.

Who Serves on the Board?

The first board often is created from the leadership group (i.e., the founder, co-founders, and the main volunteers of the organization). The board of directors becomes the program's official governing body and leadership development team. As a group the board members have full power to make decisions regarding the organization. As individuals they have no power to speak or act on behalf of the program unless the full board has given them permission.

Board members do not need to be professionals or service providers who work with children or individuals with special needs. Individuals filling positions on the board of directors may be parents of children with special needs *and* community leaders. PHP has had bank presidents and corporate CEOs who are parents of children with special needs as board members.

Parents and others who are devoted to the program, but who are not interested in business, should volunteer in the program's service activities and not become board members. They could serve on a board committee (remember, not all members on board committees have to be board members), volunteer for the day-to-day operations of the program, put together information packets, serve as supporting parents, help create newsletters and mailings, or assist with special events.

Financial Obligations of Board Members

The financial pledge of each board member can vary from $100 to $1,000 per year or more. Citizens pay thousands of dollars for the privilege and power of sitting on arts and symphony boards in major cities. Your board members should consider it a privilege to serve your program. More important, funding sources are impressed when board members make a personal financial pledge, and they are more likely to give when the board has given first. Board members are more at ease and successful asking others for funding for the program when they have given themselves. Do not let members assume that their *time* is all they should be expected to give. Their time is not commitment enough for the amount of power that they hold. Some volunteers give more time than the board members, but they do not have the power to make or break the program. As the budget grows, so should the amount of funds your board members personally provide and generate.

How Many Board Members?

How many members make the best board? If the board is too small (fewer than 11 members), then filling positions on committees can be difficult and there is not enough energy for projects. In addition, like minds working together have a tough time producing innovative thoughts for program growth or maintaining contemporary relevance to the needs of the community they serve. Board members can actually become closed-minded and less effective when they acquire a sense of knowing everything about the program and what is good for it.

Twenty-four is a good maximum number of members for an active board, but finding people who will be active is crucial. Having a smaller board is better than having a 20-member board with only 12 active members. The negative impact that flows from members who do not participate drags down the positive energy and forward movement of those who are active. With numerous poorly participating members, having a quorum, which is needed to accomplish legal business, is difficult. As stated in their by-laws, most boards function with a quorum of 50% of members plus one member.

Although an 11-to-24-member board is preferred, you may want to state in the by-laws that your board is "of no less than 7 and no more than 30." Using a broader range prevents the program from being out of compliance with its by-laws should, for example, an 11-member board suddenly drop to 10. And although you may like having 24 members, a broader range allows you the flexibility to add a 25th or 26th person should a community leader become interested in supporting your mission at the board level. Keep your options open by being careful about how quantifiable statements are made in the by-laws, lest they become too binding. Policies should be specific and detailed, but by-laws should be simple and broad in scope.

In addition, create a plan to rotate members off of the board. The roster of board members should contain not only members' names, addresses, places of business, and telephone numbers but also the expiration date of their term. Develop a schedule that allows no more than one third of the members to be completing their terms at any given time. With 3-year terms of service and with members being allowed to serve two or three consecutive terms, such a schedule can be done. Members can return after being off for 2 years to take a rest. They come back with fresh perspectives and an openness to new ideas.

Developing a Board

Developing a board begins with the production of a prospective board member packet. Several items compose the packet:

- Cover letter from the chairperson of the board and the executive director inviting the person to get acquainted with the program
- Roles and responsibilities page outlining a board member's major functions
- Agency brochure and a one-page public statement that contains information found in the brochure
- Glossy copy of program publicity information
- List of the members of all of your current boards (e.g., advisory, honorary, community associates, board of directors)
- Board grid that includes descriptive information about the board members (e.g., age, race, gender, interests, contact information, financial, political, business expertise)
- Contract to serve on the board that outlines obligations of time, number of annual meetings, number of committees on which a member must serve, the amount of a board member's annual personal financial pledge to the program and how it can be paid, term length, and the type of board or officers' liability insurance the program carries to protect board members

Approaching Prospective Board Members

If someone suggests a possible member for the board of directors, get the name, address, and telephone number of the prospect. Tell the person making the suggestion that the nominating committee, the chairperson of the board, or the executive director will get in touch with the person to explore participation. Keep the outreach for all types of board members connected to a *single point of contact*—the chair of the nominating committee or the executive director.

Nonprofit organizations use a practical series of steps for following up with prospective board members:

- The nominating committee and the CEO have an informal discussion on whether to pursue the prospect.
- If there are no outstanding objections, ask the prospect to lunch. The nominating chairperson and the chairperson of the board can attend with the executive director.
- During lunch ask the person about his or her interests in general and your mission in particular.
- Provide information about your program and your vision for growth and success, and explain what it means in terms of a board member's work load.
- Invite the person to make a site visit and tour your program.
- Provide the prospective board member with a packet to take home and peruse if there is a mutual interest in further exploring a relationship. Provide the executive summary of your long-range plan.
- Be honest and let the prospect know that you are trying to see whether your program is a fit for him or her and that you need someone who has time to help.

Do not rush the process, but do not leave good prospects dangling without contact and attention. If you are both still interested after the prospect has had some time to study the board packet and sign the contract, let the person know that you will nominate him or her for board membership. Boards often vote in new members at the agency's annual report dinner in which the state of the agency is presented.

If you and a prospective board member are interested in getting better acquainted but the prospective board member is not sure about joining the board, you might suggest that he or she join a board committee to raise his or her comfort level and to ensure a comfortable fit for him or her and the agency.

How Often Should a Board of Directors Meet?

Many boards meet monthly, and some meet quarterly. You may find that quarterly meetings are not enough because if a member misses one meeting, half a year has passed without board contact (up-to-date knowledge is key to making judicious board decisions). Every other month can work well, especially if the executive committee meets in the month that the full board does not meet. Boards of directors for programs in the early stages of development are more effective when they meet monthly. Most groups create by-laws that give the executive committee the same power to act as the full board when necessary. Remember that the executive committee is composed of all the officers (chair, vice chair, chair elect, treasurer, and secretary) of the board and the immediate past chair. Even though the executive director is an ex officio (e.g., nonvoting) member of this committee, the board should *not* meet without him or her present.

Board Committees

Boards often form committees according to their by-laws to accomplish their work. The executive committee develops the program's infrastructure, including a strong financial base and effective policies. As is true for all committees, the executive committee meets regularly to do its work and provides a written and verbal report to the board on its progress toward its objectives. The executive committee can function with the same power of the full board, especially in times of emergencies or tight deadlines.

The program committee is responsible for the program's goals, objectives, and evaluation. It works with volunteer and paid program staff to create evaluation instruments and reviews and prepares presentations on new program ideas for board approval.

The nominating committee is responsible for developing the board of directors. Its role includes recruiting, training, supporting, and conducting an orientation for new members before their first board meeting. Committee members can assign mentors from the experienced board to help new recruits learn about the program and make them feel welcome. This committee usually creates a training manual to help board members function efficiently and effectively.

The nominating committee can ask other people or agencies in the community to help them create and maintain an active and balanced board. The executive director also participates in board development to ensure that the board reflects the economic, social, geographic, occupational, racial, and educational status of the community that the agency serves.

This committee also should create and update board-of-directors' binders for all members. The board binder contains a copy of the group's by-laws, list of the members of all of the boards, and policies relating to the board, such as the audit policy, the board's roles and responsibilities, each committee's responsibilities, a summary page on Robert's Rules of Order, a copy of the latest board meeting minutes, the latest budget, the strategic plan, the annual audit, and a brief history of the agency. Also include a full board grid, which is a chart listing each board member's name and depicting with a checkmark such things as gender; race; occupational area; age group; geographic location; areas of expertise (e.g., fund-raising, law, marketing, health, education, real estate, accounting); and whether he or she is a consumer, parent, or professional.

Wise programs use the grid from the prospective board packet to evaluate the composition of the board so that they can solicit diverse members to fill particular needs of the agency. This helps an agency maintain a balanced board.

The marketing committee assumes responsibility for public awareness, logo creation, fliers, brochures, newsletters, and publicizing events and programs. The committee develops outreach and establishes the program's image in the community (e.g., local, state, national).

The fund development committee assumes responsibility for raising money to meet the budget needs of the program and creates a reserve fund for emergencies and special projects. This committee plans and implements special events, solicits major gifts, helps with proposal writing, conducts board donation campaigns, holds planned giving seminars, coordinates direct mail campaigns, and conducts membership drives.

Composition of a Board Committee

Committees are chaired by a board member, but a program staff person should be involved in each board committee. The staff person supports the committee in many ways, providing vital information to the committee about the staff's point of view, calling committee members, or sending reminder notices of upcoming meetings. This person takes the meeting notes, helps produce documents or provides background materials, and does other tasks to help make the committee successful. Until you have enough staff to involve a different person with each committee, the leader or executive director may have to serve on several or on all committees. When available, the director of fund development should belong to the fund development committee, the director of program services or program coordinator to the program committee, the newsletter editor to the marketing committee, and the executive director to the executive committee.

The executive director also needs to be on and work closely with the nominating committee, which helps build, train, and expand the board of directors. The board committees also can include community members who bring expertise to the committee.

The board leaders can create other committees as they deem necessary and as the by-laws allow. They can create ad hoc or temporary committees to accomplish particular jobs. Such committees may be disbanded or resurrected whenever needed. For instance, PHP had a personnel committee that was active as PHP embarked on creating a personnel policies and procedures manual. After they presented a copy to the board for approval, they disbanded until the next need—creation of a safety manual required by the state.

OTHER TYPES OF BOARDS

A program or agency may decide to create several other types of boards to assist the CEO and the board of directors in accomplishing the mission. These other boards are not a part of the board of directors, and their members are not members of the board of directors.

Advisory Boards

The advisory board is a completely separate entity from the board of directors, and it assists the executive director and the board of directors in making major decisions about the program. Each advisory board member provides information from his or her area of expertise. For example, if the program has a problem dealing with a legal contract, it would seek advice from the attorney on the advisory board. When preparing to sign a lease for space, the program would seek advice from the realtor on the advisory board. The advisory board's greatest gift to the program is the availability to provide professional expertise. The advisory board members do not have to attend regularly scheduled meetings but should make every effort to attend the annual long-range planning retreat and the annual report dinner at the end of the year. By attending these two functions, they get a progress report on how things went during the year, remain knowledgeable about the program, and have input into the future.

There is no set number of people for an advisory board. Such a board can consist of 6, 16, or more people. Advisory boards will be composed primarily of health, educational, legal, and social services professionals or community leaders. Obtain names from the board of directors and staff of people who might make good advisory board members. Those who helped with early development of the program may choose to serve in this capacity, or they may know people who would be good prospects. They can provide the board of directors with information so that the board of directors can decide whether the person is a good fit for the program. If someone is a great worker for another nonprofit organization, he or she may not have time for your program. Often his or her first loyalty and commitment of time, energy, and resources may go to the other organization.

People are appointed to the advisory board by the executive director and the board of directors. Their point of contact with the agency is through the executive director or the chair of the board of directors. Other staff or board members should not contact them directly. Prospective advisory board members should receive a letter that they should sign, date, and return outlining their role, responsibilities, and time obligations.

Honorary Boards

The function of the honorary board is to lend credibility and visibility to the organization, market the program, and participate in fund-raising. It often is composed of celebrities and dignitaries who lend their name recognition to your letterhead, brochures, fund-raising materials, and other documents. The members on this board often participate in special events but typically do not have regularly scheduled meetings.

Community Associates Board

The community associates board (CAB) is the vehicle for speeding the accomplishment of the program's long-range strategic goals and objectives. It meets twice a year to brainstorm about methods and people to help the agency accomplish its mission and annual strategic goals. Besides getting involved personally, CAB members, economically and socially powerful people, may involve their young adult children as well. Perhaps establishing a junior CAB could increase the CAB's efforts on behalf of the program and also could be a vehicle for creating future philanthropic volunteers for the nonprofit community.

PHP's CAB is chaired by the president of a university and includes the publisher of a major newspaper in the region, the president of a public relations company, the owner of a national brewing company, one of the largest land developers in the area, and the mother of the founder of a major computer company.

DEVELOPING STAFF

Program staff can be paid individuals or those who volunteer. Many Parent to Parent programs operate with an all volunteer staff for years, just as PHP did. When the program becomes an institutionalized organization the first person that the board of directors usually hires is the CEO or the executive director. That person often assumes the roles of all other staff people who are not yet hired and may function as the matching parent coordinator, the secretary, the bookkeeper, and the fund-raiser. As funds become available, the CEO hires other staff to take on these jobs.

There is no set rule about who to hire first, but a director of fund development is crucial to providing funds for filling the other positions. The CEO will fill positions as he or she feels the greatest need for assistance. An office manager or a financial director who understands the issues of operating a business should be hired soon after your organization is institutionalized. Although the new hire may know more than the executive director about fiscal management, keep in mind that the director knows more about the agency and makes final decisions after reviewing the financial data.

Another invaluable person to hire is a coordinator of volunteers who can bring in and properly utilize your unpaid staff. Remember, you *can* have staff without having money to pay them. Volunteers can perform every job in the program, as long as they have the skills and knowledge to do so. If the agency is paying staff but is short on funds, there is nothing to prevent staff from donating their salary back to the program after they receive their paycheck (a tax-deductible donation). Learn to produce job announcements, conduct job interviews, create job descriptions for all positions in your organization, and evaluate employees at least annually. Ask similar agencies to share these types of materials with you so that you can create your own.

Hold annual staff and board retreats for long-range strategic planning, physical and mental renewal, and building trust and friendship. Also, define your programs, evaluate your services, and create a handbook with descriptions of your program services. This handbook can be used to acquaint new hires, boards, funding sources, the general public, and volunteers with your agency.

UNDERTAKING LONG-RANGE STRATEGIC PLANNING

Long-range strategic planning is a process that will help your program to create a written document that describes *where* the organization is going, *how* it intends to get there, and *what* it will look like or be *when* it arrives. The plan allows you to capture your full vision and prioritize individual program development/expansion activities over several years.

Who Does the Planning?

The chief players in the long-range planning are the board of directors and the executive director. They invite key staff people, the agency's other boards, targeted individuals being served, and relevant community members to participate in the planning process—often in the form of a 1- or 2-day retreat. The board chair and the executive director usually invite an experienced facilitator to assist with a planning retreat; this frees them to participate more actively in brainstorming and other activities. The facilitator may also assume the responsibilities of preplanner and pull together the information derived from the planning retreat and write a draft of a plan for the agency to review. The board and CEO decide what leadership approach is best for conducting their strategic planning.

From the group of individuals assembled for the planning process, a strategic planning committee may be selected—with one person from the board, staff, families served, and community. The committee, alone or with the facilitator, takes on the job of preplanning, conducting the retreat, and creating the written plan. The strategic planning committee may present drafts of the plan to agency partners, community leaders, and volunteers for comments and input before finalizing the document for presentation to the full board for review and approval.

When Does the Planning Start?

Often the first step in strategic planning is to create an approach or process plan. For-profit businesses often create a business plan as they begin to embark on a new endeavor. Most Parent to Parent programs and other self-help nonprofit organizations realize the need for a long-range strategic plan as they see themselves start to grow in many directions. There is not a wrong time to create a plan—the key lies in matching the scope and breadth of the plan to the unique circumstances the program is experiencing at that time and the visions the leaders hold for the future.

Long-range planning retreats usually are held annually. A plan is created the first year and subsequent retreats monitor, evaluate, update, and make necessary changes to the original long-range plan. For example, perhaps the program is active and already has completed in Year 1 part of the objectives outlined for Year 2. Activities will need to be adjusted in the action plan for Year 2. The 5-year plan is not altered, but the annual action plans that are added to it each year are created to fit the changes realized from the previous year's activities and accomplishments.

How Does the Planning Occur?

Long-range strategic planning happens in three phases: 1) preplanning, 2) holding a retreat, and 3) preparing the written document—including getting input on drafts and obtaining final approval from the board of directors. Each phase is important to the success that the plan can bring to the program. Even if a written plan never materializes, the preplanning and retreat process go a long way in focusing the agency and setting it on a proper course to a successful future.

Preplanning The idea of creating a long-range plan usually is presented to the board by the CEO. Together the board and the CEO decide what the process will look like and then consider the following questions: Will they use a volunteer or paid outside facilitator? Do they want someone from the academic arena to be involved? Will they do it all themselves and test the waters by creating a simple plan? Will they create a committee to move the idea forward, or will the executive director take responsibility? Will they need to create a by-laws committee—a group of about three members to review the by-laws and bring to the board areas of concern, suggested changes, and a final draft for a vote of approval and acceptance by the full board, according to the present by-laws?

If the board and CEO decide to have a paid facilitator, will a proposal need to be written to secure the funding to pay that person? If they are going to write a proposal, should they expand it to a general capacity building grant that will provide not only for this facilitator but also for a part-time director of fund development? These are questions for the board and CEO to think about and come to a decision on according to their situation. Consulting a mentor who has completed a plan as you move forward with this preplanning phase of long-range strategic planning is wise.

The facilitator or whoever is taking the lead should meet with the executive director and the chair of the board to create a written agenda for the planning retreat. Notices about the upcoming retreat should be mailed in advance. Most agencies try to hold their retreat the same time each year so that key participants are aware of the date.

Whether your group decides to use an inside or outside facilitator, that person should continue preparing the group for the strategic planning process by interviewing staff members, volunteers, and board members to gain a perspective on the agency and people who will be creating the plan. During this preplanning phase, the facilitator should gather information on the agency's history, program service statistical facts, and budget analysis and have it available at the planning retreat.

Sending a preparation-for-planning sheet to those who will be participating and to others who express an interest in the program's planning but will be unable to attend gives people a chance to think of ideas before the retreat. People unable to attend can fill out these sheets and return them to the facilitator.

The facilitator and others should search literature for recent surveys and reports about populations in the community they serve. Foundations, the United Way, city planners, and the county Departments of Health and Social Services do surveys or studies that provide insight into needs, trends, opportunities, and threats in the external environment.

Choose an area for the retreat that is in a convenient location with ample parking. Have a variety of foods for breaks and lunch, and prepare for breakfast and dinner if it is a 2-day retreat. Nearby restaurants and hotels can be used if you are not hiring a catering service or enlisting the aid of your volunteers. Make sure that you have a flip chart and index cards to record ideas; different colored dots for prioritizing items quickly; masking tape; copies of your current plan if you have one; overhead transparencies with key parts of the plan; overhead projector; and copies of the agency's history, budget analysis, and program service statistics.

Having the Retreat Those in a leadership position should arrive early to arrange the room, set up and test equipment, locate restrooms, arrange the food, start the coffee, and ice the beverages. Have a name tag for each person, and place cards with participants' names on the tables. The leadership team should welcome the others as they start to arrive. Ask for their signatures on the sign-in sheet, provide them with name tags, start introductions, and point people toward the morning refreshments and their places at the table.

The chairperson provides a brief welcome message and logistical information. He or she thanks the committee for their work in preparation of the important task about to be undertaken. Everyone might be invited to take a 2-minute, five-question written board savvy quiz, which could include some of the following: Who is the agency's executive director? What is his or her salary? Who is the chair of the board? Who is the chair-elect? What are three board committees? How often does the board meet? What is the agency's annual budget? Each person is asked to introduce him- or herself by saying his or her name and affiliation to the agency. All of these preliminary activities allow the group to begin thinking and talking. The chair introduces the keynote speaker (optional), who delivers a brief motivational speech about long-range strategic planning.

Then the executive director thanks everyone for coming to participate and introduces the facilitator, who is now officially in charge of the meeting. This person reviews the written agenda for the day, shares the overall planning process, and defines long-range planning. The facilitator asks the executive director to share a 5- to 10-minute summary of the agency's history—its age, the number and types of programs provided, its funding or budget patterns, facility size, board size, major changes, and recent concerns and successes.

Some agencies will quickly peruse their by-laws and their organizational chart to lay a foundation for the rest of the planning. The strategic planning committee may have met with the by-laws committee during the preplanning and have specific suggestions that they want to cover. Of course, any changes in the by-laws will need to be approved by the board according to the regulations set forth in the by-laws.

Using flip charts to capture all of this vital information, the facilitator should continue to solicit information from the participants by

- Reviewing and updating the mission statement
- Gathering ideas for the future
- Brainstorming the agency's values and philosophy
- Guiding the participants through the internal and external audit
- Listing assumptions and trends

All of this information helps the group to confirm or revise the vision that they have for the program.

To save time after eliciting a vision or picture of the future for the program from the *whole* group, any and all parts of the planning can be done by smaller groups' simultaneously working on one part or another and then returning to the whole group and sharing what they have created. At that time everyone else gets an opportunity to add his or her ideas to the information that the small group has developed.

Working from the vision for the program, the facilitator has the group finalize the list of priorities they want to include in the long-range plan. The group develops a long-range goal for each priority area, selects strategies or methods to be used to approach the goal, and creates specific objectives to accomplish the goal. After the long-range strategic goal for each priority area is accepted, the facilitator can assign that goal to the members of the board committee that is responsible for that area. They can separate from the whole group and create the objectives for that particular goal. The committee members return to the whole group, share their objectives, get input, and prioritize the objectives over 5 years.

Individuals return to their smaller committee work groups and create action plan worksheets for the first year's objectives. The committees may have to schedule another meeting to complete the action plans if time is running short. After all written documents and flip chart notations are gathered for the writer of the plan (discussed in the next section), the facilitator helps the group to relax a moment before heading home. Let the group know when a draft of the plan will be ready.

Writing the Plan One person needs to take all of the information provided by the group and draft the long-range plan. The draft is presented to the planning committee or the board for review, corrections, and changes. The committee takes a draft of the plan to community members, makes final changes, and presents it to the board for their approval. The plan should be printed on quality paper and placed in a semi-flexible or soft cover. Copies of the plan to be used by the board and staff can be kept unbound and put in three-ring binders for easier and frequent use.

Elements of a Long-Range Plan

A long-range strategic plan can vary in length according to style, size of the organization, and depth or scope. Your plan may be as short as 5 pages or as long as 50 pages. A well-developed institution, such as a university or major foundation, may have a shorter plan than a newly developing agency. Why? The newer agency needs to include in its plan more goals and detailed objectives and activities around infrastructure. The written long-range plan should contain the following:

- Title or cover page that includes the title of the plan; name, address, and telephone number of the agency; and years covered by the plan
- Table of contents
- Brief history of the organization
- Introduction that includes an overview of the plan's purpose, concept, process, and approach (see Figures 8.1 and 8.2)
- Body of the plan
    1. Mission statement
    2. Targeted population (e.g., people and geographic area to be served)
    3. Vision (e.g., statements that describe the future)
    4. Internal audit (e.g., the agency's evaluation of its strengths and weaknesses)
    5. External audit (e.g., environmental analysis of opportunities and threats in the community—local, state, and national)
    6. Trends (e.g., business, community, health, education, legal, social)
    7. Philosophy and values (e.g., list of beliefs held about the program)
    8. Assumptions
    9. Priority areas (e.g., board building, program development, facility appropriateness, sufficient staff, diversified and reserve funding, management, administrative and fiscal policies, marketing)
    10. Goals, strategies, and objectives
- Outcome benefits list (see Figure 8.3)
- Multiyear long-range strategic charts (see Figure 8.4)
- Organizational chart (see Figure 8.5)
- Appendixes
    1. Program services
    2. Board committee assignments
    3. Budget percentages and program service statistical charts
    4. Diversified funders' percentage of support chart
    5. Agency's consistent public statement (see back of this chapter)
    6. Board of directors
    7. Long-range planning committee members and consultant/facilitator
    8. One year's action plan

The Strategic Planning Process

1. Review the agency's history and by-laws.
2. Create a vision for the program.
3. Develop a purpose or mission statement.
4. Conduct an analysis of opportunities and threats in the external environment.
5. Conduct an internal environmental analysis of the program's strengths and weaknesses.
6. Review assumptions and trends (local, state, national).
7. Outline philosophies and values.
8. Review the agency's financial and program data.
9. Clarify the target population and geographic area to be served.
10. Choose priority areas that the planners will address.
11. Create long-range (3-to 5-year) strategic goals.
12. Create long-range objectives for each goal.
13. Select long-range strategies for accomplishing objectives.
14. Choose outcome benefits expected from successful goal accomplishment.
15. Prioritize objectives, and distribute over 3–5 years on charts (create a chart for each goal).
16. Draft a copy of the long-range plan (include copies of the organizational chart, lists of board members, and long-range planning committee members, board committee assignments, and a one-page consistent public statement [overview of the agency] in the appendices).
17. Review the plan with planners and key people in the community.
18. Make changes and finalize the plan for presentation to the board of directors.
19. Ask the board of directors to approve and accept the plan.
20. Create an executive summary.
21. Create 1-year action work plans for each objective designated for Year 1.
22. Implement and monitor the plan.
23. Evaluate accomplishments at the end of the year as you prepare to start the process over again from Step One. At the next annual board retreat, you will begin creating the next year's annual action work plans to be added to the existing long-range plan.

Figure 8.1. The strategic planning process.

Long-Range Strategic Planning Work Plan Schedule

Activity	April	May	June	July	Aug.	Sept.	Oct.
	Potential timeline						
1. Introduce project idea	x						
2. Interview staff and board		x					
3. Project approved by board		x					
4. Prepare and review agency history, by-laws, statistical facts			x				
5. Conduct/hold/organize preretreat meeting/setting agenda			x				
6. Prepare materials for retreat			x				
7. Hold all-day planning retreat				x			
8. Prepare draft of strategic plan					x		
9. Planning committee reviews plan draft					x		
10. Finalize strategic plan						x	
11. Present plan to board for acceptance						x	
12. Board and staff create 1-year action plans							x
13. Implement the plan							x
14. Begin monitoring/evaluation							x

Figure 8.2. Sample work plan schedule. (*Note:* This time line can be completed in weeks instead of months if the group wants to push the process along faster.)

Priority Area 4: Quality Program Development

Strategic Goal 2: To provide a full complement of quality services, including information and referral with direction, family support, information, care coordination assistance, training, peer counseling, and advocacy programs in an efficient and effective manner, as well as technical assistance to the professional community on issues relating to special children and their families.

Key Strategies for Accomplishing Strategic Goal 2

- Use program monitoring and evaluation.
- Use parent to parent activities.
- Use volunteers, consultation, and collaboration with other agencies.
- Use a multisensory approach to training, presented at times convenient for families.

Objectives for Accomplishing Goal 2 by December 31, 2005

1. To provide individual advocacy assistance to at least 400 families annually
2. To perform a thorough evaluation of all programs every 3 years
3. To conduct an annual consumer satisfaction survey of at least a random 10% sample
4. To train at least 1,000 families annually about laws, advocacy, and disability
5. To provide information and referral services to at least 3,500 families
6. To provide individual or small-group education planning assistance to at least 500 parents or other family caregivers
7. To offer peer counseling training twice per year
8. To form and operate three specialty groups by ethnicity or disability
9. To create a special needs library

Measurable Outcome Benefits Expected

- 75% of families will report decreased stress and less isolation.
- 70% of parents will report increased knowledge about child's special need.
- Relevant programs will be available to meet at least four major needs of families.
- 30% increase in the number of peer helpers available to serve families
- 80% of families served will participate in child's education planning.

Figure 8.3. Sample priority area accomplishment page. Agencies choose which area of the organization to focus on during a long-range planning phase. For each priority area, a composite/summary page is created to focus on specific activities.

Administration Development Plan Years 2005–2010

Objectives	*2005–2006*	*2006–2007*	*2007–2008*	*2008–2009*	*2009–2010*
Human resources policies and procedures	Put in place	Review	Review	Review	Update
Earthquake, fire, and safety preparation	Outline	Drill	Drill Evaluate	Drill Monitor	Drill Update
OSHA requirements	In place				
Salaries and benefits	Formalize		Review		Update
125 flex plan				Available	
Job descriptions	Develop and keep on file	Update for current staff	Update for current staff	Anticipate new staff	Describe potential staff
Employee assistance program	Research	Develop	Evaluate	Monitor	Update
Records clerk				Hire at 50% time	Increase to full time
Finance/administration office manager		Hire at 50% time		Increase to 75% time	Increase to full time
Staff meetings	Quarterly	Quarterly	Six times per year	Six times per year	Monthly
Marketing Development Plan					
Agency marketing plan	Secure and research	Develop	Implement	Monitor	Review and redo
Web page	Research	Create	Monitor	Evaluate	Update
Speakers bureau	Develop	Conduct four times per year	Increase to six times per year	Increase to eight times per year	Increase to monthly
Agency fliers	Update	Add new logo and format	Develop funding flier	Develop for specific programs	Update
Media calendar	Develop media file	Create annual media calendar	Update and use	Update and use	Update and use

Figure 8.4. Sample multiyear long-range priority chart.

Organizational Chart

Board of Directors

CEO---Executive Administrative Assistant

Directors

Program services	Fiscal and administrative services	Marketing	Fund development

---

Coordinators

Health services	Facilities	Communications and public relations	Special events
Education services	Personnel		Planned giving
Social/support services	Bookkeeping		
Assistive technology			

Specialists

Trainers	Bookkeeper	Writers	Proposal writers
Counselors		Newsletter editor	Development associates
Advocates			

Assistants

Admin. assistant	Admin. assistant	Admin. assistant	Admin. assistant

---

Custodial and Other

Maintenance engineers

Figure 8.5. Sample organizational chart. (*Note:* Volunteers serve the agency on all levels.)

Executive Summary

Writing a short executive summary that can be used when a full plan is not needed (e.g., in press kits for volunteers, prospective board members, new staff) is a good idea. The executive summary should contain a cover or title page; mission statement, targeted population and geographic area served; organizational chart; reduced version of the vision; trends report; and a copy of each priority area's accomplishment sheet, which will lists goals, strategies, objectives, and outcome benefits. You might add a list of the boards, the names of the long-range planners, and the plan facilitator on a back cover sheet.

SUMMARY

Help is available in the local, state, and national community to support your efforts to institutionalize your program. See Chapter 14 for a listing of statewide Parent to Parent programs that have expertise in strategic planning. Technical assistance centers, books, training manuals, symposiums, conferences, newsletters, magazines, and other PDFRCs also can provide help and resources.

Although you are busy providing services to families, you also must be working to develop a strong infrastructure for your program so that it will last and grow into a solid nonprofit, public benefit charitable agency. A strong infrastructure for your program also includes a board of directors, staff (paid and volunteer) with clearly defined responsibilities, a professional advisory board, long-range strategic planning, well-written policies and procedures, and a diversified budget with a growing reserve fund.

RESOURCES

Applied Strategic Planning—How to Develop a Plan that Really Works, by Leonard David Goodstein, Timothy Nolan, and J. William Pfeiffer, The McGraw-Hill Companies, 1221 Avenue of the Americas, New York, NY 10020; telephone: (212) 512-2000

The Board Member's Guide to Strategic Planning: Charting the Future for Your Nonprofit, by Fisher Howe and Alan Shrader, Jossey Bass, Inc., 350 Sansome Street, 5th Floor, San Francisco, CA 94104; telephone: (800) 956-7739

The Budget-Building Book for Nonprofits: A Step-by-Step Guide for Managers and Boards, by Murray Dropkin and Bill LaTouche, Jossey Bass, Inc., 350 Sansome Street, 5th Floor, San Francisco, CA 94104; telephone: (800) 956-7739

Building Communities from the Inside Out: A Path Toward Finding and Mobilizing a Community's Assets, by John P. Kretzmann and John L. McKnight, ACTA Publications, 4848 North Clark Street, Chicago, IL 60640-4711; telephone: (800) 397-2282

How to Apply For and Retain Exempt Status for Your Organization (IRS Publication 557), by the Internal Revenue Service; telephone: (800) 829-1040; http://www.irs.gov; the web site created by the IRS provides a lot of information and numerous sources of assistance for nonprofit organizations and small businesses.

Keys to Creating, Managing, and Maintaining a Family Resource Center or Other Nonprofit Agency, a Symposium, PHP, 3041 Olcott Street, Santa Clara, CA 95054-3222

Long Range Planning Manual for Board Members, by Darla Struck, Aspen Publishers, Inc., 200 Orchard Ridge Drive, Gaithersburg, MD 20878; telephone: (800) 638-8437

Managing the Nonprofit Organization, by Peter F. Drucker, HarperCollins Publishers, 10 East 53rd Street, New York, NY 10022; telephone: (800) 242-7737; http://www.harpercollins.com; for information about the audiocassette series, *The Non-Profit Drucker,* available on 25 1-hour cassettes with listener's guide, write to Leadership Network, Post Office Box 9090, Tyler, TX 76711.

The Nonprofit Handbook, by Anthony Mancuso, Nolo Press, 950 Parker Street, Berkeley, CA 94710; telephone: (510) 549-1976; http://www.nolo.com; this book has step-by-step directions on getting incorporated, formulas for by-laws, and much more. It also is available with a computer disk to speed your activities.

Robert's Rules of Order, Newly Revised, 1990 Edition, Ninth Edition, by Sarah Corbin Robert, Henry M. Robert III, and William J. Evans; http://www.robertsrules.com

Strategic Planning Workbook for Nonprofit Organizations, by Bryan W. Barry, Amherst H. Wilder Foundation Publishing Center, 919 Lafond Avenue, Saint Paul, MN 55104-2198; telephone: (800) 274-6024; a guide to help you in your long-range planning

ORGANIZATIONS

Retired Senior Volunteer Programs (RSVP) and Senior Coalition Of Retired Executives (SCORE); call your local council on aging (COA) or United Way to find the groups in your area. COAs are great sources for volunteer or paid staff.

United Way of America, 701 North Fairfax Street, Alexandria, VA 22314-2045; telephone: (703) 836-7100; http://www.unitedway.org; the United Way uses a volunteer team of community leaders to evaluate proposals sent to them and conduct site visits at programs. That community team of volunteer citizens decides if your program should get funded. You can reapply as often as you want if you are not funded. United Way funds only a percentage of an agency's budget based on the program's need and the amount that United Way has donated to them in the past. Some programs receive as much as 30%, others as little as 3%. Talk to other agencies that receive funding to learn the corporate culture of your United Way. Properly completing a United Way proposal and preparing to meet their guidelines for becoming a United Way agency directs you toward institutionalizing your program. Therefore, applying is worth the effort, even if your agency does not receive funding. The Secretary of State, Registry of Charitable Trusts, Attorney General's Office—Charitable Trusts, State Board of Equalization, and Franchise Tax Board have applications and forms for nonprofit agencies.

Appendix
Sample Public Statement

Families Helping Families is a Parent to Parent program that serves all children who have a need for special health, education, or social services. Our services are extended to their entire family and the professionals who serve them.

OUR MISSION

Helping children become all they can be by providing them with strong families and responsive systems.

OUR MAJOR GOALS

- Happy, healthy, educated children and informed, assertive families
- Competent, caring professionals
- Accessible, coordinated family-centered systems of care

OUR PROGRAMS

- Information and referral with direction
- Training for families
- Workshops for professionals on children and families with special needs
- Special needs library
- Assistive technology for children and adults with disabilities
- Parent to Parent support services

OUR VISION

We are an agency that provides answers and resources for children with special care needs in a facility that has appropriate space for all of our programs and has a full complement of qualified, caring, and efficient staff. We are an agency that not only reaches out to all people in our diverse community, but works to take services into the community. We envision technology adding to the methods, speed, and effectiveness with which we provide our services.

OUR HISTORY

We were founded 10 years ago and became incorporated as a 501(c)3 not-for-profit public benefit organization serving Troy and immediate surrounding counties. Our agency has been a United Way funded agency for 5 years and has won numerous awards for service to individuals with disabilities. More than 3,000 families benefit annually from our services.

Funding comes to Families Helping Families from a diverse group of funders, including local, state, and national governments; United Way; individuals; corporations; and foundations. The Junior League funds two projects. Our judicious use of volunteers makes us a cost-effective program.

Our philosophy and values embrace beliefs that people have the ability to help solve their own problems. Collaborating with other organizations provides a synergy for accomplishing goals that would take more time if done alone. Those who have experience and have *been there* make excellent teachers, mentors, and guides.

Appendix
Sample By-laws

By-laws of Families Helping Families

Article I

Name of organization and principal place of business

Section 1. Name: The name of this organization shall be Families Helping Families, Inc. Doing business as FHF—the Family Resource Center. Shortened name is FHF.

Section 2. Principal Office: The principal office for transaction of business of the corporation is hereby fixed and located in Santa Clara County.

Article II

Purpose and Objectives

FHF is a nonprofit service organization operated by and for families of children with cognitive and/or physical disabilities. Its fundamental purpose is getting the family functioning independently, handling their own situation, making decisions about their child in a positive and realistic frame of mind, and helping the family return to a normal functioning unit as soon as possible. Our mission is helping children achieve their potential by providing them with strong families. Specific objectives are as follows:

1. To have the community use FHF as a source of psychosocial help for children with disabilities and their families.
2. To help new families through the stages of grieving.
3. To help each child with a disability or special need have a loving and knowledgeable family and the necessary resources to meet their needs.
4. To educate families, the public, and professionals about special needs.

Article III

Membership

Section 1. General Membership: Membership shall be open to all people without regard to race, creed, religion, sex, disability, or ability to contribute financially.

Section 2. Rights and Duties of the Membership: Members have the right to accept committee assignments, receive newsletters, attend the annual meeting, and support financial and other concerns of FHF.

Section 3. Voting: This is not a legally designated membership organization; therefore, members do not vote to effect change in the organization.

Section 4. Dues: Dues will be set by the board of directors.

Article IV
Board of Directors

Section 1. Number of Members: The board of directors shall consist of no less than 8 and no more than 30 members, including officers as listed in Article V.

Section 2. Election of Directors: The board of directors shall be elected at the annual meeting by the current board.

Section 3. Annual Meeting: The annual meeting shall take place in the month of June of each year.

Section 4. Term of Office: The board of directors shall hold office for 3 years from the date of the annual meeting at which elected. No more than one third of the current board may be added to the board at any one annual meeting. Members are encouraged to take a break from the board after two terms, but may serve as many terms as elected by the board.

Section 5. Vacancies: Vacancies on the board of directors may be filled by a majority vote of the remaining directors or by appointment to the vacant chair by the chairperson of the board. This position shall be held until the next annual meeting.

Section 6. Meetings:

1. Regular meetings shall be held at least quarterly, or more frequently if so decided by the board, at a time and place selected by the board.
2. Special meetings may be called at any time on 3 days' notice, by the chair of the board or three members of the board. The written notice should include time, place, and purpose of the meeting.

3. A majority of those currently serving shall constitute a quorum, a majority being 50% plus one. All acts or decisions made by such a quorum shall be regarded as an act of the board of directors.
4. The board shall have the power to declare the office of any director vacant if that board member shall fail to attend at least 50% of regular scheduled meetings for the year, unless a leave has been granted by the chairperson or his or her representative. That vacant position can be filled as described above.

Section 7. Powers and Responsibilities: All corporate powers of the corporation shall be exercised by or under the authority of and the business and affairs of the corporation shall be controlled by the board of directors. Without limiting the foregoing generality, the board of directors shall have the following powers.

1. To select and remove all agents and the executive director of the corporation; prescribe such powers and duties for them as may not be inconsistent with the law, with the articles of incorporation, or the by-laws; fix their compensation and require from them security for faithful service.
2. To conduct, manage, and control the affairs and business of the corporation and to make such rules and regulations therefore not inconsistent with the law, articles of incorporation, or by-laws.
3. To change the principal office for the transaction of the business from one location to another within the same county; and to fix and locate from time to time one or more subsidiary offices of the corporation within or outside of the state of California.

Article V
Officers

Section 1. Officers: The officers of this corporation shall be a chairperson, vice chairperson, secretary, and treasurer, and such other officers as the chairperson of the board may choose and other members by majority vote approve.

Section 2. The Chairperson: The chairperson shall have general supervision, direction, and control of the business affairs of the corporation. The chairperson shall preside at all meetings. In the absence or disability of the chairperson, the first vice chair shall assume the responsibilities of the chair, followed in succession by the second vice chair. The chairperson shall act as a liaison between the community and Families

Helping Families, Inc., will sign all contracts more than $2,500, and is an ex-officio member of all board committees.

Section 3. The Secretary: The secretary shall keep a full and complete record of the proceedings of the board of directors, record minutes of all meetings, handle correspondence for the group, organize and keep records, and shall discharge such other duties as pertains to the office or as prescribed by the board of directors.

Section 4. The Treasurer: The treasurer shall have control of all funds received by the corporation; shall keep, or cause to be kept, full and accurate records of all monies; shall prepare, or cause to be prepared, and present to the board financial reports as the board of directors deem necessary; shall seek fund-raising sources and shall perform such other duties as the board of directors from time to time deem necessary. Shall, with the executive director, sign all contracts more than $2,500. Shall complete or cause to be completed annual nonprofit tax forms.

Section 5. Election: The officers of this corporation shall be elected by the board of directors from its own membership.

Section 6. Powers: Nothing in these by-laws shall be interpreted to give the chairperson, any officer, or member of the board of directors the power to initiate any program or project or appoint any committee without first obtaining the approval of the majority of the board of directors.

Section 7. Term of Office: The officers shall be elected for a term of 2 years and shall hold office until the second annual meeting. It shall be the policy of this corporation that a board member shall be able to hold the same office for as many successive terms as elected by the board of directors.

Section 8. Removal of an Officer: Any officer elected or appointed by the board of directors may be removed at any time by the affirmative vote of a majority of the whole board of directors. Any officer so removed relinquishes his or her position on the board.

Article VI
Removal of a Member

Section 1. Termination: Membership in the corporation may be terminated for the following reasons.

1. Failure to pay membership dues.
2. For cause, when activities or conduct of the member brings condemnation, criticism, or dishonor to this corporation or the people with developmental disabilities generally or their families. No member shall be terminated for cause unless the member is given written notice of the conduct for which there is a complaint and is offered an opportunity to appear before and be heard by the board of directors regarding the conduct. The board of directors will terminate a member for cause only on the affirmative vote of three fourths of the members of the board present and voting at a regular or special meeting called for this purpose.

Article VII

Quorum

Section 1. Quorum: Official business may not be transacted without a quorum. A quorum will be constituted when a majority of the active board members are present. Majority means 50% plus one.

Section 2. Procedure: The rules contained in *Robert's Rules of Order, Revised,* shall govern the corporation in all cases in which they are applicable.

Article VIII

Contracts, Loans, Checks, Deposits

Section 1. Contracts: The board of directors may authorize execution of any contract instrument in the name of and on behalf of the organization, and such authority may be general or defined to a specific instance or instances. And unless so authorized by the board of directors, an officer or member shall not have the power to bind the organization by any contract of engagement or to pledge its credit or to render it liable for any purpose or any amount more than $500.

Section 2. Checks and Drafts: All checks, drafts, or other orders for payment of money, notes, or other evidences of indebtedness issued in the name of the organization shall be signed by such officer or officers, agent or agents as shall from time to time be specifically authorized by the board of directors.

Section 3. Loans: No loans shall be contracted on behalf of the organization, and no evidence of indebtedness shall be issued in the organization's name unless specifically authorized by board of directors.

Section 4. Deposits: All funds of the organization not otherwise employed shall be deposited from time to time to the credit of the organization in such banks, trust companies, or other depositories as may be specifically authorized by the board of directors.

Article IX
Amendments

These by-laws may be amended or repealed and new by-laws adopted at any regular or special meeting of the board of directors by a two thirds majority vote of the board of directors as long as a 30-day notice is given to each member and a statement of the intended changes in the by-laws.

List officers of the board of directors at time of incorporation
(full board also can be listed here)

Reminder: Have someone familiar with legal language or by-laws review your by-laws to ensure that you have not used legally binding terms in sections where flexibility is needed and vice versa. If it is written in your by-laws, then it is binding in a court of law. Do not write more than is necessary.

Appendix
Sample Articles of Incorporation

Articles of Incorporation
of
Families Helping Families, Inc.

Article I
Name

The name of this corporation shall be Families Helping Families, Inc.

Article II
Purposes and Powers

The purposes for which this corporation is formed are:

a) To offer emotional support, help, and information to families with children who have special needs.
b) To educate the public and professionals about individuals with disabilities.
c) To have and exercise all rights and powers conferred on nonprofit corporations under the laws of California, including the power to contract, rent, buy, or sell personal or real property, provided, however, that this corporation shall not, except to an insubstantial degree, engage in any activities or exercise any powers that are not in furtherance of the primary purposes of this corporation.

Article III
Organization

This corporation is organized pursuant to the General Nonprofit Corporation Law of the state of California and does not contemplate pecuniary gain or profit to the members thereof, and it is organized for nonprofit purposes.

Article IV
Principal Office

The principal office for the transaction of the business of this corporation is located in the county of Santa Clara, state of California.

Article V

Directors

The general management of the affairs of this corporation shall be under the control, supervision, and direction of the board of directors. The names and addresses of people who are to act in the capacity of directors until the selection of their successors are

Names Titles Addresses

Article VI

By-laws Provisions

a) Directors: The manner by which directors shall be chosen and removed from office, their qualifications, powers, duties, compensation, and tenure of office, the manner of filling vacancies on the board, and the manner of calling and holding meetings of directors shall be as stated in the by-laws. The directors of this corporation shall have no liability for dues.

b) Members: The authorized number, if any, and qualifications of members of the corporation, the filling of vacancies, the different classes of membership, if any, the property, voting, and other rights and privileges of members, and their liability to dues and assessments and the method of collection, and the termination and transfer of membership shall be as stated in the by-laws.

Article VII

Dedication and Dissolution

a) The property of this corporation is irrevocably dedicated to charitable, educational, and scientific purposes, and no part of the net income or assets of this organization shall ever inure to the benefit of any director, officer, and member thereof or to the benefit of any private individual.

b) On dissolution or winding up of the corporation, its assets remaining after payment of, or provision for payment of, all debts and liabilities of this corporation shall be distributed to a nonprofit fund, foundation, or corporation that is organized and operated exclusively for charitable purposes and that has established its tax-exempt status under Section 501(c)3 of the Internal Revenue Code. If this corporation holds any assets in trust, or a corporation is formed for charitable purposes, such assets shall be disposed of in such manner as may be directed by decree of the superior court of this county in which the corporation has its principal office, on petition therefore by the attorney general or by a person concerned in the liquidation, in a proceeding to which the attorney general is a party.

Article VIII

Limitation on Corporate Activities

None of the activities of this corporation shall consist of the carrying on of propaganda or otherwise attempting to influence legislation, nor shall this corporation participate in, or intervene in (including the publishing or distributing of statements), any political campaign on behalf of any candidate for public office.

Execution

In witness whereof, the undersigned and above named incorporators and first directors of the corporation have executed these articles of incorporation this ______ day of __________________, 20 .

______________________________ ______________________________

Chairperson of the board Secretary of the board

______________________________ State of California

Treasurer of the board County of Santa Clara

On this ______ day of _________________, _______________(year), before me _____________________________,

a notary public for the state of California, with principal office in Santa Clara County, personally appeared ____________________________, ____________________________, and ____________________________,
known to me to be the people whose names are:
Harry Jones, Sara Quinones, and Martha Smith, subscribed to the within articles of incorporation, and acknowledged to me that they executed the same.

In witness whereof, I have hereunto set my hand and affixed my official seal on the day and year first above written.

____

(signature)

Notary Public

(seal)

9

Funding Your Program

Getting and Staying Afloat

"A good cause and a good tongue:
and yet money must carry it."

—Thomas Fuller

Although Parent to Parent programs can and do exist with little or no funding, there is no question that secure funding contributes to program stability and capacity. In this chapter you will learn about typical Parent to Parent program budgets and funding sources and the successful fund-raising strategies used in Parent to Parent programs nationally. Because money is a necessary vehicle for accomplishing your mission, goals, and objectives, it is important not to treat fund-raising as separate from your other program services. The executive director and the board of directors must make fund-raising their first priority, whereas program staff make quality services their highest priority. Funds should always be tied to the programs they allow you to create for children with special needs and their families.

When a program becomes serious about its future, fund-raising grows into what the nonprofit world calls *fund development.* The main difference between fund-raising and fund development is that the latter is broader, has a planned and well-organized approach, and includes a marketing plan. Fund development involves developing long-term relationships in the community to generate significant financial support of the program over time.

Parents Helping Parents Fund-Raising Story

Because receiving funding to start a program has both risks and benefits, we were thankful that Parents Helping Parents (PHP) started as a nonbudget program. Some program coordinators are able to leverage start-up funds into a stable ongoing program, but others become frustrated when the start-up funds are not renewed and other funding has not been found. Then the future of their program is at risk. Because PHP had no initial funding, we were forced to learn many valuable lessons for keeping our program alive, and we doubt that PHP would be around today if it had been securely funded during its start up years. PHP's success, despite the lack of initial funding, gave us the confidence we still have today about our program's staying power. Visitors to PHP often get the courage to start a program because they see what can happen from such meager beginnings. Although we started as a nonbudget program, we were spending about $2,000–$3,000 per year out of our own pockets. We learned to find funding from a diverse base of supporters and that there is extended program life in that diversity.

For our first 8 years, money came mainly from parent contributions, cupcake and cookie sales in front of grocery stores, hot dog and nacho sales in the park, and proceeds from Christmas and Halloween family boutiques. Volunteer staff, friends, and families served, and others brought their favorite crafts and baking and canning products to a central site to be sold. All goods were donated and all funds collected went to support the program. The leadership team visited social service clubs to ask for small donations, and we participated in a survey project that paid us for tasting and evaluating foods for a local research group. We also charged a $2 membership fee to belong to PHP. These schemes brought in only small amounts of money.

In 1983 when the leadership team decided to institutionalize the program so that it could survive, we embarked on more lucrative funding methods. We had done a good thing by becoming incorporated as a 501(c)3 nonprofit state and federal tax-exempt organization a few years earlier.

All of the steps we took to institutionalize the program were perfect precursors for the enhanced fund development we needed to do to move the program forward. We updated our long-range plan, clarified our budget needs, and vigorously pursued funding from many sources. We increased *our membership fee from $2 to $20 with the surprising result of a tenfold increase in members. We concluded that people did not like to take the time to write a $2 check.*

We wrote 10 proposals, and none received funding. We reviewed them with our retired executive volunteer (REV) consultant and decided that the mission statement did not correctly reflect our program's goal of helping children. We changed the essence of the mission from helping parents to helping children get the resources to achieve their potential by providing them with strong families and dedicated professionals. With this new emphasis, we attained about an 80%–90% success rate on proposals submitted. We sought and received community; corporate; foundation; and local, state, and federal government grants; as well as United Way funding.

PHP continued to diversify its budget by creating two major fund-raisers, a Boys Choir Christmas Musical and a CuisineArt Show and Auction. The latter brought in about $20,000, and the musical became a break-even event that was more of a friend-raiser than a fund-raiser. The board and staff had become serious and successful fund-raisers.

PARENT TO PARENT PROGRAM BUDGETS

It is difficult to outline a typical budget for any particular Parent to Parent program because it will vary according to size, the state in which it is located, the number of volunteer and paid staff, and whether funds are spent on marketing the agency. Most programs start without a budget, and they gradually increase their income as they grow and add paid staff. Parent to Parent program annual budgets range from $0 to $500,000. Table 9.1 in Appendix A at the end of this book gives you additional information about the annual budgets of local Parent to Parent programs. The fact that the greatest percentage (35%) of local Parent to Parent programs have annual budgets of less than $1,000 is a reflection of the commitment Parent to Parent program coordinators have to making the parent to parent matched opportunity available to other parents—even with very little funding to do so.

It is wise to diversify the sources of your income, regardless of the size of your budget. Prospective funding sources get nervous and are less likely to give when they see that 50% or more of the program's funding comes from only one source, especially if that source is one governmental agency. Funding sources prefer a large grass roots financial involvement. Most autonomous Parent to Parent programs do have more than one funding source, and Table 9.2 in Appendix A describes these different funding sources. As you might imagine, if a Parent to Parent program has a sponsoring agency, its budget is provided primarily by the sponsoring agency.

FUNDING SOURCES

The many sources for funding for Parent to Parent programs include

- Individuals—they contribute more money than foundations do. Asking your family, friends, other individuals, and philanthropists is the most effective fund-raising strategy you can use.
- Foundations—there are private, family, community, and corporate foundations. Get a copy of your local, state, or national *Foundation Guide Book* to learn more about foundations and what they fund. Libraries, hospitals, universities, county offices of education, social services, and the attorney general's office can supply information about these guides, as well as about other funding opportunities. Use the Internet, grantsmanship offices, and technical assistance groups in your area to learn more about foundations.
- Corporations—call, visit, and get acquainted with businesses in your area. Read the business section of your newspaper. Someone at PHP read an article about a company that was putting on a golf tournament and was looking for a charity to share the profits. PHP was happy to share! Recruit board members from corporations—companies give more money when their employees are involved with your program. Document the occupations of families that you serve, and ask for permission to use their names in proposals or when you approach their place of employment for funding or donations of supplies, furniture, and equipment.
- Membership fees—families served by the program can usually afford to pay a small membership fee. Services are never denied at Parent to Parent programs because a family does not have a membership, but funding sources are impressed and give more freely if the grass roots group is doing its share. Offer different levels of memberships: individuals with special needs ($10), families ($20), professionals ($30), special friends ($50), silver circle supporters ($100), gold circle supporters ($250), and corporate memberships ($2,500).
- Government grants—city, county, state, and federal grants are available throughout the year. Check with your city and county about community development block grants, and ask to be put on their

mailing list to receive their requests for proposals (RFPs). Call the mayor's office for help in getting to the right department for various funding sources. Get a copy of the *Federal Register,* which lists RFPs from U.S. Government departments such as the U.S. Department of Education and the U.S. Department of Health, Maternal and Child Health's Special Projects of Regional and National Significance grants.

- United Way—United Way will send you the necessary guidelines and forms for applying for funds that are usually ongoing. They are a good source of information about other funding and technical assistance as well. Even if your application is rejected, you will no doubt learn much about creating a strong program with a stable infrastructure.
- Combined Federal Campaign—this is a funding mechanism that allows federal employees to give to your program through their local United Way. You must complete forms and provide documentation about your program and its nonprofit status to United Way. If approved, your program will be assigned a number to designate your nonprofit status. Your program name and identification number will be included on the information forms that are checked by employees as they decide which programs they will donate to.
- Combined Health Appeal—this funding source includes only health agencies. Organizations apply by submitting a proposal, and the application process is similar to United Way's. If you receive United Way funding, Combined Health Appeal will not give you funding.
- In-kind funding—this is a vital but often overlooked source of income that involves donations of needed services or goods from organizations or individuals. For example, PHP asked a cleaning service to clean the office each week without charging the usual $250. The yearly cleaning services equaled a $13,000 donation. Because the best legal and auditing paper trail for such transactions is full documentation, the cleaning service submitted its monthly bill for the services they provided and then PHP wrote a check to pay them. The cleaning service then wrote a check in that same or a larger amount as a donation to PHP. In this way the cleaning service could legally claim a tax deduction on its income taxes, and the PHP bookkeeping was in good order for the auditor. To be a valid in-kind donation the service must be needed and necessary for the operation of the nonprofit organization. A Parent to Parent program could not claim $500,000 of valuable paintings hanging on its walls as an in-kind donation. The $13,000 cost for cleaning services, however, is

legitimate and should be included as both an expense and contribution income in the budget.

- Special events—these are the most time-consuming source of funds, so limit the number of special events for your program. The best special events are those that are planned and carried out by others who then donate the funds to your charity. There are all types and sizes of special events, and there is even the nonevent, in which people stay in the comfort of their own home and write a check to your program to help children achieve their potential.
- "Thons"—telethons are usually long but can be short television programs to solicit funds. PHP held a 2-hour telethon after its annual Boys Choir Holiday Musical and also tried a "phonathon" by gathering a group of board members, staff, and other volunteers to call people from the database of families, professionals, and friends.
- Sales to the public—nonprofit charities can sell items that relate to the services they provide. The Parent to Parent program can sell the training manuals it uses to teach parents about education planning. These sales are documented as a part of the program service fees. If it costs you $6 to produce a training manual, you can sell it for $10 and use the extra money to support that program service.
- Planned giving funds—these kinds of donations are now being sought more often by smaller nonprofits. A planned giving program is a way of allowing supporters of your agency to remember the program in their wills, in their estate plans, and through insurance policies. The donor benefits from tax savings, and the program services gain stability and prestige in the community. You can learn about developing a planned giving program by attending seminars put on by other nonprofit organizations and by reviewing and reading materials sent to you seeking your planned support for other established nonprofit agencies.
- Direct mail campaign—the first campaign should be a small, targeted one. *Targeted* means that the letters requesting funding are accompanied by a return envelope sent to families, friends, professionals, and agencies you know. After you are experienced with the process, expand it. Many programs send direct mail requests to prospective and former donors about four times per year. Offer funding sources a choice of either sending one lump sum or providing a small amount monthly.
- Coins—Find a way to collect nickels, dimes, and pennies. Put canisters in shops and stores, or put a request in your newsletter and have an open house quarterly for people to drop off their coins.

- Endowment funds—these are funds that are donated or invested; only the interest generated is used to support the program. The original endowment funds keep giving.
- Investments—carefully invest reserve funds and other nontargeted donations so that they can provide funds for the program's needs. Accept stocks and bonds from donors who prefer to give in this manner.
- Fees for service—there is nothing wrong with charging program service fees. When concerned about families who cannot afford to pay, add a sliding scale down to zero, and do not use any criteria for determining eligibility except the family's word that the fee will be a financial hardship. If a grant pays for a training program, the funded agency may still have to charge a fee for the training materials if they are not covered in the grant. PHP's national symposium on parent-directed family resource centers (PDFRCs) is in its seventh year as a fee-for-service program since the 3-year government grant expired. Demonstrating the ability to convert a program to a fee-for-service entity is a great way to assure a funding source that a program will last into the future.
- Unit or chapter dues—if a statewide or national umbrella agency is providing services to local units, small dues are in order. Be cautious, however, if an umbrella agency takes a large share of local dues and provides little in return except perhaps a quarterly newsletter.
- Miscellaneous sources—plan a small amount of miscellaneous income in your budget's income column. These unexpected dollars arrive so often that most budget worksheets and forms leave a space for them. PHP received funds from another agency going out of business, a high school musical group, a collaborative funding pot in which they were included, major items donated before budgeted money was spent to purchase them, and a windfall that United Way shared with its agencies.

After you have identified some possible funding sources, then, as part of your fund development plan and your long-range strategic plan, create a proposed template of 10 funding sources with the percentage of funding your program will try to secure from each (see Figure 9.1). If your agency's annual balanced budget is $50,000, the fund development committee would be wise to create a fund development plan that could bring in at least $75,000. Overestimation means that even with a 33% failure rate of the plan, your program will still bring in the total amount needed for that fiscal year. The next section gives you some ideas about how to raise this $75,000.

Fiscal Year 7/1/01–6/30/02

Potential funder	Amount	Percentage of budget
United Way	$5,000	5%
County Department of Social Services	10,000	10%
State Department of Health or Developmental Disabilities	20,000	20%
U.S. Department of Education	25,000	25%
Membership dues	5,000	5%
Special events (CuisineArt Show, holiday musical, and Day at the Races)	5,000	5%
Contributions (corporate, foundations, etc.)	20,000	20%
Board of directors' pledges	5,000	5%
Direct mail campaign	5,000	5%
	$100,000	100%

Contingency plans		
Bingo	$20,000	20%
Flea markets	3,000	3%
Major donors campaign	10,000	10%
Program service fees	3,000	3%
Speaker's bureau (social services clubs)	2,000	2%
	$38,000	38%

Figure 9.1. Sample diversified budget template.

FUND-RAISING STRATEGIES

- An important first step in fund-raising is to recruit volunteers whose only job is to concentrate on fund-raising for the program. Creating a volunteer "Friends of (agency's name)" group frees the hands of staff to care for families while the volunteers help the board with important fund development activities. The board of directors must approve the volunteers' activities because they perform under the nonprofits' 501(c)3 tax-exempt status.
- When seeking funds be enthusiastic about your program, and don't broadcast any program limitations. The CEO's or the director of fund development's office should promote the program as well-organized and of high quality. Your program's documents (e.g., brochure) are a reflection of the program and should be brief and error-free.
- The most important function of the board of directors is to be involved in fund-raising, and a board member should always accompany the program director or director of development when the program approaches an individual for a funding request.
- Fund-raising and administrative costs can be less than but should not be more than 25% of your program's total budget, so be sure to include all program services costs in your budget's expense column. Do not forget audit costs, insurance for the program and for the board, utilities, rental fees for copiers or other items, depreciation costs, and items related to in-kind services. A larger, more accurate budget decreases the percentage of funds being spent on fund-raising and administration of the program (see Table 9.2 in Appendix A).
- Programs also can gain funding through subcontracts from their networking partners' proposals. Subcontracting is a mechanism whereby one agency receiving a grant contracts with another for the other agency to do part of the proposed workload. The second agency is given appropriate funds from the grant to accomplish their piece of the work. Subcontractors must keep good quantitative records of objectives completed, as well as good bookkeeping documentation on money spent, so that they can provide proper evidence to the lead agency as they seek their share of the funds. The lead agency is still responsible for the accomplishment of the work and proper use and auditing of the funds. Remember to send a copy of the audit to the address specified on federal grants. In Arizona, RAISING Special Kids and Pilot Parents of Southern Arizona offer a good example of fund sharing through subcontracts. Subcontracts go back and forth between them depending on who has the project lead. The two organizations have the same mission, and trust and respect between them has been built over the years. They

both realize that the significant factor is that they accomplish their mission and that who leads the way is secondary.

- Once your fund-raising strategies are successful, don't forget to ask families who have benefited from your program to write a note of thanks to the funding source. Although the Maternal and Child Health Bureau no longer funds PHP's National Center, the trainees in its annual national symposium on PDFRCs write to the bureau to thank it for past support of the project.

All of the fund-raising strategies can be summed up in the words of the leadership of RAISING Special Kids of Arizona:

> *There are four basic parts to any request for funds. It is no different from someone asking you for money. You would want to know 1) what the person wants to do and how he or she will go about it (goals, objectives, methods, or strategies), 2) why is it important to do this activity (needs), 3) how much money will be needed and why (budget and budget justification), 4) how you will know if the money was put to good use and accomplished what you set out to do (evaluation).*

Using a New Language

Sometimes obtaining funds for a Parent to Parent program can be difficult because others don't know the significance of parent to parent support to a child's welfare. Parent programs must learn to frame their requests for funding around the child rather than the parent. Funding sources want to fund *direct services* to children, so use language in your proposals that presents your program as providing direct services to children. For example, write, "We provide children with trained advocates to help them acquire an education," instead of, "We train parents in advocacy skills."

Look through your materials and begin revising them using this child-oriented language. Move away from language that says, "We support and strengthen families," to language that says, "We provide children with strong families." As you continue to use this approach, it will become familiar to funding sources, the community, and yourself.

A national funding and nonprofit consultant spoke of the importance of using language that includes tangibility, specificity, and immediacy (TSI) in fund-raising requests. *Tangibility* is the degree to which your program has easy-to-grasp features and benefits. *Specificity* is the degree to which your program meets the needs of individuals with whom the prospective donor has a high affinity. *Immediacy* is the degree to which the need is urgent and your program can have an immediate impact. The consultant noted that these are the three things to which funding sources most readily respond, so you may want to evaluate your funding requests with these criteria in mind. TSI is found in the following two statements: "A little boy needs shoes or his feet will freeze and may require amputation." "Children cannot wait for early intervention services or the critical time for brain development will have passed." Use child-oriented and TSI language in your funding requests to get better results.

Grantwriting

A grantwriter for Parent to Parent programs proposes a series of activities for a potential funder to consider funding. Many Parent to Parent programs rely on grantwriting to fund at least some of their program activities. You might find it helpful to take one or more proposal writing classes to help you learn more about grantwriting. Also, find a mentor to help you as you write your initial proposals.

Preparing to Write a Proposal

Before you start to write, gather a full copy of the request for proposal (RFP) if one is being used, the funding source's guidelines, application forms, application process, annual report, and previous grant proposals. Write to the directors of the foundations to introduce yourself. Call to find out whether they are interested in the project you are proposing.

Before preparing a full proposal, find out if your funding sources will accept a letter of inquiry. If they do not request or require one, feel free to test the waters by creating and sending one. An inquiry letter is a 1- or 2-page document that introduces your idea to a potential funding source and tests the funder's interest in a full proposal (see sample inquiry letter at the end of this chapter). The letter starts with how much money you are seeking, why you want it, how you'll use it, who you are, and your credibility. It includes a brief problem description, as seen not only by you but also by experts in the field. If the funding source is interested, he or she will ask you to submit a full proposal.

Although some grant writers create their proposal abstracts last, do it first and then do a potential budget to match its objectives. The abstract and budget drafts clarify the project in your mind, provide you with ready references, and then are available to send to those from whom you are seeking support letters. By matching the budget and the abstract, you are less likely to propose too large a scope of work or request insufficient funds in the budget. By doing the budget early, you will know how much personnel will be available to carry out your action plans.

The best proposals are written specifically for a particular funding source. Do not send a boilerplate proposal (i.e., one using the same wording) to several funding sources. You may request funds for the same project from different sources, but make each proposal specific for the part you want them to fund. When one project is being funded by several grantors, the body of the proposal will look the same, but the cover letter, scope of work, and the part of the budget you are requesting will vary according to the funding priorities of the potential funding source.

PARTS OF A PROPOSAL

There are about a dozen key parts to a thorough proposal. The length and depth of each part will depend on the guidelines from the potential funder. Each part should relate in a relevant way to the others. For example, the budget should adequately reflect the scope of the work plan, and the objectives should respond to the needs.

Introduction

The introduction provides an opportunity for you to give a brief history and overview of your program or organization. For example, highlight your agency's age if that is one of its assets. Depending on the funding source being pursued, being old and experienced or new and just starting can be equally valuable. Government agencies prefer the tried and true, whereas some foundations want to be in on the creation. Make them aware of your accomplishments, your uniqueness, the breadth of your support in the community, and your ability to survive in the future. Introduce the problem or issue with which you are concerned. A large part of having a successful proposal includes having a great organization and a dynamic principal investigator (e.g., project director) behind it. An example of an introduction follows:

PHP is a 23-year-old local, state, and federally funded, uniquely parent-directed family resource center serving children with all types of physical, mental, emotional, and learning disabilities. It is housed in a facility that provides ample space for its multiservice one-stop system of support, training, information, technical assistance, and assistive technology services for children and families. Accomplishing its mission of helping children achieve their potential by providing them with strong families, dedicated professionals, and responsive systems of service has earned PHP many awards, including the prestigious Senator Lloyd Bentsen Award for family-centered care. PHP is a tax-exempt nonprofit United Way agency easily accessed by public transportation in the heart of Silicon Valley.

Need Statement

In the need statement you will describe your project's main area of concern; the gaps in services; people's suffering, pain, and lack of opportunities; and hurdles faced by the targeted population you intend to serve. Outline the breadth, width, and depth of these problems—how many people, how they are being affected, and what systems are dysfunctional or have gaps in their service procedures. Search the literature for and include statistics and other data from experts in the field that support your statements. Remember to add these sources to your list of references or bibliography that is attached to the proposal. An example of a need statement follows:

Children with disabilities often need many different services to support their growth to their fullest potential, and their parents are their most important advocates. However, many parents lack information about available resources and special education laws, as well as the assertiveness skills needed to advocate for their child. Too often young children with special needs don't receive early intervention services either because their parents do not know about these services or there is too great a time lag between the identification of the need and the provision of the services. Too many parents are not attending their children's individualized family service plan (IFSP) meetings, so their perspectives are not taken into account in the planning of the child's early intervention program. Because there is a brief 3-year eligibility period for early intervention, young children with special needs can't wait.

Through contact with other parents who have children with special needs, parents gain relevant information and skills and the motivation to handle their role of parent and advocate for their child. Research validates the effectiveness of a parent to parent match in meeting the emotional and informational needs of parents. However, there is no formal system in place for providing parent to parent matches for the children identified in this county as needing early intervention services, and professionals have a difficult time reaching parents who can serve as mentors for other parents.

Note that this need statement does not say "parents need information packets," nor does it say that "parents need training." Those are not need statements; they are answers. An additional sample need statement appears at the end of this chapter.

Vision, Mission, Goals, and Objectives

The beginning of the vision, mission, goals, and objectives section is sometimes called the project narrative, especially in federal RFPs. This is the main body of your project.

Vision Statement A vision statement describes what you hope your program or specific project activity will look like in the future. The founder or executive director often creates the vision statement, then requests the support of the rest of the leadership, board, staff, and community. Their buy-in usually results from their participation in programs or in planning and having an opportunity to add pieces to the picture or means for accomplishing the vision. An example of a vision statement follows:

We envision a 4,000 square foot facility that is specifically configured for children and families—with a play yard for kids and a meditation room for parents. A competent staff will operate our 10 major quality programs centered around enhancing children's chances and broadening their horizons through a compassionate Parent to Parent program.

Mission Statement The *mission statement* is a *brief, global* statement about why the program exists; it is *not* a statement of *what you do.* A good mission statement has three key parts: 1) who ultimately will benefit from the program, 2) what will they gain or receive, and 3) how the program will uniquely cause it to happen. PHP's mission statement follows:

PHP's mission is helping children get the resources, education, health care, love, hope, and respect that they need to achieve their full potential, by providing them with strong families, dedicated professionals, and responsive systems.

In this mission statement, "children" are the *who;* "achieve their full potential" is the *what;* and, "by providing them strong families, dedicated professionals, and responsive systems" is the *unique how.* The training, support, collaboration, and other interactions that a Parent to Parent program has with professionals, service systems, and parents are only the vehicles by which Parent to Parent cares for children.

Goals *Goals* are *broad* statements of what you will have if your vision and mission are accomplished. A goal is not what you do, it is what you want to exist. An example of PHP's goals follows:

- Goal A: Well-informed, emotionally supported, caring, active families function as equals in a partnership with children's care providers.
- Goal B: Children have prompt access to state-of-the-art care and resources.
- Goal C: Professionals provide family-centered, culturally competent care and work collaboratively with parents on behalf of children.
- Goal D: Service systems are responsive to children and families' ongoing developmental, financial, and emotional needs.

There is one major goal for each key area of the group's concern—the family, child, professional or care providers, and service systems. One or more objectives are written for each of these goals.

Goals and Objectives *Objectives* are *specific* statements of what you do to accomplish the *broad goals* that keep you progressing toward your *global mission,* which may never be finished in one group's lifetime. There are process objectives and behavioral objectives. *Process objectives* are simple statements of what you intend to do in broad terms but do not contain specific time frames or quantities. *Behavioral objectives* must be *specifically focused, timed, quantifiable,* and *doable. Outcome benefits* or a statement of the anticipated results are sometimes included in behavioral objectives. You might have a process objective that states, "We will train parents," or, "We will provide training." To put that in the form of a behavioral objective with outcome benefits, one would state, "We will train 50 parents of children who need special services in education planning by September 20, 2001, thus increasing their participation in parent–teacher meetings by 25% within 3 years."

Whereas process objectives are broad, behavioral objectives are specific and can be helpful to you as you evaluate your program. Are you doing what you said you were going to do, for the population indicated, in the amounts, and by the time frame proposed? And, last, if you did accomplish your objective, was there an outcome that benefited the population in question (e.g., outcome benefit)? This is why you brainstorm needs, issues, and concerns before creating your objectives. The outcome benefit should read like a partial resolution of a need or problem that the program is attempting to address. "Increasing parents' participation in their child's planning meetings" is the outcome benefit in the example above.

A group that is seeking funding for its Parent to Parent program might start with mission, goals, and objectives that resemble the following:

Mission: Helping children with special needs acquire services by providing them with active parents

Goal A: Well-informed, active parents

Objective A-1: Match a veteran parent with referred parents.
Objective A-2: Provide an information packet on child disability rights.
Objective A-3: Create a newsletter and a special needs library.

Goal B: Children receiving state-of-the-art care

Objective B-1: Reach out to the professional community to invite family referrals.
Objective B-2: Train supporting parents and match them with referred parents.
Objective B-3: Hold parent support group meetings to provide family emotional support.
Objective B-4: Set up an information, referral, and direction program to connect parents to resources.

Goal C: A strong, viable, well-funded Parent to Parent program

Objective C-1: Create a board of directors.

Objective C-2: Get incorporated as a 501(c)3 tax-exempt nonprofit organization.

Objective C-3: Create, implement, and monitor a 5-year strategic long-range plan.

These process objectives can be turned into behavioral objectives by adding quantities and time frames.

Methodology

Inexperienced proposal writers often confuse objectives with methodology. *Methodology* is the manner in which you will go about accomplishing the objectives. Several examples of methodology statements follow:

- *This project will use dynamic, multisensory (e.g., lecture, role playing, audiovisual) teaching strategies during workshops.*
- *Technology will be used to make parent to parent matches.*
- *A broad breadth of knowledge and experience will be provided compassionately from parent to parent to ensure children's care, growth, and development.*
- *The staff will collaborate with care providers to bring services quickly to children.*
- *We will utilize committees to increase the board's performance.*
- *Free consultants from the REV program will facilitate completion of the 501(c)3 application.*
- *Staff will collaborate with a local university to carry out an outside evaluation of the project.*

Action Plan Worksheets

Action plan worksheets describe the activities for completing each objective (see Figure 9.2). This section of the proposal often takes the most time to prepare, as detailed activities are presented in a sequential time frame for accomplishing them. But when you receive the grant and start to implement the proposal, the action plan worksheets will be the most useful. They will be a direct guide for any staff that you hire to carry out your proposed activities.

Evaluation Arm

In the evaluation section of your proposal, you will describe the methods by which the project will be appraised and how your successes will

Action Plan Worksheet				
Objective C-2: Get incorporated as a 501(c)3 nonprofit tax-exempt group.				
What's to be done	By when	How	Who	Milestone evaluations
Get incorporated	12/31	Reserve name	J. Smith	Called Secretary of State 6/13 and reserved name and requested incorporation application.
		Draft articles of incorporation	J. Smith	Original and four copies mailed 6/29 with payment check. Approval received 12/15; 90% of payment refunded.
		Draft by-laws	Board	Reviewed and accepted by board 6/25. Mailed with application forms 6/29.
Gain federal tax-exempt status	12/31	Contact the IRS for Form 1023	A. Jones	Contacted IRS 6/13. Forms received 7/1. Forms completed 7/15. Forms mailed 7/25 with payment check.
Gain state tax-exempt status	12/31	Contact the state for Form 3500	A. Jones	Called Franchise Tax Board 6/13; forms received 7/1. Forms completed 7/15. Forms mailed 7/25 with payment check.
Get employer identification number	1/30	Contact the IRS for Form SS-4	A. Jones	Contacted the IRS for forms 12/1. Forms received, completed, and mailed by 1/2.
File annual state Statement of Domestic Nonprofit Corporation (verifies leaders and agency address)	1/30	Automatically sent annually by the state to the agency	J. Smith	One-page form completed and mailed 6/30.
Plan to meet deadlines for filing tax forms (no payments)	1/30	IRS and State Attorney General automatically sends	J. Smith	Filed annual forms. Registered with Registry Charitable Trust 6/30.

Figure 9.2. Sample action plan worksheet.

be defined. The efficacy of your program accomplishments is tested (e.g., determining the significance or worth of the program). Be sure to include in your evaluation section how you will monitor the accomplishments of the project and the funds. Some evaluation statements follow, and additional information about program evaluation appears in Chapter 13:

- *At their regular meetings, the board of directors will receive quarterly reports from the executive director on the progress of the activity plan.*
- *The program coordinator will meet monthly with the project director to review objective milestones.*
- *Formative (e.g., identifying changes and other knowledge gained) and summative (e.g., counting quantifiable data) methods will be used to evaluate program services.*
- *At least 85% of the project's objectives must be completed for this project to be a success.*
- *Pre- and posttests will be used to assess skills learned in the training.*
- *Satisfaction surveys will be sent to a randomly selected 20% of the families who used the program services.*
- *Typical nonprofit bookkeeping tracking of money will be done.*
- *Checks written for more than $500 will require two signatures.*
- *An annual outside audit will be performed by a reputable auditing firm.*
- *Dr. Doe and several research students at the University of ABC will collaborate with the staff on overseeing and accomplishing this evaluation.*
- *Evaluation data will be used to change, retain, or improve program services and will be used in short- and long-range planning.*

Budget

Funding sources usually request a detailed annual budget of the specific project for which you are seeking funding, and the budget you submit may not be your entire agency budget. Sometimes funders want to see both the project budget and your overall program budget to evaluate how the project budget fits into the overall budget and how it compares in size. If you are submitting a proposal to help fund the total agency, as may be the case with a United Way proposal, then the total agency budget should be submitted.

Complete a balanced budget with income and expense columns (see Figure 9.3). Include an indirect cost figure, which covers such costs as audits, insurance, rent, bookkeeping, and other critical costs that are indirectly related to the accomplishment of the program. Have your indirect cost percentage rate calculated. An acceptable figure for indirect

Budget Worksheet

Fiscal Year: ________

Expenses	Total budget	Fund-raising and administration	Program A	Program B
Salaries				
Employee benefits (fringe)				
Payroll taxes, etc.				
Professional fees (including audit costs)				
Supplies				
Telephone				
Postage and shipping				
Occupancy (lease/rent)				
Rental and maintenance of equipment				
Printing and publications				
Travel				
Conferences, conventions, and meetings				
Specific assistance to individuals				
Program membership dues				
Awards and grants to others				
Miscellaneous expenses				
Insurance (board and liability)				
Allowable depreciation				
Payments to affiliated groups				
Total expenses				

Income				
Contributions (include in-kind)				
Special events				
Legacies and bequests				
Collections from local units (e.g., affiliated support groups)				
Contributions from associated groups				
Federated fund raising				
Government grants (federal, state, county, city)				
Membership dues				
Program service fees				
United Way				
Sales to the public				
Investment income				
Miscellaneous				
Funded from reserves				
Total income				

Figure 9.3. Sample budget worksheet. (*Note:* Nonprofit agencies should present a balanced budget—total income matches total expenses.)

costs for small agencies is 10% of personnel costs before fringe benefits are added. Check with funding sources for their guidelines on indirect costs. Some ask that you spell out what the indirect dollars will be used for; others do not. Be prepared to know how you expect to spend the indirect funds.

In your budget be sure to itemize all of the expenses related to completing your proposed activities, including expenses for personnel, payroll taxes, and fringe benefits. If your funding request does not include the cost of the space (i.e., rent) you are providing to carry out your program, then include the rent cost in the *expense column* of the budget for the program. Be sure to include your program as a source of funding for the rent in the *income column,* and attach the rent cost as your agency's contribution. Including your program as a source of funding shows funding sources that you are doing your part to support the project.

ATTACHMENTS

Most funding sources request that you attach certain basic items to the proposal as you prepare it for mailing. They also may put a limit on the number of such documents. *Send only what they request.* Use labels and titles as they are referred to in the RFP or application to help the evaluators easily identify each piece of the proposal. These attachments are generally found at the back of the proposal and usually include the following (keep extra copies easily accessible for use with your proposals and other documentation activities):

- IRS letter—a copy of the program's nonprofit 501(c)3 tax-exempt status letter
- Letters of support—letters from relevant people who support your proposal. A letter of support should indicate a person's willingness to do the part that has been indicated in the proposal, his or her knowledge of the need outlined in your proposal, and his or her enthusiastic support for your methodology. Be sure that letters highlight past, present, and future collaborative efforts between your program and him- or herself or his or her agency. When requesting letters of support, send the individuals writing the letters a copy of your abstract so that they are informed about the project. Federal grantors will indicate in the RFP whether it is necessary for the grantee to include a letter of support from a relevant state department.
- Curriculum vitae or biographies of key staff attached to the project (e.g., project director, program coordinator, major trainers)

- List of the board of directors, with addresses, occupations, and term expiration dates
- Organizational chart of the program and an organizational chart of the project (e.g., how the project fits into the organizational chart)
- Financial statements or a copy of the latest audit
- Map with directions to your facility
- Publicity about the program (e.g., newspaper articles, magazine articles)
- Program documents (e.g., newsletters, fliers, brochures)

Proposals also usually include some attachments at the front as well.

- Abstract (e.g., your proposal in one to four pages)—a good abstract provides a limited definition of your program, its credibility, the need or problem addressed, the mission, goals, and objectives, the population to be served, your methodology, and your evaluation approach. Be sure that the abstract captures the essence, enthusiasm, and uniqueness of your project in a clear, concise, and factual manner (see the abstract of a proposal at the end of this chapter).
- Cover letter—contains the title of the project, the agency's name and address, a brief description of the project, the target individuals and geographical area being served, and the names of and contact information for key people serving as the point of contact for this grant. A statement of board approval for the proposal can be included in the cover letter. The statement is usually signed by the chairperson of the board, the executive director, or the director of development. If more proof is required, then provide a copy of the minutes of the board meeting during which the approval occurred. The board can provide an umbrella permission for the fund developer and the executive director to seek governmental, corporate, and foundation funding to support programs and operations.
- Transmittal letter—contains the amount of funds being sought, the level of support that the agency has from the board and the community, brief statements on needs, and how the project will help resolve those needs. Include in the transmittal letter how the project fits with the mission, goals, and objectives of the funding source if possible. An RFP may provide grant seekers several choices of categories for applying under the same general area of funding. So, if the funds are being requested under a particular segment of an RFP, make note of that and be sure that you are submitting under the correct segment. Some proposals have been rejected because they were submitted under the wrong segment.

SENDING THE PROPOSAL

Now that the proposal is written, proofread it twice and let someone else proofread it as well. Complete and sign all forms attached to the RFP as requested, make the appropriate number of copies, package it as requested by the funding source, and mail it via certified mail. Most funding sources let you know immediately that they have received your proposal and indicate when their board will be meeting to review and decide on funding. Some funding sources request that you send a stamped, self-addressed postcard along with the proposal so that they can easily let you know that they have received the proposal.

Once a decision has been made, the funding source will send you a letter informing you of the acceptance or rejection of your proposal. Some funding sources request a visit to your site before making their final decision. Choose a day when your programs are active so that the visitors can get the truest picture of your activities. Some funding sources will send you their evaluation comments along with their decision letter. If not, call or write and ask them for evaluation comments, especially if your proposal was not funded.

If your program is funded, send a thank-you letter indicating your acceptance of the grant. You may still have to negotiate the budget and may even be able to negotiate for more money. The proposal becomes a contract to be honored between the funding source and the nonprofit organization. Do not make major changes in the scope of work, and do not bring in a new director of the project without letting the funding source know. Make a note on your calendar to send the grantor a *brief* interim report on your progress in 6 months, and note due dates for all required reports to the funding source. If it is a multiple-year grant, send an annual report thereafter. A final report is usually due to the grantor 30–90 days after the last day of funding. Many funding sources will fund an agency for 3 consecutive years for the same area or for a new program area. After those 3 years, however, you often must wait a few years before seeking more funding from that particular funding source.

RECOMMENDED PRACTICES

There are recommended practices that programs should follow as they seek funding and work with funding sources.

- If a funding source is providing 10% of your program budget, that source should not be telling you how to run the other 90%. Some want too much control over the entire agency for the small amount of funding they are providing. Pass it up; it is not worth the hassle and loss of control and dignity.

- Securing funding is an ongoing process. Parents of children with special needs tend to understand unending needs better than most. Hiring a fund developer or director of fund development early in the organizing of the program is wise, but this does not relieve the board of directors and the executive director of their fund-raising responsibilities.
- Choose funding that fits your mission, goals, and objectives. Making your program fit the funding RFP distorts the focus of your program. Seek funds to cover what you already do, otherwise your variety of program services will become overwhelming and staff may begin to complain about reaching out in too many directions.
- Many funding sources will not support operating expenses, so be sure that they do before requesting them. Funders typically want to pay for a program service or a special project. They like to be a part of creating a model that can be replicated locally, statewide, or nationally.
- If you send several proposals for one project to many different funding sources and they all get accepted, write to the grantors and tell them of your good fortune. Ask if you can use their funds for another part of your program or to broaden the scope of work, enhance the amount or quality of some major equipment, or extend the life of the project another year or two beyond its present deadline.
- Learn to use space-based or staff-based allocations when your program is funded by several sources. With such an arrangement, each grant pays a part of the budget items, such as rent, supplies, insurance, or telephone bills. For example, if you have six employees and three are involved with Project A and one each with Projects B, C, and D, then a staff-based allocation would have Project A paying for 50% of the supplies, insurance, and the telephone bill because three employees are 50% of your total number of employees. Projects B, C, and D would each pay 16%–17%. But, using a space-based allocation, if Projects A, B, C, and D are each housed in only 25% of the total space, all projects would be charged 25% of the rent each month. Auditors find these very acceptable allocation methods. Do not arbitrarily choose an amount for a project to pay.

SUMMARY

Money is available. In preschool we learned to say, "Hi," "What's your name?" and, "Do you want to play?" This is what fund-raising is all about. You have to initiate a contact on the telephone or in writing to find out about the company, foundation, or person and to make your mission known to see if it is something they are interested in. Look for a proper fit before seeking finances.

Get prepared to seek funding. Do your homework. Get incorporated. Create a long-range strategic plan. Build a board of directors. Separate board and staff.

Hire a fund developer not as a consultant but as staff. Funding sources often give a capacity building grant that can include the salary for a full- or part-time fund development staff person for 1–3 years.

Go to fund-raising school. Take proposal writing classes. Locate a mentor. Read your local newspaper. The executive director and the fund developer should read the newspaper daily to obtain ideas for fund-raising and to stay up-to-date about the community in which you function.

Although funding sources want to help a good cause, they want to be sure the cause is meeting a community need and has a good infrastructure and a sound future. Most funding sources also want to be sure that they are not the only one interested in funding the program. There isn't any project that funding sources would rather give money to than one that helps children. Therefore, it behooves Parent to Parent programs to be sure that the message they send and the language they use in their written and verbal communications reflect how Parent to Parent helps children with special needs get education services; obtain state-of-the-art health care; and receive resources that speed their development and enhance the quality of their lives as well as provide them with the one thing that children need most to achieve their potential—knowledgeable, assertive, caring parents. Nothing increases successes like exuding enthusiasm and passion for your mission.

RESOURCES

Allen, J. (2000). *Event planning: The ultimate guide to successful meetings, corporate events, fundraising galas, conferences, conventions, incentives and special events.* New York: John Wiley & Sons.

Colvin, G.L. (1993). *Fiscal sponsorship: 6 ways to do it right.* San Francisco: Study Center Press.

Drucker, P. (1990). *Managing the nonprofit organization, principles and practices.* New York: HarperCollins Publishers.

Flanagan, J. (1999). *Successful fundraising: A complete handbook for volunteers and professionals.* Lincolnwood, IL: NTC Publishing Co.

Keegan, P.B. (1994). *Fundraising for non-profits.* London: HarperCollins Publishers.

Kouzes, J.M., & Posner, B.Z. (1995). *The leadership challenge.* San Francisco: Jossey-Bass.

Poyadue, F.S. (1991). *Steps to starting.* Santa Clara, CA: Parents Helping Parents.

Organizations

Discover Total Resources; telephone: (412) 234-3275

The Fund Raising School, Indiana University, Center of Philanthropy, 550 West North Street, Suite #301, Indianapolis, IN 46202; telephone: (800) 962-6692. The Fund Raising School offers a 5-day, intensive, comprehensive, down-to-earth training program. It also offers several 2- to 3-day training programs on the various aspects of fund-raising.

Parents Helping Parents: The Family Resource Center, Department: Technical Assistance and Training, National Center on Parent Directed Family Resource Centers, 3041 Olcott Street, Santa Clara, CA 95054-3222; telephone: (408) 727-5775; http://www.php.com. PHP's annual national symposium on the Keys to Creating, Managing and Maintaining a Family Resource Center or Other Nonprofit offers an exciting 5-day training adventure that covers issues from getting incorporated, to fund-raising, to long-range planning, and more. Inquire about other training, materials, and technical assistance offered at PHP.

Appendix

Sample Inquiry Letter

September 22, 2001

ZYX Foundation
123 Main Street
Somewhere, USA 12345

Dear Ms. Smith:

Family to Family, Inc. (FTF) is seeking $30,000 from the ZYX Foundation in order to transition from a volunteer agency to a combination of paid staff and volunteers. On August 27, 2001, our board of directors unanimously agreed that we should seek this grant. *(Key information is included here: your agency's full name, the funders full name, the amount you are seeking, why you want the funds, and your board's awareness of and approval of this request.)*

FTF was formed 8 years ago by professionals and parents who were concerned about children with special needs and the financial, social, and emotional problems confronted by their families. *(Key information: brief history and key participants whom funder perhaps respects)*

There were, and still are, many fine agencies available to give services and expert care to these children. Few, if any, assist with giving them the one thing that they need most—parents who feel supported and prepared to care for their children. *(Key information: clarifying your point of service and your position in the community)*

FTF strives to provide these children with parents who are informed about their children's rights; who know how to advocate for them to get the best services; who are emotionally stable and able to love and accept their children; and who can maintain a loving home. *(Key information: children highlighted as the ultimate beneficiary of your services and of their funding assistance. Note how language states "providing these children" not "providing parents")*

We accomplish these goals through direct services to the children and families of Humane County, and they include but are not limited to

1. In-home, in-hospital, or telephone peer counseling
2. Training in coping, advocacy, and counseling skills
3. Information packets on services and agencies
4. Family rap or guidance sessions
5. Conferences for siblings
6. Information and referral with direction services

(Key information: short list [no more than six items] of specific, easily understood activities and the specific geographical area to which the service is pinpointed)

Whereas one agency may use its funding to provide the child with speech-language therapy for 1 hour a week to help him or her learn to talk, FTF uses its funds to assist the child's parent with the child's speech and language development the other 167 hours during the week when he or she is not with the therapist. *(Key information: highlighting your agency's or services' uniqueness and clarifying how you are different from agencies that the funder may believe are doing what you are proposing or doing)*

We accept referrals from agencies such as Special Children's Society, developmental centers, schools, hospitals, and others. We also offer training for professionals who are interested in better ways of working with families. Our speakers' bureau is active at schools, churches, clubs, and homes to increase public awareness about the special needs of these families. *(Key information: You are letting the funder know that you are aware of similar agencies or agencies that provide services to the same customer you are serving; and you are informing the funder that you are a collaborative player with these other providers, how your services and your work with these agencies serves and benefits the broader community, and that it is not an unnecessary duplication.)*

We make a difference where others cannot. One doctor called us exasperated. He had tried unsuccessfully for 8 months to get a mother to get her child into an early intervention program. In less than 8 hours, we saw the mother and 8 weeks later the child was in therapy. For that mother, getting information from someone who had "been there" made the difference and gave her the confidence to trust others and herself to become involved in helping her child. Our program of experienced parents can connect with families to offer real examples of what has worked and to support overwhelmed caregivers. *(Key information: You are providing the funder with a poignant, short, and emotional true story that shows the value of your services.)*

We envision a solid financial base in the future, as the Developmental Center believes in the value of our work and supports us by providing space for us to carry out our business and activities. The county is working with us to complete an application for ongoing funding. And we are proceeding with our application for United Way funding. *(Key information: You are letting the funder know that there is a financial future for your program and how you plan to make that future happen; and you are informing them that there are others interested in supporting your activities—most funders do not like to fund alone.)*

Your support now, and hopefully for the next 2 years, will go a long way in helping us to obtain our United Way funding and achieve our goals. United Way will not fund an agency that does not have a full-time, paid executive director. We need your support to make this happen. *(Key information: you are informing the funder that you hope to build an ongoing relationship with them; and you are showing them how you are planning to leverage their funds into bigger things as their funds boost your chances for other major funding or activities.)*

Thank you for considering our application.

Sincerely,

Aidan Gabriel
Executive Director
(Key information: inquiry letter should be no more than two pages in length, unless the funder has specified that they are open to more. Some major funders ask for four pages, which often is called a concept paper)

Appendix
Abstract of a Proposal

Project title: Parents Activating Family Centered Care
Organization name: Family to Family, Inc.
Address: 456 Elm Street, Somewhere, USA 12345
Project director: Jane Smith
Project coordinator: Ann Jones
Contact person: Jane Smith
Telephone: (408) 777-5755
Fax: (408) 777-0982
Project period: 4 years
From: 7/1/02 to 6/30/06

Problem: Managed care health plans have been around for a long time, often functioning in isolation from other community-based care providers. Now, managed care is at the heart of Medicaid cost containment and health reform (Delotte & Fransen, 2001). The problem is how family-centered, culturally competent care can be introduced into this well-established system of coordinated care with its emphasis on critical pathways, that is, setting time lines for care and cost containment as patients move through the system. These plans reflect a lack of knowledge about incorporating family-centered care and a lack of contact with consumer issues as they concentrate on third-party contracting payers. The public, local, state, and federal health providers lack knowledge about, and do not have a connecting link to, managed care health plans. Professionals and families lack familiarity with the elements of family-centered care and family–professional collaboration skills (Knight, et al., 2001) needed for state-of-the-art care for children. Parents lack assertiveness to function as equals in a partnership with care providers. The bottom line is that children suffer.

Goals and objectives: The mission of this project is to ensure family-centered, culturally competent care for children with special health care needs in managed care health plans through parents helping parents. Our major goal is to have a national model for introducing this family-centered, culturally competent service for children with special health care needs through a collaborative consumer–provider partnership between a parent-directed family resource center (PDFRC) and a well-established managed care facility. Our objectives are to achieve the following by June 30, 2006.

1. Create a collaborative working relationship between FTF, a PDFRC, and Stone Creek, a managed care health plan.
2. Establish and operate a new position at Stone Creek entitled Parent Liaison for fostering family-centered, culturally competent input into the health plan's evaluation, implementation, and planning system.
3. Train 40 doctors in family-centered ways of breaking diagnostic and other news to families.
4. Train 100 nurses in family-centered, culturally competent manners of caring for children who have special needs.
5. Train 240 parents and professionals in family–professional collaboration skills.
6. Provide emotional support to at least 360 parents and professionals via small-group process and parent to parent and professional to professional mentors.
7. Create a computerized directory system for health reform information, resources, and networking for parents and professionals.
8. Provide outreach, training, information, and support to Hispanic and Vietnamese clients via parent to parent visiting community resource parents from those cultures.
9. Create and disseminate a document on replicating this model, to be co-written by parent and physician.

Methodology: Building on an 18-year relationship, FTF, a parent-directed nonprofit organization, will create a consumer–provider partnership via a memorandum of understanding with Stone Creek, a managed care health company. A new position at Stone Creek, called a Parent Liaison, will be cocreated, cosupervised, and coevaluated. This person will provide family-centered input into Stone Creek's planning, implementation, and evaluation of services for children with special health care needs and will also provide support, information, and training to professionals. Cross-training in family-centered health reform for doctors, nurses, and parents will be cotaught by FTF and Stone Creek staffs. Rubio University will conduct the evaluation process and provide personnel to coteach parent–professional collaboration with FTF. A computer disk of the FTF's database and training methods will be provided to Stone Creek. Stone Creek staff will spend time at

FTF as they volunteer for community outreach. A neutral overall consultant, Dr. Roman Alexander, will nurture the consumer–provider partnership and coauthor a replication document. A satellite office of FTF will be located at Stone Creek and operated by Parent Liaison.

Evaluation: The overall evaluation of this project will be carried out by an external team to conduct process and outcome studies under the direction of an independent team in research methods at Rubio University. Before starting the project, we will establish baseline data related to specific recommended practice behaviors in providing family-centered care, and analysis of outcomes will be in terms of behavioral changes toward family-centered methods. Process evaluation will assess the extent to which the project was implemented according to its conceptual plan. We will utilize the family-centered individualized family service plan (IFSP) rating scales created by Harrell, et. al. at the Park Center on Children and Disability at the University of Dean as a guide. We will use the up-to-date products of the national Family Centered Care Project and the Parent/Professional Collaboration project at the University of Islas to create investigator-designed questionnaires and follow-up studies to measure family–professional collaboration and satisfaction. Pre- and posttests will be used in all training classes. Satisfaction feedback forms will be included in the main product and in materials sent to families and professionals.

Appendix
Sample Need Statement

The Beach Center has developed this statement, complete with references, that can easily be adapted to fit any grant written for local or state funding.

Caring for a family member who has a disability is an experience that few parents anticipate and plan for and one that comes with many strong emotional responses and day-to-day challenges. Families that have a relative with a disability must not only cope with the typical demands of family life but also with a host of disability-related issues that accompany their transition from a world without disabilities to a world with disabilities. They must learn about the disability itself and what it means for the individual as well as for the whole family; they must learn the languages of the medical, legal, financial, and special education worlds; they must find their way in a service system that may or may not provide appropriate support opportunities; and they often must face the loss of their more familiar social supports as relatives and friends distance themselves out of fear or misunderstanding.

Several studies document the challenges faced by families of a person with a disability. For families that learn that their child has a disability at birth, the experience often is emotionally overwhelming, shattering many of their hopes and expectations for the future (Pearson & Sternberg, 1986). Parents may feel guilty, angry, depressed, numb, lonely, or confused (Seligman & Darling, 1989). Intensifying many of these feelings are the day-to-day logistics of caring for a child with special needs. These realities often include multiple visits to medical centers and the resulting bills, demanding and time-consuming home caregiving responsibilities, little opportunity for respite, managing the concerns of family and friends, and juggling personal needs as well as the needs of other children (Gallagher, Beckman, & Cross, 1983; Schell, 1981). Each of these challenges will be present throughout the child's lifetime and will be augmented by additional needs as the family moves into and through the services system.

In the past, strong family networks existed that often helped families meet the challenges of family life, but today's increased mobility and decreased interdependence means extended family often lives far away (Kazak & Marvin, 1984). As a result, many parents face these challenges alone.

When asked who would best be able to support them emotionally, families that are dealing with these challenges often mention other parents who are sharing their experiences (Boukydis, 1984; Summers et al., 1990). Apparently sharing family experiences with someone who is in similar circumstances is an important source of social support.

The idea that social support may be helpful to families that are involved in parenting has been documented in family research. Crnic, Greenberg, Ragozin, Robinson, and Basham (1983) found that when mothers of young children received social support from a variety of sources—neighbors, friends, extended family members—they reported more satisfaction with the parenting experience and more positive parent–child interactions. Pilon and Smith (1985) observed that parents become better health care managers for their young children (as measured by the child's weight gain, hospital usage, use of the educational system, and self-ratings) when they participated in weekly parent support groups. Parent social support systems therefore can be a coping support under the various stressful conditions that accompany the parenting experience.

Social support opportunities often occur naturally and spontaneously for families that do not have a member with a disability—over the backyard fence, in play groups, and through community programs. Those who have a family member with a disability tend to have fewer naturally occurring opportunities and smaller social networks (Dunst, Trivette, & Cross, 1985). For these families, finding a family with similar experiences and needs often is very difficult. Parent to Parent programs have evolved to meet the special needs of families that are challenged by disability.

Since 1975, Parent to Parent programs have been providing a unique form of support to families that have a family member with a disability. Emotional and informational support is provided to parents by matching a trained veteran parent with a referred parent in a one-to-one relationship. Because veteran parents have *been there* and know from personal experience the challenges and special joys that come with parenting a son or a daughter with a disability, they are able to provide uniquely qualified support.

Parent to parent matches are made quickly, often within 24 hours of the referral, and are based on similarities in disability and family issues. Often, at the time of the match, the referred parent has just been given the diagnosis or is just beginning a new era in the life of the child with a disability. Once matched, each relationship evolves individually, depending on the needs and preferences of the referred parent. For some parents, the match is short term and involves primarily the exchange of information; for others, the match endures for years and develops into a lifelong friendship. Because the two parents share so many experiences, the match offers a unique form of support that is different from that provided by professionals. Because the relationship between the parents is one to one, the nature of the support is different from that found in parent support groups.

Parent to Parent programs emerged in the United States in the early 1970s. The first organized Parent to Parent program, the Pilot Parents Program, was established at the Greater Omaha Arc in Nebraska and was soon being replicated in 33 sites in four midwestern states (Smith, 1978). In 2000, Parent to Parent programs that are modeled after the Pilot Parents program exist throughout the United States and in Canada, Australia, New Zealand, England, and Denmark (Boukydis, 1987; Hornby, 1988; Hornby, Murray, & Jones, 1987; Iscoe & Bordelon, 1985; Santelli, Turnbull, Lerner, & Marquis, 1993; Santelli, Turnbull, Marquis, & Lerner, 1993; Santelli, Turnbull, Marquis & Lerner, 1995; Smith, 1993).

In an effort to learn more about Parent to Parent programs, the Parent to Parent National Survey Project at the Beach Center on Families and Disability at The University of Kansas conducted a national survey of Parent to Parent program coordinators and the veteran and referred parents who are participating in these programs. The data from the programs participating in the survey describe 374 Parent to Parent programs serving approximately 30,000 families in 47 states. The vast majority of these programs are cross-disability, matching parents whose children have a wide range of physical, mental, and emotional disabilities, including chronic illness and acquired disabilities. Parent to Parent programs range in size and age from newly developing programs serving fewer than 10 parents to programs that have been operating for 20 years and are serving several hundred families. Most Parent to Parent programs are low-budget efforts energized by volunteer parents, fewer than half of Parent to Parent programs have a paid coordinator, and all of the veteran parents who are matched with referred parents are unpaid (Santelli, Turnbull, Lerner, & Marquis, 1993; Santelli, Turnbull, Marquis, & Lerner, 1993).

At the very heart of Parent to Parent programs is the one-to-one match; all of the programs responding to the national survey reported that the matched opportunity is the foundation of their program. Because the quality of support that will be offered in the match is dependent on the relationship between the referred parent and the veteran parent, great care is taken when making a match. Programs reported using an average of six different factors when making a match, with similar disability issues and similar family issues being mentioned the most often.

Another hallmark of Parent to Parent programs is the training component for veteran parents. In 78% of the responding Parent to Parent programs, at least 1–3 hours of formal training is provided to veteran parents before they are placed in a match. Many programs also offer veteran parents ongoing training opportunities and informal support from the program coordinator once they are matched with newly referred parents.

Although a variety of supports and services are provided through the one-to-one match, more than 90% of the responding programs reported offering each of the following: someone to listen and understand, information about the disability, information about community resources, assistance with referrals, and problem-solving support. These key support opportunities, delivered through a match between a trained veteran parent and a newly referred parent, are the very essence of Parent to Parent. Although some programs reported other program activities beyond the one-to-one match, the delivery of these key support opportunities is the common denominator among all Parent to Parent programs that responded to the survey (Bassin & Kreeb, 1978; Brookman, 1988; Iscoe & Bordelon, 1985; Porter & Dean, 1979; Santelli, Turnbull, Marquis, & Lerner, 1993; Smith, 1978).

In response to requests from parents and program directors at local, state, and national levels for efficacy data on Parent to Parent, a participatory action research team consisting of parents, program administrators, and researchers submitted a field-initiated proposal to the Office of Special Education Programs to conduct a national efficacy study of Parent to Parent (Santelli, Singer, DiVenere, Ginsberg, & Powers, 1998). In 1993, funding for this 3-year study was granted, and from 1994 to 1996, data were collected from 400 referred parents in five different states to determine the impact of the Parent to Parent experience on parents who are referred to Parent to Parent programs for emotional and informational support. The results of this study indicate that parent to parent support increases parents' acceptance of their situation and their sense of being able to cope. Moreover, parent to parent support helps parents to make progress on the need they present when they first contact a Parent to Parent program, and more than 80% of the parents found parent to parent support to be helpful (Singer et al., 1999). Interviews with parents suggest that the kind of support that Parent to Parent offers is unique and cannot come from any other source (Ainbinder et al., 1998). Based upon significant data, the research team recommends that parent to parent support should be one essential component of a comprehensive family support system.

Parents and professionals who are participating in or connecting parents to Parent to Parent programs also have provided compelling anecdotal evidence of the importance of the emotional and informational supports that are offered through the one-to-one match between parents. One matched parent shares:

Without question, my match with my pilot parent was my single most valuable resource since my son was born. She and her husband listened to our questions about the immediate and the future and didn't give us too much information but enough to help us cope at each stage. The value of talking to a parent 3 years down the road is immeasurable, and I wish that every parent would take advantage of this unique, valuable resource—critical to raising a child with a disability.

Another parent who coordinates a Parent to Parent program relates:

I think Parent to Parent is the most important thing in my life. It helped me so much when my daughter with Down syndrome was born. I ran the program without funding for 6 months, and then with limited funding for 9 months—I believe in it!

A professional adds:

When the Parent to Parent program was established, we knew that the program would be of assistance for families, but we didn't realize until later that it also would be of great assistance to the staff. As professionals, we often feel inadequate because we cannot truly understand what families are going through since we haven't actually experienced what they have. Our staff became aware that this program could fulfill a need for families that they as professionals could not. In this way, the program supports the role of the professional as well as supporting the family.

Since 1975 Parent to Parent programs have been providing this support without much funding, without much national visibility, and until recently, without any research data to give credibility to their efforts, is evidence of the commitment of the parents involved with the programs.

REFERENCES

Ainbinder, J., Blanchard, L., Singer, G.H.S., Sullivan, M., Powers, L., Marquis, J., & Santelli, B. (1998). How parents help one another: A qualitative study of Parent to Parent self-help. *Journal of Pediatric Psychology, 23,* 99–109.

Bassin, J., & Kreeb, D.D. (1978). *Reaching out to parents of newly diagnosed retarded children: A guide to developing a parent-to-parent intervention program.* St. Louis: Association for Retarded Children.

Boukydis, C.F. (1984). *The importance of parenting networks.* Paper presented at the Parent Care Conference, Salt Lake City.

Boukydis, C.F. (1987, October). *An overview of parent support groups.* Paper presented at the Fourth Parent Care Conference, Philadelphia.

Brookman, B.A. (1988). Parent to parent: A model for parent support and information. *Topics in Early Childhood Special Education, 8*(2), 88–93.

Crnic, K.A., Greenberg, M.T., Ragozin, A.S., Robinson, N.M., & Basham, R. (1983). Effects of stress and social support on mothers and premature and full-term infants. *Child Development, 54,* 209–217.

Dunst, C., Trivette, C., & Cross, A. (1985). Roles and support networks of mothers of handicapped children. In R. Fewell & P. Vadasy (Eds.), *Families of handicapped children: Needs and supports across the life-span* (pp. 167–192). Austin, TX: PRO-ED.

Gallagher, J., Beckman, P., & Cross, A.H. (1983). Families of handicapped children: Sources of stress and its amelioration. *Exceptional Children, 50*(1), 10–17.

Hornby, G. (1988). Launching parent to parent schemes. *British Journal of Special Education, 15*(2), 77–88.

Hornby, G., Murray, R., & Jones, R. (1987). Establishing a parent to parent service. *Child Care Health & Development, 13,* 277–288.

Iscoe, L., & Bordelon, K. (1985). Pilot parents: Peer support for parents of handicapped children. *Children's Health Care, 14*(2), 103–109.

Kazak, A.E., & Marvin, R.S. (1984). Differences, difficulties, and adaptations: Stress and social networks in families with a handicapped child. *Family Relations, 33,* 67–77.

Pearson, J.E., & Sternberg, A. (1986). A mutual project for families of handicapped children. *Journal of Counseling & Development, 65,* 213–215.

Pilon, B.H., & Smith, K.A. (1985). A parent group for the Hispanic parents of children with severe cerebral palsy. *Children's Health Care, 14*(2), 96–102.

Porter, F., & Dean, S. (1979). *Pilot parents manual: A design for developing a program for parents of handicapped children.* Omaha: Pilot Parents—Greater Omaha Arc.

Santelli, B., Singer, G.H.S., DiVenere, N., Ginsberg, C., & Powers, L. (1998). Participatory action research: Reflections on critical incidents in a PAR project. *Journal of The Association for Persons with Severe Handicaps, 23*(3), 211–222.

Santelli, B., Turnbull, A.P., Lerner, E., & Marquis, J. (1993). Parent to Parent programs: A unique form of mutual support for families of persons with disabilities. In G.H.S. Singer & L.E. Powers (Eds.), *Families, disability, and empowerment: Active coping skills and strategies for family interventions* (pp. 27–57). Baltimore: Paul H. Brookes Publishing Co.

Santelli, B., Turnbull, A., Marquis, J., & Lerner, E. (1993). Parent to parent programs: Ongoing support for parents of young adults with special needs. *Journal of Vocational Rehabilitation, 3*(2), 25–37.

Santelli, B., Turnbull, A., Marquis, J., & Lerner, E. (1995). Parent to parent programs: A unique form of mutual support. *Infants and Young Children, 8*(2), 48–57.

Schell, G.C. (1981). The young handicapped child: A family perspective. *Topics in Early Childhood Special Education, 1*(3), 21–27.

Seligman, M., & Darling, R.B. (1989). *Ordinary families, special children: A systems approach to childhood disability.* New York: The Guilford Press.

Singer, G.H.S., Marquis, J., Powers, L., Blanchard, L., DiVenere, N., Santelli, B., & Sharp, M. (1999). A multi-site evaluation of Parent to Parent programs for parents of children with disabilities. *Journal of Early Intervention, 22*(3), 217–229.

Smith, P.M. (1978, April). *Early family intervention: How to develop a child's best advocates.* Paper presented at the meeting of the International Cerebral Palsy Society, Oxford, England.

Smith, P.M. (1993). Opening many, many doors: Parent to parent support. In P. Beckman & G. Beckman Boyes (Eds.), *Deciphering the system: A guide for families of young children with disabilities* (pp. 129–141). Cambridge, MA: Brookline Books.

Summers, J.A., Dell'Oliver, C., Turnbull, A., Benson, H., Santelli, E., Campbell, M., & Siegel Causey, E. (1990). Examining the individualized family service plan process: What are family and practitioner preferences? *Early Childhood Special Education, 10*(1), 78–99.

10

Adding Program Components

Other Supports for Families

"The strongest principle of growth lies in human choice."

—George Eliot

Because families are complex units of individuals who have multiple levels of interactions and needs, agencies serving them often become involved in providing more than just one service. For these same reasons, Parent to Parent programs find it difficult to limit themselves to one type of service when other needs are obvious. Programs that start by serving families through parent to parent matches soon begin to add other components. Many parent leaders see parent matching as the foundation for a variety of activities that will bring parents together in different ways.

This chapter describes many program activities beyond the parent match that Parent to Parent programs provide. It also offers guidelines for making program expansion decisions as well as for containing a program's scope of work so that the program remains focused and manageable.

The following program stories illustrate how Parent to Parent programs provide a multitude of program services. Because most program coordinators are family members themselves, they know and feel the same needs as the families being served and they are more than ready to add components as these family needs are identified.

PHP Program Story: Providing Additional Support

For the first 10 months, we concentrated on providing a match for every parent referred to us. But because families also were asking for information, we soon developed information packets. First we had one general information packet that we used for all families. Then we created specialized packets for specific disabilities, for types of services needed by the child, for particular issues facing children, and for various ages and stages in the lives of children and families.

Later, when my sister sent me a box of clothes and toys for my son, her gift made me think about adding a program component that would provide other families with this same kind of gift. We started the infant gift bonding component, and it allowed us to send a gift to newborn referrals.

We found that a newsletter was the most efficient, effective, and inexpensive way to stay in touch with families. A newsletter provides a continuous stream of stories, updates about changing laws and trends, and relevant information that is helpful for successfully parenting a child with special needs.

Parents were concerned that sometimes the way they were informed of their child's diagnosis made it harder for them to bond with their child or left them with little hope for the future. So, programs for training health care and educational professionals were a natural outgrowth of this parent interest in educating professionals about the family perspective.

Parents mentioned their concerns about not being treated fully as collaborative partners in their child's individualized education program (IEP) process. Because the information parents were trying to provide was not reaching the table, children were not receiving the appropriate services they needed for optimum development. So we added IEP training for parents.

We knew that parents could not find child care or opportunities for their "special" kids to interact with kids without disabilities, so we collaborated with nurses to create a course of study to train child care providers on how to include children with special needs in child care and preschool centers.

When I was told that my son had Down syndrome, one of my first concerns was for my other children. When other parents expressed similar concerns, we decided to start a program called sibling therapeutic fun to address issues of siblings of children with special needs.

As our program became better known in the community, calls to come and speak at clubs, schools, churches, and universities were a catalyst for us to develop a speakers' bureau. We felt that the more the community knew about our kids, the easier their lives would become.

A volunteer respite program for parents evolved from a collaborative effort between Parents Helping Parents (PHP), a college student, and the Council on Aging (COA). The student coordinator interviewed prospective baby sitters, who were senior citizens referred to the program by the COA, and arranged training for them through local schools serving children with special needs. This program recruited and maintained a roster of trained volunteer baby sitters whose names and telephone numbers were available to families seeking relief from the constant care of their children. Families interviewed several volunteers, made a selection, and taught the volunteer how to take care of their children.

An assistive technology program for children with special needs called Introduction to Technology Easing Children's Handicaps (iTECH) was a natural outgrowth of the impact of computers and other assistive technology. Computers and assistive technology (any physical, electrical, manual, or automatic device that can be used to increase, maintain, or improve functional capabilities of individuals with disabilities) boost the ability of a child to accomplish life's tasks through something as simple as a switch on a toy that makes it tumble or as complicated as a computer that responds to the blink of an eye to provide a voice for a child who cannot speak. iTECH provides information about technological products, funding, and referrals to assessment services. Monthly workshop topics include assistive technology entitlements under the law, using technology in the classroom, and assistive technology vendor fairs. As a member of Alliance for Technology Access, more than 80 vendor partners provide equipment to iTECH, which in turn allows a family to test equipment before purchasing something that might or might not work for their child.

Within 8 years we had developed more than 12 other program services that benefited children with special needs through support, information, and training given to their parents.

PROGRAM COMPONENTS

From the other program stories presented in this chapter, you will learn about some of the unique additional service components that Parent to Parent programs create to meet the needs of families and children with special needs. Typical additional program components include but are not limited to the following:

- Information and referral with direction services
- Support groups (e.g., heterogeneous, language, disability, issue specific)
- Information packets
- A special needs library
- Newsletters
- Training for parents
- Training for professionals
- Sibling support
- Respite care
- Assistive technology for children with special needs
- Speakers' bureau

See Table 10.1 in Appendix A for data about the many different program activities that are provided by local Parent to Parent programs. Chapter 14 also has information about the additional program components that *statewide* Parent to Parent programs have developed.

The Parent to Parent of Vermont Story

A prime example of programs that have grown out of the needs expressed by families is our child care program. A staff person was invited to speak to undergraduate physical therapy students about Parent to Parent and family-centered care. After hearing some family stories, one of the students asked how to help. From this initial question and the volunteer efforts of student coordinators, the child care program evolved. Physical therapy students volunteer 3–5 hours of child care per week for families. At the beginning of the fall and spring semesters, a gathering is held for interested families and students. The program is explained in detail, families and students meet, and parents have the opportunity to observe how different students interact with their children. The child care program's get-acquainted evening becomes a time to meet other parents and children, share stories, and feel a common bond.

After signing a waiver form that explains that the students providing the child care have received no formal training, the parents are given a list of students who are willing to provide child care. The list includes telephone numbers and addresses of students, as well as other information such as class schedules, available transportation, CPR training, and other special interests. Each year two students work with a staff member from Parent to Parent of Vermont to coordinate the program.

Another program that was started in response to an expressed family *need was a flexible funding program, now called the Brookes Baker Family Support Fund. Families can request as much as $200 for needs that are not covered by traditional sources such as insurance, Medicaid, schools, or respite funds. Requests can be made to cover costs of telephone bills, transportation, lodging to travel to another city or state for hospital stays, adaptive beds, bathing facilities, child care for an evening out, clothing, holiday gifts, camp fees, computer programs, exercise equipment, or car repairs. A committee looks at all requests, provides funding whenever possible, and suggests other sources of partial funding when the request is larger than $200.*

ArtsAbility is a community-based arts program cosponsored by Very Special Arts and Parent to Parent of Vermont that provides ongoing movement and poetry workshops for children with special needs and their friends and families. It is used to excite the imagination, spark the intellect, and empower children through the exploration of dance, poetry, song, storytelling, and the visual arts.

ArtsAbility, Medical Education Project/Community Faculty (see Chapter 14), Sibshops, and a library are all additional program components that have been made feasible because of our basic program of one-to-one support. The Parent to Parent program that provides emotional support and information to families also helps them to find ways to continue into other child advocacy roles and to reach out for other programs for their children. Although disability concerns and issues may change over time and demand different measures of energy, they usually do not go away. For that reason the heart of the program, one-to-one support, needs to be continually nurtured.

Though the one-to-one matching is the heart of our program, coordinators and staff must be prepared to provide ongoing support each time they receive a telephone call from a parent. What may begin as an informational call can become a longer conversation when the staff person shows enough interest in the situation.

Most expansion components are created in response to the needs of the families being served. Program components also are created to fill gaps in family services that are left by professionals, service providers, or agencies. What is clear is that family-identified needs are driving the development of these ever-growing program components.

ADDING THE COMPONENTS

Eventually there will come a time when there are so many program activities that program leaders begin to question their ability to add another program component. The program's leadership team must then begin to develop and utilize criteria for deciding which activities the Parent to Parent program can provide and to create a policy that will guide program expansion.

The leadership team needs to determine whether the new program component fits with the mission statement of the program. For example, a hospital called a Parent to Parent program about developing a support group for women who had had miscarriages and were grieving. That group would not fit under the program's mission of *helping children* become all they can be because there were no children to help. Although this support group did not fit the program's mission, the program leaders decided to provide technical assistance and mentoring to help the hospital develop its own program of support.

After evaluating whether the new component is relevant to your mission, there are many other questions to consider:

- How many parents or professionals are requesting the service? Is there a big enough need to warrant the creation of another component?
- Can the need be taken care of by an existing program within your organization?
- Is there another program in your community that is providing or that can be approached to provide the services being considered? Is there another agency with whom you could collaborate to do the program?
- How much will the new component cost?
- Where can the group find the funding to support the new component?
- Can the program activity be accomplished by using volunteers?
- Is there space available, or is there a place to house activities elsewhere?
- Has the program leadership or board of directors approved proceeding with this program?
- How will this new component have an impact on staff and current services to families?
- How does this new component fit with the long-range strategic plan? If it can't be done now, would it be appropriate at a later time?

After considering these questions, you might create an abstract of the idea and a budget for the proposed component. Having a document that is similar to a proposal abstract with a proposed budget attached is a way for your program leadership to evaluate the idea, share it with other potential collaborators, or use it when approaching prospective funders. After funding is secured, plan to hire more staff or add extra, paid hours to your current staff's workload. With this kind of research and planning, the new program should be off to a good start and a successful future.

PROGRAM COMPONENTS FOR CHILDREN AND FAMILIES

- Training for families through workshops can be offered by your program. Workshops can be scheduled throughout the year to explore such topics as parent–professional collaboration, working with children who have autism, facilitating a support group, school-to-work transitions for high school students, child assessments, creating children's IEPs, creating goals and objectives for children, understanding children's legal rights, individualized family service plans (IFSPs), positive behavioral support, and assistive technology. The workshops are often facilitated by parents or professionals.
- A program might add an activity that provides a parent mentor who supports other parents at due process hearings, team planning, and any time a parent might benefit from a reliable ally. Parents who have been trained as mentors volunteer to accompany other families to hearings when they contest an agency's decision to deny a child a service or sit with a family and provide support or information at other meetings with service providers.
- Educational and disability awareness programs, such as interactive educational puppet shows, can be presented to the community to enhance ability awareness and acceptance of children who have disabilities, illness, or other special needs.
- Inclusive playgroups for children are started when parent coordinators encourage children in their neighborhood to gather for games so that they may get acquainted and gain knowledge about people who are different. Summer picnics and holiday parties are popular with grass roots support groups. The groups usually have gatherings in which whole families participate. These affairs are usually potluck, and group leaders handle the logistics for these events. During the winter holiday season, there is usually a photo session with gifts for all of the kids.
- Many programs develop special needs libraries that have books, films, magazines, audiotapes, videotapes, and other materials focused on children with special needs. These libraries often start as a few boxes of books but expand quickly due to parents' thirst for in-

formation about their children's disabilities or illnesses, their search for contemporary resources and services, and their own generosity in donating books. Computer software is offered to families of children with special needs who use the computer to collect information, find answers, and connect with other parents. Moms on Modems (MOM) was started at PHP to enhance mothers' comfort with using the computer and to increase their ability to help their children take advantage of all that technology has to offer.

- Respite care programs allow parents to take a break from caring for their child by providing an alternate caregiver. Some states have agencies that pay for respite care as a service to the child.
- Some Parent to Parent programs offer local or statewide conferences and symposiums that focus on a specific disability or provide technical assistance strategies to parents who want to start, manage, or maintain a Parent to Parent program or a parent-directed family resource center.
- Different statewide Parent to Parent programs coordinate a 3- to 5-day international Parent to Parent conference that is held every other year in a different part of the United States.
- Legal advocates for children complete a training course to prepare them to support and help children who are wards of the state or are involved in the legal system. Families are supplied with the name of an agency and its telephone number when they call the parent program for help, and the parent coordinator takes time to explain what the agency is, what it does, how best to gain access to its services, what to do first, and what to bring to an appointment.
- Parent liaisons are *experienced* parents who have completed training to prepare them to help families and professionals understand each other's perspective, work together, and connect with other resources in the community. Parent liaisons can work in many settings, including hospitals and state departments of health or education. From the hospital site, they provide the same information, emotional support, and direction given from their Parent to Parent program. Parent liaisons can work in other service agencies to link families and providers with coordinated, family-centered, state-of-the-art care for children with special health care needs.
- Grief counseling provided in small-group sessions may be held for families whose children have died. Families who have experienced this same loss conduct the regularly held sessions.
- The U.S. Department of Health and Human Services and the American Academy of Pediatrics are supporting the development of *med-*

ical homes that provide a central care coordinator or care coordinating place for children with special health care needs to enhance the collaboration between care providers. Some Parent to Parent programs are working with health providers to create the medical home and to make family and professional communities aware of this concept of care. Parents are seen as an integral part of this process, and they often take the lead on transporting their children's health information from one care provider to the next.

- Coordination assistance for child care and services is sometimes provided by Parent to Parent programs to families after they arrive home with instructions from professional offices or agencies and need to talk with someone who has experience with the same plan of care in the home.
- Grandparent programs offer support, information, and training to grandparents who may be parenting their grandchildren. These programs also provide emotional support to grandparents who are going through the grief process for grandchildren born with disabilities or who have a chronic or terminal illnesses.

PROGRAM COMPONENTS FOR PROFESSIONALS

Parent to Parent programs also often provide important services to professionals through training, information, and assistance to professionals in their effort to provide emotional support and information to families. Parent-directed agencies provide services in a relaxed, less formal, family-friendly atmosphere, and professionals often are pleased to meet new families for the first time at a parent-run agency. Meeting families at parent-directed agencies is one way that professionals can enhance family-centered principles in their care of children, reduce parents' feelings of anxiety, and increase parents' participation.

- Training for physicians often is available through workshops conducted by parents, and this training often includes information about delivering the diagnosis—what families prefer to be told, how, where, with whom, and by whom. For example, if the family is more familiar with their obstetrician than with their child's pediatrician, the obstetrician may be the best person to tell the family about the diagnosis. Training also helps physicians to get in touch with what families may be feeling during these situations and introduces them to the parent to parent process.
- Training for nurses and other allied health professionals on the family perspective often covers the grieving process, professional

reactions to disability, sources of help in the community, interaction with families, elements of family-centered care, principles of family–professional collaboration, indicators of cultural competence, and parent to parent support and its presence in their community (see Figures 10.1, 10.2, and 10.3).

- Consumer–provider partnerships involve parents' collaborating with health care providers to activate or enhance family-centered care at their facilities. Activities include creating Parent to Parent programs at health care sites; training personnel; and participating in policy, planning, implementation, and evaluation of health services.
- Parents can and do provide assistance to attorneys and judges to help create protocols and policies that serve children with disabilities and help them connect with other service providers for a coordinated system of care when a child is involved with the law. The parent coordinators also may provide training or join committees to enhance the legal system's knowledge about disability and other service systems.
- Some parents are working with university professors to create internships for students and develop and implement preservice curricula and programs to educate professionals (e.g., teachers, nurses, social workers, physicians) so that they can provide better care for children (see Chapter 14). Parents can be guest speakers and lecturers at these same schools, colleges, and universities.
- Because a Parent to Parent program has more experience than other service providers in creating support groups, teachers may ask a Parent to Parent program to help them form a support group to address teacher and parent concerns and issues. For example, providing training and support on contemporary approaches to teaching children with learning disabilities or autism becomes a joint venture between parents and professionals. With such a group in place, teachers find that they can return to the classroom renewed, refreshed, and better prepared to teach children with disabilities.
- Parents also have created simulation workshops that allow educators to experience what it is like to have a disability. By "feeling the disability," professionals gain a greater understanding of disabilities and increase their ability to interact effectively with children. Parents in Florida created a wonderful simulation game called "Agencyopoly" to help professionals understand what children and families endure as they go from agency to agency seeking services.
- Parents also can be supported by a Parent to Parent program to serve as consultants to professionals. Decisions about children with special health care needs are clarified or made with input from these expe-

Key Elements of Family-Centered Care

1. Recognize that the family is the constant in a child's life, whereas the service systems and personnel within those systems fluctuate.

2. Share completely unbiased information with parents in a supportive and ongoing manner.

3. Recognize family strengths and individuality; respect different coping methods.

4. Encourage and facilitate family to family support and networking, and honor the racial, ethnic, cultural, and socioeconomic diversity of families.

5. Facilitate parent–professional collaboration at all levels of service provision: services for an individual child; program development, implementation, and evaluation; and planning and policy formation.

6. Design accessible service delivery systems that are flexible, culturally competent, and responsive to family-identified needs.

7. Implement comprehensive policies and programs that provide emotional and financial support to meet the needs of families.

8. Incorporate developmental needs of children and families into service delivery systems.

Figure 10.1. Key elements of family-centered care.

Principles of Family–Professional Collaboration

1. Families and professionals work together to ensure the best services for the child and family.

---

2. Recognize and respect the knowledge, skills, and experience that families and professionals bring to the relationship.

---

3. Acknowledge development of trust as an integral part of a collaborative relationship.

---

4. Encourage open communication so that families and professionals feel free to express themselves.

---

5. Create an atmosphere in which cultural traditions, values, and diversity of families are acknowledged and honored.

---

6. Recognize that negotiation is essential in collaborative relationships.

---

7. Bring to the relationship the mutual commitment of families, professionals, and communities to meet the needs of children and their families.

Figure 10.2. Principles of family–professional collaboration. (Courtesy of the University of Vermont.)

Key Indicators of Cultural Competence

1. Recognize the power and influence of culture in shaping values, beliefs, and experiences.

2. Understand your own cultural values, beliefs, and behaviors and how you respond to individuals whose values and beliefs differ from your own.

3. Learn about the cultural norms of the communities with which you engage and about the extent to which individual families share those norms.

4. Approach each family on its own terms, with no judgments or preconceptions, and enable each family to define its own needs.

5. Help families learn about how the mainstream culture is reflected in the service system so they are able to use the system to meet their needs.

6. Acknowledge that many families have experienced racism and other forms of discrimination that affect future interactions with service providers.

7. Eliminate institutional policies and practices that, deliberately or inadvertently, exclude families from services because of their race, ethnicity, beliefs, or practices.

8. Build on the strengths and resources of each child, family, community, and neighborhood.

Figure 10.3. Key indicators of cultural competence. (From the National Maternal and Child Health Resource Center on Cultural Competency; reprinted by permission.)

rienced parent consultants. This type of consultation has been used by education, health, developmental disability, and social services agencies. Parental input and assistance with planning, implementation, and evaluation is provided by having parents participate on boards, planning committees, research surveys, and task forces. Sometimes professionals call parent programs for help with issues they and their clients face. Professionals find that experienced parents are often more familiar with extended services in the community and how to gain access to them for the child.

- Professionals doing research often need to find parents to participate in their research projects. Parents are being invited to participate as members of action research teams (see Chapter 13) to design research. Many parents also agree to participate in research by responding to surveys or being a part of focus groups. Parent to Parent programs help researchers to gain access to families who are willing to participate in their research projects.

STAYING GRASS ROOTS AS YOU GROW

How does a program that begins by simply offering the one-to-one parent match keep the heart and soul of its program as the organization branches out and becomes larger? One of the best ways to stay grass roots is to maintain a strong and vigorous organizational infrastructure for your program—one that continues to support a strong parent matching component while adding new program activities slowly and carefully.

Parent to Parent programs consist of the services they provide and the organizational infrastructure that supports the provision of the services. As programs grow, parent-directed agencies should keep the heart, soul, and flexibility *in their services* to children and families. But at the same time, the program also must tend to the organizational or business activities. The physical layout of your program office can be arranged to reflect these two important sides of a Parent to Parent program. For instance, space for the bookkeeper, office manager, executive director, and fund developer can be separated from the program services areas such as the library, the family room, and the early intervention play room.

Another way to be sure your program remains true to your grass roots beginnings is to continually evaluate the level of grass roots support for your program activities. Don't be afraid to charge reasonable fees for your services and memberships, with a sliding scale for families who cannot afford to pay as much. When you have solid grass roots support that is evident through donations of time and money, then you will know that the families for whom the program was started value its growth and development.

Be sure to keep the grass roots families that you are serving informed and ask them to participate in planning, implementation, and evaluation of your program. They may not be able to participate, but they will still appreciate being asked, they will know what you are doing in the community, and they can spread the word whenever an opportunity presents itself. Keep some grass roots representation on your boards, on your committees, and involved in your strategic planning, fund-raisers, and other community events. To maintain your connection to your grass roots families, provide good services and ongoing promotional campaigns and continue to be available first and foremost for the needs of families.

SUMMARY

Over time, you will probably want to add other service components to your Parent to Parent program because families have other needs that must be addressed. Evaluating the new program components' fit with the program's mission, goals, and long-range strategic plan and figuring out where to find funding for the appropriate staff to implement the new program activity are critical to the success of any new program activity. The goodness of fit and the sources of funding for the new activity will be important factors in the board of directors, and the executive director's decision.

Parent to Parent programs offer numerous services to children and families that include support, training, technology, technical assistance, social activities, information, and direction. And Parent to Parent programs make an effort to ensure that all of their program activities provide culturally competent services for the families they serve. Many Parent to Parent programs also offer services to professionals, including those in the health, education, social, judicial, legal, and political systems; and families are becoming more involved in the preservice curricula and training of people in these helping professions. The more collaboration between parents and professionals, the more likely it is that children will receive quality care that is coordinated and family centered.

Creating too many different components makes it difficult for Parent to Parent programs to clarify a single, focused identity to the public. Perhaps this is why many Parent to Parent programs are moving toward promoting themselves as being one-stop shops for families. But as programs add components and grow, they also have concerns about staying grass roots and maintaining the warm, friendly atmosphere their programs started with. By making a conscious effort to separate the *business side* of the program from the *service side*, most programs are able to function effectively as multifaceted organizations and maintain their unique family atmosphere. To keep the grass roots programs active, it is important to include them in program activities and planning, as well as to provide a mechanism for seeking their financial and volunteer support. New program components often add to the success of the parent to parent matching services and help the program to stay grass roots.

RESOURCES

Bishop, K., Woll, J., & Arango, P. (1993). *Family/professional collaboration for children with special health needs and their families.* Burlington: University of Vermont, Department of Social Work.

Blanchard, K. (1997). *Mission possible.* New York: McGraw-Hill.

Jackson, D. (1998). *Parent liaison training manual.* Santa Clara, CA: PHP, Inc.

Johnson, B., Jeppeson, E.S., & Redburn, L. (1992). *Caring for children and families: Guidelines for hospitals.* Mount Royal, NJ: Association for the Care of Children's Health (ACCH).

Poyadue, F.S. (1983). *Better ways of breaking diagnostic news.* Santa Clara, CA: PHP, Inc.

Poyadue, F.S. (1998). *Facilitating support group meetings.* Santa Clara, CA: PHP, Inc.

Poyadue, F.S. (1998). *Parents activating family-centered care.* Santa Clara, CA: PHP, Inc.

Roberts R.N., Barclay-McLaughlin, G., Cleveland, J., Colston, W., Malach, R., Mulvey, L., Rodriguez, G., Thomas, T., & Yonemitsu, D. (1990). *Developing culturally competent programs for families of children with special needs.* Washington, DC: Georgetown University Child Development Center, The National Maternal and Child Health Resource Center for Cultural Competence.

ORGANIZATIONS

Institute For Family-Centered Care, 7900 Wisconsin Avenue, Suite 405, Bethesda, MD 20814; telephone: (301) 652-0281; fax: (301) 652-0186

11

Promoting Your Program

Connections in the Community

"Doing business without advertising is like winking at a girl in the dark. You know what you are doing, but nobody else does."

—Steuart Henderson Britt

Promoting your program to the community often is described as marketing, public awareness, or publicity. Promoting a program is the process you use to make others (e.g., corporations, foundations, the families served, the general public, the professional community) aware of what you have to offer and to make contacts for keeping what you have to offer contemporary, available, and desirable to your customers.

Parent to Parent programs, like other nonprofit agencies, need to recognize that they have a product to sell. A Parent to Parent program's product is the set of services that it provides to children with special needs, their families, and professionals. Because the product is a service, the staff of nonprofits become an integral part of their product. So, if a nonprofit is going to improve its product, it must find ways to enhance, nourish, and keep good staff (see Chapter 8).

Sometimes it is difficult for Parent to Parent programs to define themselves to the public because they are not disability-specific organizations, such as United Cerebral Palsy, nor are they focused on a single issue, such as Mothers Against Drunk Driving. Understanding that emotional support and information for a parent benefits the child's well-being, growth, and development can be a hard concept for the public to grasp. Because most Parent to Parent programs offer a multitude of services, effectively marketing them is not an easy job.

Sometimes a program's staff and volunteers put time and energy into creating a quality program activity or a special fund-raising event and then fail to apply the same time and energy to marketing the event. Without sufficient marketing, participation in and income from the activities are likely to fall short of expectations. Unfortunately, the people planning these events often go back to the drawing board, review, evaluate, and change the *event*. They do not see that their poor success rate was due to poor marketing. Changing a program event without evaluating the effectiveness of your marketing strategies can put your program in a vicious cycle of unproductive change.

This chapter 1) examines why and how to promote your program and the relationship between maintaining a contemporary, quality program and marketing, 2) provides marketing strategies and tips from parents and professionals, and 3) prepares you to create a formal marketing plan.

WHY PROMOTE YOUR PROGRAM?

Marketing your program is important because it advertises your services to families and helps you to continue to provide services that families need and want. One of the very first promotional activities of most Parent to Parent programs is the creation and dissemination of a brochure to let the community know about the program and its services.

Marketing is defined as planning, producing, and promoting a product that the customer wants and is satisfied with. Promoting your program starts before your service is created and continues after your services have reached their destination—families. Activities for promotion should be coordinated throughout all aspects of your program because proper marketing can bring many benefits, such as referrals, funding, board members, volunteers, collaborative opportunities, public awareness, wiser consumers, and greater acceptance of and sensitivity to the special needs of the children.

Although a profitable sales volume is important in the for-profit business world, Parent to Parent programs are not-for-profit organizations. For Parent to Parent programs, successful *sales* volume equates to successful *service* volume. Funding sources want to know how many families are being served, in what ways, and for how long.

Parent to Parent programs promote themselves in the community for many reasons. These reasons reflect the leadership's concern for 1) its customers, 2) its competition, and 3) its program.

Marketing and Your Customers

Who are Parent to Parent programs' customers? Customers include families who are or will be served, professionals who refer families to the program, and funding sources that you hope will support the program. Program leadership must determine for each of these customers what they want and how the program can satisfy their needs. Gathering customers in focus groups to discuss their needs and level of satisfaction, encouraging customers to complete survey forms immediately after receiving services or perhaps annually, and determining what your customers want can be accomplished by finding opportunities for customers to be involved in policy making, planning, implementation, and evaluation of program services, as well as in the design of the facility that will serve children and families.

Parent to Parent programs find that promoting their programs to their customers helps them to accomplish the following:

- Reach out to find families who need their services.
- Inform professionals about their services so that professionals can refer families and take advantage of programs provided for professionals.
- Gain input from the community so that program services remain relevant.
- Educate and inform the public.
- Create consumer–provider partnerships on behalf of children and families.
- Make sure issues affecting children with disabilities and special health care needs are included in the discussion when community changes are in progress or when state and national problems are being addressed.

Marketing and Your Competition

Because the nonprofit world is concerned with public benefit, it is hard to imagine that competition plays a part, yet there exists competition for money, resources, and customers. Therefore, it is necessary to promote your program in order to 1) highlight its uniqueness, 2) enlarge its visibility, 3) heighten public and professional awareness, and 4) define your program and its position in the community.

Some Parent to Parent program competitors are fee-based centers, such as family counseling centers, social services departments in hospitals, and early intervention centers, that may see a conflict of interest in referring patients to parent programs. Professionals in these agencies may not understand how a parent to parent match is different from the services that professionals provide. However, Parent to Parent programs have worked hard to get to know other agencies and to help them to understand how Parent to Parent program services are different from professional services. These awareness efforts have helped professionals to understand that Parent to Parent programs provide services that are unique and complementary to services provided by professionals.

Competition also can come from disability- or issue-specific agencies that have an emphasis on research and prevention. Referrals to Parent to Parent programs may not be forthcoming from these agencies because parent support is not high on their agendas and because they do not want to lose their relationships with the family.

Even within the parent movement, there is sometimes competition between parent training and information centers (PTI) and Parent to Parent programs as they vie for funding and families. Competition between PTIs and Parent to Parent programs is beginning to fade because the emphasis is now on collaboration, networking, and partnerships among those providing services to children with special needs and their families. PTIs and Parent to Parent programs recognize more readily how their services are both unique and complementary.

Marketing and Your Program

Developing your program includes growing and stabilizing your infrastructure as well as your services. Promoting your program in the community is a tool that assists you with the capacity building of your agency and helps you to

- Reach potential board members, volunteers, and donors
- Enhance opportunities for collaborating with other organizations
- Gain partners for producing services and materials
- Get letters of support for proposals

Parent to Parent of New Hampshire Promotion Story

We started in November of 1989, and the referrals poured in, mainly from parents and professionals involved with the developmental disability service system. In fact, the original networking brochure that we use today was developed by our state's developmental disabilities agency. We had written them a note to advertise the existence of our network, and they responded with a brochure that carried their endorsement to more than 3,000 parents. We have used that design numerous times to reach out to parents with children who have other special needs.

Advertising our toll-free telephone number in the media turned out to be a good way to promote our programs to families. Building a good relationship with our state's Title V program allowed us to widely disseminate through their contacts and distribution mechanisms a booklet we had written on parenting premature babies. Having the printed word circulating in the community not only created awareness of our existence but also gave others a tool to use to tell others about us.

By including our university affiliated program in a proposal we were writing, we could provide an evaluation component to increase the university staff's awareness of our program. This increased knowledge about what we did, and their personal involvement with us gave them confidence to spread the word about our program activities. The staff could use our program as an example of care and services to families, thus promoting our program to their colleagues and the students they were teaching. The students, in turn, shared information about our program among their personal and occupational acquaintances.

PHP Promotion Story

We promoted PHP in the community by creating a brochure about our program and what we had to offer. It was mailed to schools, hospitals, social services agencies, churches, nonprofit organizations, disability organizations, and our local politicians' offices. We complemented this brochure with a newsletter that we mailed to families and to all types of agencies serving children and families.

We accepted all invitations to speak and focused on speaking to college and university classes that were not only training the next generation of service providers but also training current providers in continuing education or graduate-level or master's degree-level classes. And we reached out seeking opportunities to address different groups through our speakers' bureau.

We wrote and sent exciting one-page letters introducing our program to specific individuals in relevant leadership positions in key organizations or agencies. For example, in hospitals we sent letters to the director of nurses, director of medical education, and coordinator of nursing education instead of to the chief of staff or to the administrator of the hospital.

We contacted radio and television stations to secure spots on the news and to be guests on local talk shows. We created 30-second public service announcements (PSAs) and aired them live on radio. Whenever an article appeared in the newspaper about disability, birth defects, or other special needs, we wrote letters to the editor to get our name in front of the public. We also advertised our programs in the community calendar of events section of major newspapers. All of these techniques were free and worked well.

When we started to do workshops to train professionals about improving interactions with families, our services to the professional community became a large part of our outreach to that segment of the community. We saw our special events as other ways to reach the community, showcase our wares, and become known to those who needed our services.

Local, state, and national keynote addresses provided an opportunity for publicity about PHP and its programs, whereas our written products increased knowledge about and use of PHP services. These materials included our manuals for training professionals and families, as well as other books and booklets about providing technical assistance to other programs that were creating or operating a Parent to Parent program or a parent-directed family resource center (PDFRC).

After PHP was institutionalized and had an annual budget of more than $500,000, we believed that we were doing a lot of things right, and yet we were still told that there were people who had never heard of us.

Because the number of families and professionals whom we were serving was growing rapidly, we also needed a rapid growth in our financial income, which was not yet forthcoming. We knew we had to change the public's perception of us as just a parent support group and show them we were a comprehensive, multiservice, one-stop family resource center that needed larger sums of money to succeed.

We also needed to show the public and professionals that PHP served a broad group of people, including children with Down syndrome and spina bifida but also children with sickle cell anemia, asthma, severe allergies, learning disabilities, attention-deficit/hyperactivity disorder, and those who were born prematurely, to name a few. We knew that a limited view of the individuals we serve might curtail the numbers and types of families that were referred for help and limit the view of grass roots, funding sources, and the general public about how much money we needed to operate PHP.

Even though our efforts at promoting our program had worked well in the beginning stages, as we grew we became more aware of these problems and decided to seek outside help in marketing our agency. We felt that through a marketing evaluation and plan, we would be able to clarify who we were, what we did, how to better reach potential families needing our help, how to secure necessary funding, and how to increase awareness of our program.

Our marketing specialist suggested that we aim one brochure toward funding sources, another toward service providers, and another toward the families we served. We also would need several brochures for our various programs, as well as an overall agency brochure.

We decided to consult a local university's business development association (BDA) to ask for help in creating a marketing plan for PHP. The BDA links business students with local entrepreneurs, owner of small businesses, and nonprofit managers for "real world" projects. We had to put in a comprehensive but concise proposal outlining our needs, goals, and objectives. BDA selected us to be one of the projects that their team would work on that year.

HOW TO PROMOTE YOUR PROGRAM

Marketing a Parent to Parent program or a nonprofit agency is more difficult than marketing a for-profit business because a business is selling a tangible product, whereas a Parent to Parent program is marketing its services. Because children with special needs are involved with numerous service systems (e.g., health, legal, social, recreational, educational), marketing efforts must be targeted to these different systems.

Creating Targeted Approaches

You need to create targeted approaches to a wide range of customers and differentiate your approach for funding sources, service providers, and the families that you serve. For each you will highlight your area of emphasis and the unique way in which you provide services. When other agencies proclaim that they provide emotional support and information to families, Parent to Parent programs must show how their support from people who *have been there* is their unique specialty.

Remind all of the program's boards, staff, families served, and professionals of their obligation to act as ambassadors in the community for the program. All of these formal and informal agency representatives should take every opportunity to speak or write about the program as they interface with city councils, school boards, and other community groups.

Be sure that these ambassadors work toward transferring the loyalty and support that they have from others in the community to your program. They should include your name on letters that they send to friends seeking help for the program, take you to lunch with those friends, and encourage you to talk about your program. When they plan meetings with foundations seeking funds or other support for your program, they should take you along and be enthusiastic about your program and your vision and leadership.

Another promotional approach that has worked for many Parent to Parent programs is to incorporate the promotion of the program into family routines and daily activities. For example, consider leaving your program brochures and a business card when you go to houses of worship, schools, shopping malls, doctor's offices, or the beauty parlor or barbershop. You may get calls from these groups to speak about your program's services.

To keep your program known throughout the community, take advantage of every opportunity to do the following:

For your family customers

- Publish and disseminate your own newsletter
- Publicize awards and recognition your program receives in the newspaper and in your newsletter
- Use all forms of the media (e.g., radio, television, Internet, newspaper) to sell your program and your products

For your referral source customers

- Put articles in other agencies' newsletters
- Exhibit your program materials during poster sessions at conferences
- Wear your program's buttons to work and throughout the community
- Produce business cards for staff and board members to use
- List your program services down one side of your letterhead so that each time you send a letter, you send a message about what you do and whom you serve
- Give awards to local celebrities

For your funding customers

- Volunteer at your local United Way to talk to corporations; you can use these speaking opportunities to represent your program as well
- Create and circulate an annual report that describes your program and its activities
- Participate in other groups' fund-raising efforts
- Serve on local, state, and national government agency committees, proposal evaluation teams, or advisory boards
- Produce publicity about your program and place it in newspapers or magazines

The best promotion for your program comes from providing ongoing quality services. Quality services will create satisfied families who tell other families that you are in the community and that your staff does a great job. But you must also learn how to control damage and handle dissatisfaction with your program when something goes wrong. Get in touch with the person who is dissatisfied immediately to let him or her know that you want to hear about what has happened. Seek any suggestions they may have for remedying the situation.

Nothing sells your program like your enthusiasm and passion for what you do. Your vision and mission statements should be catchy and accurately reflect your program's reason for existence. Be sure that they are well defined in your spoken and written words, and be sure to keep the child at the center. Talk and write about the benefits to children from your interactions and services to parents and professionals.

For example, in some school districts, special services are still not readily given to children who need them, so parents have to know the laws that support their child's rights to a free, appropriate public education in the least restrictive environment and how to advocate for their child's rights. Many Parent to Parent programs provide parent training in individual education planning, and Parent to Parent programs need to promote that they are a part of the mission to help children through education. And when Parent to Parent programs provide simulation training for teachers, they must emphasize that their goal is to improve children's educational services—to provide students with qualified teachers to enhance learning experiences. Parent to Parent customers (families, professionals, and funders) can then more easily see these program components as direct services to the child.

RECOMMENDED PRACTICES

Although agencies such as the American Heart Association and the American Cancer Society are widely known, Parent to Parent is not as widely known. Parent to Parent programs have faced the challenges of promoting their services in the community and are making progress in this area. The following story describes one program's success.

Dare to Be Different

Our quarterly reports reflect activities that are a part of our contract requirements with the North Carolina Department of Maternal and Child Health. The format for these reports, however, was not doing justice to our other pro-

gram pieces such as parent matching and community outreach. So, on our final report we decided to outline our programs' highlights on each program's letterhead and attach a brochure. The final report was presented in a colorful notebook with a cover that included a photograph of our program coordinators. These efforts brought a personal touch to the bureaucratic nature of our reporting systems. Eventually the report notebook was sent to the chancellor's office to become part of a statewide display of university-based programs. We learned that taking risks and daring to be different could pay off.

The most effective message for Parent to Parent programs to convey is that their services are provided by parents of children with special needs; and that, therefore, Parent to Parent programs fully understand the needs of their customers. It is a different level of understanding than that held by health care, educational, or social services professionals who have studied the experience but have not lived through it themselves.

In your promotional literature, define *special needs* broadly and provide a list of specific family problems for which the agency can provide help and specific services your program offers (e.g., referrals to specialist agencies, library, peer counseling, on-line database). Describe your services in enough detail that physicians, social workers, and teachers can decide for which children your services would be appropriate.

Reaching the Professional

Sometimes your plans work out successfully, although perhaps not in the way you anticipated. One of the most difficult marketing activities for Parent to Parent programs is to successfully reach physicians and effect a positive change in their referrals to the program. One Parent to Parent program encouraged parents to take "physicians' packets" to their own doctors. The packets contained program brochures and other program information to let the doctors know about the availability of parent support, lists of other community resources, and articles to educate them about issues for children with special needs and their families. This marketing effort ran very smoothly and helped to create a strong bond between the physicians and the parents.

Not long after this marketing activity was initiated, the program coordinator found an unexpected benefit from another activity—the outreach program. Although not a formal part of the original marketing plan, the outreach program contributed in a very significant way to the marketing efforts of the program. Here is how it happened:

The Parent to Parent program set up an outreach program that included placing an elaborate set of materials (including the physicians' packets) at a nearby hospital. There were files for the nurses' station and the social services department; specific information for the neonatal intensive care unit (NICU), the nursery, and the pediatric department; posters for the different areas; and mail-back cards for parents. A presentation was given at a specified time so that as many nurses and social workers as possible could attend, and a tape recording was made of the presentation for the nurses and staff working on different shifts.

Although the outreach program was directed primarily to nurses and social services staff, the personal contact that the Parent to Parent program made with nurses meant that the nurses could then promote their program to others as well. Soon, the program was able to enlist the nurses to tell physicians, social services staff, and parents that the program was available—a multilevel marketing approach.

Seek opportunities to speak at medical staff meetings at hospitals and at large physicians' group practices. Work with editorial staff of local chapters of the American Academy of Pediatrics to reach pediatricians through newsletters and conferences and other events.

Make sure that social workers are on the agency's newsletter mailing list. School nurses are a good focal point for reaching older children with subtler needs. Provide them with brief articles about the program that can be placed in school newsletters to parents and with quarterly mailings of your program's newsletter.

Advertise your services through publicity materials that have a single focus and that always highlight your agency and logo. Publish press releases to be sent to funding sources, partners, or staff, especially those who have children with special needs (see Figure 11.1).

Consider whether certain people will respond better to an organization that is run by parents of children with special needs or by professionals who also are parents of children with special needs. Let the public, and especially the professional community, know about the higher education of parent leaders. To further enhance the comfort level of professionals and increase referrals from professionals, emphasize that supporting parents are trained and that each match is carefully followed.

Value of Sharing Stories

When given the opportunity to give a presentation about your program, always use your personal family story. You will find that potential donors and referral sources understand more when they are presented with a real-life story. Marketing a Parent to Parent program may not be easy, but when someone hears parents tell their own story about what Parent to Parent means to them, the rewards are evident. Telling personal stories influences funding sources' decisions about whether

For Immediate Release
September 21, 2001

Families Helping Families, Inc.
2829 Young Street
Santa Maria, CA 33421

and

Stone Creek Health Center
24 Maco Drive
Santa Maria, CA 33487

Families Helping Families, Inc. (FHF), the family resource center that serves children who have a need for special education or health care, has received a 4-year grant of $600,000 from the Bureau of Health.

FHF will be working in a collaborative partnership with Stone Creek Health Center to create a national model. This pilot program introduces the concepts of family-centered care for children through a consumer–provider collaborative partnership.

Family centered care provides quality, state-of-the-art care for children, with parent–professional satisfaction, through parental involvement in a partnership with health professionals in planning, implementing, and evaluating care.

The project is based on the principles of family–professional collaboration. The major project components include

1. Co-training of health care staff and families
2. Support outreach to diverse populations
3. Use of a local interagency network communications system
4. Counseling and parent to parent support during and after a child's hospitalization
5. Parent-directed family resource center (PDFRC) satellite facilities at health care sites
6. Opportunities for family input into policy, planning, and evaluation of the site

Stone Creek Health Center's point of contact is Dr. Aidan Rubio, chief of genetics. Dr. Jay Quinn, of Santa Maria University, is the consultant for the evaluation. Antonia Symone, Ph.D., said, "I am excited and honored to co-author a book for replication of this national model."

FHF is a United Way agency, established as Point of Light #416 by former President George Bush. Stone Creek leads the nation in providing state-of-the-art managed care. Dr. Rubio says, "This time, children with special care needs are the winners of this consumer–provider partnership between these two community leaders."

Dean Keith of FHF is the project director, and Jill Stewart is the program coordinator. For more information on this exciting national model, write to Mr. Dean Keith, FHF—The FRC, 2829 Young Street, Santa Maria, CA 33421, call (406) 777-0099 ext. 123, or e-mail dk@fhf.com.

Octave A. Salvador, Chair of the Board FHF Representative	Turhan Michaels, Medical Administrator Stone Creek Medical Representative

Figure 11.1. Sample joint press release.

to support a Parent to Parent program. They like to see that the program has had a positive influence on families and that their access to services and resources has improved. Of course, some funding sources seek facts to back up your story. Fortunately, there are now research data to corroborate parent stories about the effectiveness of parent to parent matches. Family stories, combined with these research data, provide a powerful tool for promoting Parent to Parent programs. See Chapter 4 and Appendix A for additional information about research that validates the effectiveness of the parent to parent match.

Promotional methods also have been devised to help others experience parents' feelings about having a child with special needs and thus gain a greater understanding for the value of parent to parent support. Some groups use a simulation activity in which a sighted person is blindfolded and tries to negotiate a room. Another simulation activity involves distributing new fliers to some workshop participants and crumpled fliers to the other participants. When asked to describe their feelings after receiving crumpled fliers, participants provide a similar list of emotions that parents experience when they learn of their child's special needs: sadness ("Why me?"), shock ("She didn't do that, did she?"), and anger ("How dare she do that to my flier?"). As the discussion progresses, they try to smooth out the flier and compare it with the others—the same actions that parents take as they work to improve their child's abilities and potential. This activity can lead to a meaningful discussion as both groups of participants share their reactions and feelings. A parent facilitator can help participants see the connection between their feelings and those of parents who have a child with special needs and can stress the importance to parents of support provided by another parent.

Another activity that works well to help others understand the value of Parent to Parent programs involves the simple task of sorting a group of various brochures. Participants are divided into two groups, given a set of brochures, and then told to "hobnoy" them. One group is provided with a mentor who knows that the word "hobnoy" means "sort by color." That group finishes quickly. As the second group struggles, they are asked if they would like to talk to someone who has been through this before. This second group is asked to describe their thoughts and feelings before and after being provided a mentor. The final questions that is asked is, "What are your views now on providing parents as mentors?"

Promoting in Underserved Communities

Underserved refers to those communities whose residents are socially, economically, educationally, occupationally, linguistically, or geographically challenged. Some people may think that these underserved populations' cultures prevent them from gaining access to services. But lack of money and knowledge, and their isolation due to these challenges, has more to do with their inability to gain access to Parent to Parent program services than their race or ethnicity does.

Parent to Parent programs strive to reach out to underserved communities so that no children or families are left without information, resources, and support. Because underserved families often lack the transportation and financial resources to gain access to the program, special efforts to reach and involve underserved families must be made. Because of their past experiences with service systems, some families may be hesitant to approach Parent to Parent programs.

Be especially conscious of treating everyone with dignity and respect when reaching out to underserved communities. Think about ways that you can make your program more open to diverse groups of people. Have your telephone greeting in more than one language. Put articles in your newsletter in languages other than English. Create your agency brochure in multiple languages. Create language-specific support groups for those who do not speak English or whose preferred language is not English. Find ways to take your services to the families in their communities. Promoting your program in underserved communities can be both challenging and rewarding, and it is essential to ensuring that Parent to Parent is available to all families in all communities.

Terry Tafoya, a Native American family counselor, stated that one of the best ways to make families feel welcome is for them to see themselves reflected when they arrive at your program. Pictures on the walls, the color of furnishings and walls, artifacts and items that represent different cultures, and even mirrors on the walls so that people can see their own reflections as they come in often are helpful.

One of the best ways to reach underserved families, provide them with services, and make them feel welcome is to have people from underserved communities as part of your paid staff. You will then have staff who know their issues, know their neighborhoods, speak their language, and understand their culture. You will be learning from them and they will be learning from you.

CREATING A MARKETING PLAN

There are three steps to producing a promotional or marketing plan.

Step 1: Gathering Information and Data

The board's marketing committee or the program leadership should gather program data to help you 1) analyze the program's current resources (e.g., annual budget, reserve funds, funding sources, fund-raising trends), 2) analyze current program services (e.g., who is served, through what programs), 3) define the program's main line of business, and 4) develop survey forms to assess your presence in the community (see Figures 11.2 and 11.3).

Step 2: Creating Marketing Goals and Objectives

Parent to Parent programs should create an overall marketing goal and related marketing objectives. For example, a marketing goal for the year might be to achieve a 5% awareness rate of the program among the citizens of the county, with 1% donating funds or volunteering. Another goal might be a 20% increase in services provided to families. Specific marketing objectives can then be identified to accomplish these marketing goals. Marketing objectives to increase the awareness rate of the program might include dissemination of your program brochure to new segments of your community or establishing linkages with nondisability agencies.

Step 3: Refining Goals and Objectives

The final phase of the marketing plan is to refine the goals and objectives for your program by identifying the elements of an effective marketing message. For example, suppose you have decided to promote your program to a certain service provider sector, such as the chronic health care community. To identify messages that will resonate with the chronic health care community, conduct interviews with the target sectors of this community (e.g., families, health care practitioners). Then seek out effective channels to reach these sectors, and promote issues that could have an impact on the effectiveness of any appeals you might make. Be sure to identify the implications of increased awareness of the program and the increased activity it will generate.

By interviewing representatives of the corporate community, you might learn that corporations in your area

- Support local organizations first
- Support organizations in which the corporation's employees are involved
- Support groups that have one of their corporate executives on the boards
- Support the same organizations over time
- Want agencies to be held accountable for any assistance received and for results
- Rely on referral clearinghouses for national support

Marketing Survey Form (for Families)

We are trying to reach more people who need Parent to Parent services. Please take a few minutes to complete this survey. When you have finished, please drop it in the mail. Thank you in advance for your valuable help.

1. How did you first hear about Parent to Parent?
2. What is your child's special need?
3. Which people and/or organizations did you first turn to for assistance in addressing the needs of your child(ren)?
4. How would you describe Parent to Parent to other people?
5. Do you read the Parent to Parent newsletter? Regularly?
6. Do you share the Parent to Parent newsletter with anyone else? If yes, with whom?
7. Do you tell other people about Parent to Parent? If yes, how and when?
8. Do you have any suggestions about how Parent to Parent can tell more people about the services it provides?
9. How do you receive health care (employer's health care plan, Medicare or Medicaid, or self-insured)? Which plan are you covered under (e.g., Kaiser Permanente, TakeCare, Blue Cross)?
10. How old are your children?
11. Are they in public or private school?
12. What city do you live in?
13. Are you male or female?

Note: All replies are confidential. Please do not sign your name.

Figure 11.2 Marketing survey form for families. (Courtesy of Parents Helping Parents, Santa Clara, California.)

- Are unlikely to fund a Parent to Parent program unless their corporate employees submit the request
- Focus their newsletters on issues that apply nationally; local interest stories must have a corporate employee connection

Fortified with information from the previous steps, the marketing committee or program leadership is now positioned to develop a focused campaign to meet their needs. Examples of focused campaigns include the following:

Corporate campaign: Focus efforts on a few local corporations that employ people from your program. Approach corporations with the intention of educating them about your program services. Recruit families to approach their corporate employers for financial and marketing support or donations of equipment. After making a donation, most corporations want an accounting of how donated funds are used, how they are translated into good deeds, and how children benefited from the program services. Funding corporations also often want a summary of their employees' contributions of money and time to your program. And companies always appreciate a thank you, preferably in a form that they can use in a public relations capacity, such as a letter from the program's CEO or board chairperson that can be printed in the corporate newsletter.

Health community campaign: Create an opportunity to improve the program's ability to reach parents of *children with less obvious special needs,* and aim an awareness-building effort at professionals who focus on general health care, *not just those who concentrate on children with more involved special needs.* Develop a mechanism for increasing efforts to reach general pediatricians, hospital social workers, school nurses, and parent education groups while focusing on the idea of being an information clearinghouse by doing the following:

- Simplify your position to focus on just two of your program services (e.g., parent support, information clearinghouse).
- Identify your clearinghouse services as offering one-stop shopping for families seeking a comprehensive list of resources for children with special needs and as being a free service that does not require approval for referral from insurance companies.
- Define parent support services as offering one-to-one emotional and pragmatic support from *parents who have been there,* as well as providing specialized support groups for specific needs.

Develop and implement an advertising campaign to the general public: Remember that you are a part of the general public, so think about what

Marketing Survey Form (for Corporations)

1. When you hear of a child with special needs, what kinds of "needs" do you think the child might have?

2. If you had (or have) a child with special needs, which individuals would you turn to for help or advice?

3. What organizations would you contact for help or information?

4. Where have you seen information or advertisements on resources for families with children who have special needs?

5. Have you ever heard of any of the following organizations? Please check all that apply.

____ United Way
____ State Children's Services
____ Perinatal Substance Abuse Newborn Recovery Program
____ Parent to Parent
____ Special Education Local Planning Area
____ County Office of Education
____ Crippled Children's Care
____ FTF—The Family Resource Center
____ Public Health Nursing
____ Regional Center

6. If you had a child with a special need, do you think that an organization called Parent to Parent might provide you with some of the assistance that you needed? Yes___No___Don't know___

7. If you had a child with a special need, do you think that an agency called *FTF—The Family Resource Center* might provide you with some of the assistance that you needed? Yes___No___Don't know___

Figure 11.3. Marketing survey form for corporations. (Courtesy of Parents Helping Parents, Santa Clara, California.)

Figure 11.3. *(continued)*

8. If you have a child with a special need, have you ever heard of or contacted Parent to Parent? Yes___ No___

9. If you have a child with a special need, have you ever heard of or contacted FTF—The Family Resource Center? Yes___No___

10. How old are your children?

11. Are your children in public school? Yes___No___ Private school? Yes___No___

12. What city and state do you live in?

13. Are you male or female?

14. What is your approximate annual household income?

    _____ $0–$24,000
    _____ $25,000–$49,000
    _____ $50,000–$74,000
    _____ $75,000–$99,000
    _____ $100,000–$199,000
    _____ More than $200,000

15. What ethnic group do you identify with?

16. What religion do you identify with?

17. What health care plan are you covered under (e.g., Kaiser Permanente, Aetna, Cigna, TakeCare, Lifeguard, Travelers, Blue Cross)?

Note: Information is confidential. Please do not sign your name.

captures your attention and makes the marketing activities of other agencies worthy of your time and money. The general public usually wants information in concise sound bites, visually colorful, and presented where they are—in their homes watching television, in their cars listening to the radio, or seeing billboards as they travel.

- Define your objectives: Your job is to sell an idea, so define your objectives clearly. Make them simple, precise, and direct for easy understanding.
- Choose people both inside and outside of your program to carry out the campaign.
- Develop a theme for the campaign: Use words and visual aids that can communicate your services' *benefits* in about 1 minute.
- Spread the word: You can advertise through television, radio, newspapers, billboards, magazines, city and county transportation vehicles, brochures, direct mail, and cooperative mailings with other agencies.

SUMMARY

Promoting your program in the community is a necessary challenge that allows your program to grow and be successful as a service for families. You need to be aware of what your customers (e.g., families, professionals, funding sources) want and when, where, and how they want it. Remember that because your program is a nonprofit organization, your program services are your product.

It helps to plan, integrate, and coordinate your marketing activities throughout all aspects of your program. Watch and track trends that influence your program and your customers so that what you offer is current and desired. To be noticed and remembered as a service provider, focus your marketing efforts. Dare to be different by highlighting what is unique about your product; use a personal approach; and use family stories to help funding sources, professionals, and the general public understand your position in the community and the services you provide. And remember that marketing can be done with a minimal amount of funding by taking advantage of the free or inexpensive opportunities provided through newsletters, radio, television, and newspapers.

You also may find that promoting your program produces new volunteers. The job of managing the efforts of volunteers will grow as you do more effective marketing of your program. So you will need a well-thought out and meaningful work plan for volunteers. Adding a formal, paid coordinator of volunteers to a growing program helps ensure that volunteers are utilized and nurtured.

Some general marketing tips you might want to remember include six steps to help you succeed at promoting your program in the community:

1. Set objectives: Whom do you want to reach? What do you want them to do?
2. Identify content areas: What do you want to tell your community? What does your community want to know?
3. Identify communication channels: Which media will reach your audience most effectively?
4. Establish a budget: How much can you afford to spend? What compromises do you need to make? How can you get it done without paying or just paying very little?
5. Establish an overall plan and timetable: What needs to be done? How long will it take? Who is responsible for each action item? Who are the key decision makers, and what are the potential obstacles?
6. Plan your follow-through: How will you measure effectiveness? How will you gather feedback? What is your plan for maintaining forward momentum?

Each advertisement that you create needs to focus on a single message; that is, market a single problem and solution at a time. Keep in mind that agencies that are bigger and wealthier can and will claim to provide the same services that you do, even if they only provide them at a minimal level. Be sure to highlight your unique services that support children with special needs by helping their parents—these are what people will remember. Sell the characteristics of your program services as being provided by people who have been there and the idea that your program offers a one-stop shop focus for meeting families' needs.

Promoting your program in the community is essential to your program's success, and you will find that promotional activities will increase your services to the community, educate the community, find underserved families in the community, and become an asset to your funding efforts.

RESOURCES

Drucker, P.F. (1990). *Managing the non-profit organization.* New York: HarperCollins.

Jeppson, E.S., & Thomas, J. (1995). *Essential allies: Families as advisors.* Bethesda, MD: Institute for Family-Centered Care. (Available from the publisher, 7900 Wisconsin Avenue, Suite 405, Bethesda, MD 20814; telephone: [301] 652-0281)

Knauft, E.B., Berger, R.A., & Gray, S.T. (1991). *Profiles of excellence.* Washington, DC: Independent Sector. (Available from the publisher, 1828 L Street NW, Washington, DC 20036; telephone: [202] 223-8100)

Staff Leader (monthly journal), Aspen Publishers, 7201 McKinney Circle, Frederick, MD 21701; telephone: (800) 638-8437

Stokes, G. (1993). *Please be brilliant! An alternative way to view staff development and your organization.* Chicago: Family Resource Coalition. (Available from Family Support America, 20 North Wacker Drive, Suite 1100, Chicago, IL 60606; telephone: [312] 338-0900)

ORGANIZATIONS

National Resource Center for Family Support Programs, 200 South Michigan Avenue, Suite 1520, Chicago, IL 60604; telephone: (312) 341-0900; fax: (312) 341-9361

Appendix
Tips for Promoting Your Program

1. Have people with public relations expertise on all of your boards, and make friends with advertising agencies to gain access to their knowledge and resources.
2. The three key words for success in promoting products are *fast, easy,* and *painless.* What you offer and how you present it to the community must fit this criteria.
3. To gain a quick and free lesson in marketing, take time to study promotional materials created by well-run, highly respected, and well-known organizations. Find the formula they are using, and transfer it to your materials.
4. Make good use of novelty giveaways, such as balloons, stickers, pens, pennants, cups, and bookmarks, by placing your logo and message on them.
5. Study advertisements in magazines and newspapers. See what captures your attention, and replicate it in your materials.
6. You probably miss at least 10 opportunities every day to promote your program. Look at your materials. Do you have your program's name on as many pages as you should? Do your staff and boards wear agency pins or have bumper stickers?
7. Helping other organizations further promotes your program because you are getting your name out in the public.
8. Build a media file, which is a list of sources with detailed information on the various news media in your area (e.g., address, telephone number, names of key staff, publication dates, deadlines). Get to know key staff. Having this information readily available encourages use of the media to promote your program.
9. Create a basic press kit. This is an attractive packet of materials that is provided to the media and others in the community. The folder should have your name, logo, copy of your brochure, newsletter, historical page, annual report, and glossy copies of publicity about your program.
10. Learn to create press releases. See Figure 11.1 for an example of a joint press release.

12

Building Partnerships

The Benefits of Collaboration

"The first thing to learn in intercourse with others is non-interference with their own peculiar ways of being happy, provided those ways do not assume to interfere by violence with ours."

—William James

The basic growth and ultimate survival of Parent to Parent programs depends largely on collaborative relationships. Parent to Parent programs quickly realized the benefits of partnership, and programs have developed partnerships to make their programs work; the stories in this book include numerous examples of these partnerships. Need breeds leadership, collaboration, and partnerships.

This chapter explores 1) the importance of partnerships to a Parent to Parent program's development, growth, and survival; 2) the development and maintenance of different types of partnerships; and 3) the skills for negotiating a successful collaborative relationship.

IMPORTANCE OF PARTNERSHIPS

A Parent to Parent program's development, growth, and survival may hang on the successful partnerships it creates. Because many programs start with little or no money, they learn to barter their unique parental expertise to get things done. Exchanging the services of one agency for the space and money of another is a common and useful form of partnering. This basic exchange leads to further collaborative projects. These partnerships often bring funds, skills, and knowledge to the parent program and to its partners. The synergy and clout of increased numbers of people involved in a project enhance its prospects for successfully accomplishing its goals and objectives. Partnerships also

1. *Increase access to people and information:* Partnerships immediately put Parent to Parent programs in contact with the broader community. These contacts provide programs with more referrals, information about resources that are available for families, and ways to gain access to these resources.
2. *Enhance program infrastructure:* Collaborative efforts save programs money by using shared resources and by increasing financial income for their services to families through subcontracts. Agencies gain access to equipment, space, and larger pools of potential board members to further enhance their growth and stability. All of these shared resources strengthen the infrastructure of programs and give them the ability to start, grow, accomplish their goals, and survive.
3. *Expand benefits for families and the community:* Through partnerships, services are better coordinated and the speed at which children are served is improved. Parents, the public, and professionals gain a greater knowledge of the laws, and parents have more opportunities to advocate for their children and more responsive services. Unnecessary duplication of services is eliminated, and the financial burden on communities decreases through parent–professional collaborative relationships. There also is an improved usage of community services and resources by all agencies involved. Partnerships can lead to the creation of new organizations that bring new approaches to serving children and individuals with special needs, thus increasing service opportunities for consumers and families.
4. *Strengthen the program's marketing component:* When Parent to Parent programs partner with other agencies, the shared activities increase public awareness about their program. Partnerships also allow the partnering programs to improve their service to families by helping them remain contemporary and relevant through co-training of service providers and collaborative research. The col-

laborative activities become a vehicle for mutual input to the partnering programs—input into planning, policy, implementation, and evaluation of the programs.

WHO PARTNERS WITH PARENTS?

Parent to Parent programs have created partnerships with likely and unlikely partners, including education, health, legal, and social services systems; other parent organizations; service providers; corporations; funders; and local, state, and national governmental agencies, including the military. Some partnerships evolve to help the program's development, while other partnerships start on behalf of the children. Parents are important partners because they have knowledge about different service systems, whereas most professionals have knowledge about one particular area of expertise. Parents bring to the meeting or planning group this broad knowledge base, actual experience with service systems, a collaborative spirit, and a passion for helping the group to focus on the whole child.

Partnerships with Parents

Often the first partnership developed by a Parent to Parent program is the one between the program leaders and the parents who become volunteer support parents. This kind of partnership often is a simple verbal agreement, but some programs have a written Memorandum of Understanding that summarizes the expectations that the program and the support parents have for each other. The program expects the volunteers to participate in the program's support parent training and provide support services to families in an efficient and confidential manner. The support parents expect the program to provide ongoing information and emotional support to help them celebrate, appreciate, and become effective in their volunteering.

Parent to Parent programs also have created partnerships with other parent-directed support groups. Whereas Parent to Parent programs provide one-to-one emotional and informational support, parent support groups provide small-group emotional benefits, and they concentrate their efforts on one disability or issue. Often the Parent to Parent program becomes incorporated as a 501(c)3 nonprofit public benefit organization. A parent-directed support group that decides to partner with a Parent to Parent program that is a 501(c)3 organization does not have to get its own 501(c)3—a process for which few have the expertise, time, or money. The support group helps to provide support to families and becomes an available source of support parents for the Parent to Parent program. Support group members are given training by the Parent to Parent program and are more confident and able to facilitate their own meetings and gatherings. These support groups also help the Parent to Parent program stay anchored to grass roots needs, and they can become extra hands for fund-raising. In return, the Parent to Parent program provides the support group with all of the benefits of a 501(c)3 organization.

Partnerships with Professionals

Individuals in the helping professions often work collaboratively with parents to help them create support programs. These professionals volunteer their time and sometimes even risk negative reactions from their colleagues for working with self-help programs that are seen as outside their usual occupational frame of reference. Psychologists and counselors may co-facilitate support group meetings with parents until the parents gain confidence and skills to facilitate alone. Social workers and educators also may help with the training of support parents and the development of the training curriculum. Professionals may partner with the Parent to Parent program to conduct valuable research or to provide an evaluation component to various parent program projects. As you will remember from Chapter 4, the first Parent to Parent program was started by a parent who partnered with two professionals. Although they may have their differences, professionals and parents working collaboratively often produce the best outcomes for children.

Partnerships with Staff

The leadership of the Parent to Parent program develops a collaborative partnership with the paid staff of the program. The board of directors makes a commitment to plan for and hire competent executive staff and maintain a financial base from which the staff can launch its services. The board also undertakes the responsibility to provide for the staff's well-being by providing a safe and healthy workplace, as well as fringe benefits such as health and dental insurance and retirement packages. The staff fulfills its half of the partnership by providing quality services in an efficient and effective manner. In the nonprofit world there also is a close partnership between the board and the chief executive officer (CEO) of the program because they work hand-in-hand to accomplish the program's mission.

Partnerships with Agencies

Parent to Parent programs have created partnerships with agencies of all types, including universities; public, private, and government agencies; hospitals; regional centers; schools; and juvenile justice systems. Most of these partnerships are created to enhance family-centered, culturally competent, coordinated care for children with special needs. These collaborative efforts are typical win–win situations in which the parent programs bring their personal experiences and lessons learned from their hours working with families to the agency's services and planning, policy, and evaluation components. These partnerships include the exchange of services for money, staff, space, training, curriculum building, internships, research, program development, and more.

Partnerships with Funding Sources

The United Way; corporations; foundations; individuals; and local, state, and federal governments all come to mind when considering parent to parent partnerships with funding sources. Each of these funding entities has its own agenda of goals and objectives, and each has found a partner in parent programs to help them accomplish their mission. Funders provide the money, and the parent programs provide the strategies, methods, and energy to complete the objectives of the funders that match the program's mission of helping children and families. These partnerships are established most often when the funder issues a request for proposals (RFP) and the parent program submits a competitive proposal.

Partnering Program Stories: Insight from Parent to Parent of Pennsylvania

Pennsylvania's Department of Education, Department of Public Welfare, and Department of Health collaborated to help establish Parent to Parent of Pennsylvania. By working together with these three agencies, we were able to realize our dream of creating a parent support program. This was a successful public–government partnership.

Our partnership with the Department of Health gave us the opportunity to collaborate with the Special Kids Network on housing, and we benefited from a huge advertising campaign already planned for that agency. The Department of Health's advertising company also suggested that the Special Kids Network and Parent to Parent of Pennsylvania share a toll-free telephone number. After 6 months of negotiating a better understanding of what was required of each agency, the individual roles began to crystallize and the partnership was formed.

Today the programs operate independently yet work together—they are autonomous agencies collaborating to accomplish mutual goals. Public presentations are given jointly by personnel from both programs, and agency-to-agency referrals help keep both programs alive in the community—refer-

rals to Parent to Parent regarding special needs services are sent to Special Kids Network, and referrals to Special Kids Network regarding parent support are passed to Parent to Parent of Pennsylvania.

Parents Helping Parents Partnerships

Parents Helping Parents' (PHP) first partnership was with the Parents of Down Syndrome (PODS) support group. We decided to work together to accomplish our goals under one 501(c)3 incorporation instead of having PODS become incorporated as a separate entity. That partnership still thrives today, along with similar partnerships with more than 40 other specialty parent support groups. PHP gained access to hundreds of potential support parents by partnering with these disability- and issue-specific support groups. The program also benefited from the financial grass roots support of these groups. We gained access to more volunteers to help with special events and other service activities, as well as connections to community leaders already attached to the support groups.

We also created partnerships with military families who were stationed in our county to help provide support and training and help them set up their own Parent to Parent program that would be implemented under PHP's umbrella. And we partnered with other agencies to produce an annual symposium on children with special needs. Because of our numerous collaborative relationships, we became involved in Santa Clara County's Interagency Coordinating Council for early intervention services. We created collaborative partnerships with several other agencies to find solutions for the lack of housing for families' adult children seeking supported and independent living. This partnership included the regional center that provides service coordinators and funding for individuals with developmental disabilities, agencies that provide job training and recreational services, and organizations that provide supported/independent housing programs and independent living instructors. For the first time, we talked with the Adult Independent Living program that tends to concentrate its efforts mainly on individuals who have physical disabilities. A new independent nonprofit organization concentrating on housing issues was born of that partnership.

We developed a contractual partnership with the state of California and Santa Clara University (SCU) to teach a course on parent–professional collaboration. A PHP parent and an SCU professor co-taught the program. The course was a year of studies that culminated with students' receiving some of the first Collaboration Specialist Certificates from the state of California. Further partnerships were encouraged by having parents and professionals attend the class as student partners and complete a final project for a system's change in a local agency serving children or adults with special needs.

One of our greatest partnerships was created in 1994 with Kaiser Permanente, a managed care health provider. This mutually beneficial, consumer–provider partnership has now been extended to include three more hospitals—a Kaiser Permanente facility that is a nonprofit health care facility; Columbia Good Samaritan Hospital, a for-profit managed care agency; and Valley Medical Center, a governmental managed care facility. These partnerships allow PHP to set up satellite parent-directed family resource centers at the hospitals to provide parent to parent services for families and training for hospital staff in family-centered, culturally competent care. The Kaiser Permanente hospitals provide PHP funding (the other hospitals are still funded by PHP's maternal and child health grant) to pay the parent liaison staff who operate the centers, and they also provide space, equipment, and furniture to outfit the centers. PHP sets up the satellite sites; hires, trains, and evaluates the staff; and evaluates the program by having families and hospital staff complete surveys. Families and hospital staff attend workshops provided by the project. The hospitals now find it easier to include parent input into their planning, implementation, and evaluation and into new policies and procedures of care for children with special needs. For hospital staff, parent liaisons also have become a link to the broader community.

PHP looks forward to setting up Parent to Parent programs on school campuses and at businesses in the future. Partnership satellite sites are constant visual reminders of the need for parent to parent services—never out of sight or mind and working together for the common good of children and families.

TYPES OF PARTNERSHIPS

Partnerships can be formal or informal. Many years ago an agreement might have been sealed with a handshake. Today, formal legal partnerships are sealed with a Memorandum of Understanding, Declaration of Unity, or a merger pact.

Informal Partnerships

Informal partnerships often occur as the result of a meeting in which one or more parties verbally agree to accomplish a mutual objective. Partners agree verbally that each person will contribute his or her part and that no one has acquired a legal responsibility for the outcome of the complete project.

Partnerships also can follow a family structure, with one party taking on the responsibilities of a parent or primary partner and the other assuming the child's role or secondary partner. Although one partner bears the greater responsibility, the important factor is to be sure that each partner understands the common ground to which both are committed and their respective roles. Each partner's function is important to the success of the partnership, and building a win–win situation from the beginning increases chances that another partnership will take place.

Some partnerships are merely close collaborative efforts, such as participation in a local government assessment and planning for children's health care or youth services, a United Way campaign or evaluation, the YWCA's family education advisory board, an elected official's annual conference on families, a national Head Start conference, or the local schools' strategic planning and evaluation.

Being involved in these partnerships takes time, but you will find that partnerships provide learning opportunities, increase contacts with important people, and offer a chance to get your agency's name and programs known in the community.

Formal Partnerships

A *Memorandum of Understanding* is a formal partnership that is legally binding when properly signed and sealed by the parties involved. To protect your program, do not enter into any binding legal agreement without first consulting an attorney. Have the attorney review the Memorandum of Understanding, explain its implications, and ensure the appropriateness of the language being used for the obligations expected.

As you develop a Memorandum of Understanding, remember that sample Memorandums of Understanding and other legal documents can be attained from stationery stores, and you can use or adapt these for your program. Basically, these memorandums spell out who the partners are, what is expected of each, the length of the agreement, how the parties can be relieved of their responsibilities, and how disputes will be settled. Finalize the process by affixing the signatures of both partners, imprinting the program or agency seal, and dating the document. A Memorandum of Understanding is binding without having witnesses to the signatures or notarization, but some partners may prefer and/or require these two additional steps.

If you decide to proceed with a formal merger with another agency or program, seeking legal help also is important. Consult an attorney who is experienced in this area so that all local and state laws are strictly adhered to. Before you commit to a merger, carefully consider your reasons and look at potential benefits and drawbacks. Some smaller agencies might consider merging if they are having difficulty maintaining a stable financial base or if the founding executive director is leaving and wants to better position the agency for survival. The leadership of the larger agency should consider whether the new partner's programs fit its mission, whether the agency is familiar with the new partner, whether it has a good reputation in the community, whether the services are needed, and whether people in the community want to see those services maintained. Having similar program activities and goals makes the transition easier for both agencies.

Before the merger happens the two agencies will need to meet and begin discussions to get to know each other. Several informal luncheons and other meetings should happen between the two agencies' executive directors. The two board chairpeople meet and then the full boards create a merger committee. After several months of discussions, the committee may make an initial recommendation for the merger. After the merger is finalized, programs or agencies often have someone serve as a transition liaison to help the two programs or agencies grow in a positive manner and prevent the forming of an "us versus them" attitude. This transition position may need to be filled for 3–12 months according to how well the two merging agencies know each other and how similar they are in programs, products, philosophy, and structure.

Networking Partnerships

The nature of both formal and informal partnerships varies according to the people involved and the purpose of the collaboration. Networking partnerships consist primarily of mutual sharing of information with another agency. Networking partnerships are easy to develop and maintain, and they are essential to a program's visibility and credibility. For example, the vast majority of statewide Parent to Parent programs have a program newsletter that they share with parents and agencies as a way of networking ideas and needs. Statewide Parent to Parent programs also share promotional literature from other agencies with parents who are involved in Parent to Parent.

Coordinating Partnerships

Coordinating partnerships allow each of the partners to modify its own agency behavior on behalf of the families it serves. For example, most statewide Parent to Parent programs share a system of mutual referrals with other local and statewide agencies. The statewide Parent to Parent program shares information about and refers parents to the partnering agency and vice versa. Several statewide Parent to Parent programs have coordinating partnerships with universities and university affiliated programs (UAPs). Parents involved with Parent to Parent of Vermont serve as community faculty at the University of Vermont Medical School. These parents teach medical students in university classrooms and also are matched with medical students for meetings in a family's home. Similar opportunities exist through the University of Vermont UAP for

Vermont parents to be matched with graduate students preparing for careers in early childhood special education, nursing, and occupational and physical therapy.

Coordinating partnerships require ongoing nurturing, particularly of providers who are working directly with families. The staff turnover rate is high in social services professions, and for referrals to be made and received, there must be strong links among people who are meeting and talking with families on a daily basis.

Cooperative Partnerships

A cooperative partnership exists when agencies work toward a common vision or purpose and each is allowed to do what they do best. In this type of partnership, there is little change in the configuration, style, or manner of operation of the partners. Each is obligated to provide a separate part of a total plan or project for which either or neither is responsible for the overall outcome. For example, many statewide Parent to Parent programs work closely with other agencies to bring early intervention services to young children and families. Some of these statewide programs also receive contracts from Part C of the Individuals with Disabilities Education Act (IDEA) Amendments of 1997 to serve as the statewide early intervention resource providing information and referrals to parents who have infants and toddlers with developmental delays. The parent program is not responsible for the state's early intervention program but is held responsible for providing the information and referrals. Some Parent to Parent programs work in cooperative partnership with other county agencies, such as the county office of education, to provide the family resource centerpiece of the county's total early intervention package. The cooperative partners come together to develop a plan for dividing and implementing the work, they sign an agreement, and then they return to their respective agencies to fulfill their obligations for which they receive a comparable share of money allocated to the total project. Here are some examples of cooperative partnerships:

The Family Connection of South Carolina was awarded a contract to develop and implement the Family Partner program, which provides parent to parent support for parents of children who are eligible for BabyNet, the state's early intervention program. Family Partners are parents of young children with special needs who are already trained as supporting parents and who receive additional training so that they are prepared to support parents of infants and toddlers who are eligible for early intervention services. Since 1992, trained Family Partners have provided more than 55,000 hours of parent to parent support to more than 2,500 families.

The Family Support Network of Michigan enjoys a cooperative partnership with Michigan's Title V program that is administered by Children's Special Health Care Services (CSHCS). In 1988, CSHCS created the Parent Participation Program (PPP) to provide ideas and opinions for enhancing the system of services. From the efforts of parents involved in the work of the PPP, the Family Support Network of Michigan emerged as a source of emotional and informational support for parents who have children with disabilities or special health care needs. More than 50 network chapters in Michigan offer emotional support and practical suggestions for day-to-day living, information about available services, and ideas for working with others to meet families' needs.

The Parent to Parent Support Program of Washington also has a cooperative partnership and state contract with its Title V program. The contract to the Parent to Parent Support Program came as a result of the state's response to the federal mandate to involve parents in planning, program, and policy development. The Parent to Parent Support Program and the Washington State Department of Health, Office of Children with Special Health Care Needs, established parent–professional collaboration and family-centered practices. Parents who participate in the program provide input on a variety of issues, tasks, and projects being considered and implemented by the Office of Children with Special Health Care Needs.

Parent to Parent of Vermont has established multiple cooperative partnerships with several different state entities—the Title V program, Part C (early intervention), the Vermont parent training and information center (PTI), and the Network of Parent Child Centers—to develop a peer support model for all families, not just those of children with special needs.

Collaborative Partnerships

Another type of partnership is a collaborative partnership. Collaborative partnerships occur when individuals or agencies are willing to enhance the capacity of others, even with some tradeoffs. In this type of partnership, there are likely to be changes in the role and function of the partners. A collaborative partnership occurred when Florida's PTI and its statewide Parent to Parent program realized that greater strength and capacity could be achieved by merging the two organizations. The Family Network on Disabilities of Florida emerged as the statewide organization in which families could obtain the training and advocacy that PTIs provide and the information and emotional support through the one-to-one matches of Parent to Parent. The capacity of the agencies to better serve families happens through enhanced shared knowledge and increased human, financial, and material resources.

Building Statewide Partnerships

You have read about many partnerships that have been forged by statewide Parent to Parent programs, and most statewide Parent to Parent programs do have partnerships with other statewide agencies. Table 12.1 in Appendix A describes these partner agencies. The majority of statewide programs are functioning in partnership with their state's agencies, such as health, education, and social services agencies; early intervention programs; developmental disability councils; and state disability organizations. More than half of statewide parent programs have formed partnerships with UAPs, PTIs, hospitals, school districts, and state rehabilitation agencies.

DEVELOPING AND MAINTAINING PARTNERSHIPS

To develop and maintain partnerships, you will need to work with everyone whose activities will help you accomplish your mission, goals, and objectives. Be involved with a variety of agencies from Head Start, to the Council on Aging, to local universities. Universities may appreciate an offer for students to do internships at your agency, and you can work with educational facilities to create family-centered curricula and train with them. The more you are in the community helping others accomplish their goals, the more you will accomplish your own objective of promoting your program and making the community aware of your mission of children with special needs and of the families you serve. Work with others to create symposiums and conferences and to form panels to speak to various groups. Offer your services as fiscal agent for a program that is not yet incorporated. All of these are ways that you can develop informal partnerships to help yourself and others grow.

To be successful at partnering requires the skills, attitudes, and behaviors necessary for collaborating, being assertive, and negotiating. Collaborating and negotiating are both skills that can be easily taught and/or learned. Don't hesitate to attend a class or conference on these topics (see Figure 12.1 and the resources at the end of this chapter).

When two or more people intend to work collaboratively, they should start by defining the problem on which they intend to work. Too often disagreements resurface when only one partner or one side has defined the problem or need. Collaborators also must be allowed to disagree and have different points of view. Coming to a consensus opinion when there are differences is one of the hallmarks of good collaboration.

Collaboration requires working closely with other partners, and in any collaborative relationship you can choose your response—a passive response, an assertive response, or an aggressive response. People who behave in a *passive* manner may not care enough about themselves to speak up for themselves. People who behave *aggressively* may care only about themselves and their needs. People who behave *assertively* care enough about themselves to speak up but also care enough about the other person to do so without attacking that other person. The middle ground of assertiveness is a productive route to improved communications and interactions in partnerships. Some ideas for being assertive in your discussions with potential partners include the following:

- Keep the discussion short and simple (KISS).
- Persist.
- Repeat your need to be sure that it is understood.
- Avoid insulting or attacking the other person.
- Do not overuse the phrases, "I think," "I feel," "I believe," and, "I hope."
- Seek common ground on ideas.
- Avoid switching the focus of the conversation.
- Define only yourself and how you are feeling.
- Ask for specifics or details.
- Gather facts and information.
- Write, plan, and rehearse.
- Learn from the times when you are not assertive.
- Be aware of how others use conversation to their advantage.
- Dress for the occasion.

NEGOTIATING

Negotiating is a process that involves coming to an agreement in which both parties win. If you are negotiating with someone and his or her needs are not met but yours are, then the negotiation has not been successful. According to Fisher and Ury (1981), there are four main strategies to a successful negotiation:

1. Separate the person from the problem. Put yourself in the other person's shoes, and don't blame the person for the problem.
2. Establish interests, goals, and priorities. Each party needs to define the problem as they see it and identify their goals and desired outcomes. Look for things you agree on and be flexible and open to compromise.

Are You a Collaborator?

Circle the number that best matches your skill level.

Skill	Needs improving		Adequate		Well developed
I am self-confident.	1	2	3	4	5
I know my strengths and weaknesses.	1	2	3	4	5
I make a conscious effort to improve my skills.	1	2	3	4	5
I am open to differences (e.g., cultures, personalities, ideas).	1	2	3	4	5
I have a clear set of values.	1	2	3	4	5
I am assertive in expressing my values.	1	2	3	4	5
I am self-directed.	1	2	3	4	5
I am interdependent (cooperative yet independent).	1	2	3	4	5
I have a systems perspective (looking at the whole picture—family, community, society).	1	2	3	4	5
I am able to tolerate ambiguous situations.	1	2	3	4	5
I am flexible.	1	2	3	4	5
I have good observation skills.	1	2	3	4	5
I am able to negotiate in conflict situations.	1	2	3	4	5
I possess good communication skills.	1	2	3	4	5
I like to help others.	1	2	3	4	5
I understand group process and dynamics.	1	2	3	4	5

My two greatest skills are

1.

2.

My two weakest skills are

1.

2.

(Write or discuss plans to enhance weak skills.)

Figure 12.1. Self-evaluation collaboration quiz. (From Cegelka, P., & Mendoza, J. [1986]. *Parents and professionals advocating for collaborative training: Component I.* San Diego: San Diego State University; reprinted by permission.)

3. Generate options that can achieve a win–win position. Based on the goals of each party, brainstorm for options to solve the problem, and don't make premature decisions.
4. Strive for agreement. Evaluate your options in terms of effectiveness in meeting both parties' goals.

When these four negotiation strategies are used in an assertive manner, the chances for a successful outcome will be improved.

SUMMARY

Partnerships are a way of life. Our potential list of partners is enormous. As Parent to Parent programs expand beyond local relationships to state, national, and international relationships, so will their collaborative relationships. Size does not hinder the capacity of a program or agency to develop or benefit from partnerships with individuals, funders, agencies, or the government.

Much can be accomplished in less time when one is willing to create partnerships with others who have a common mission and goals and objectives. To make these collaborative relationships work requires an attitude of respect for each individual. Being competitive is no longer the main path to success in the nonprofit or for-profit business world.

Partnerships help Parent to Parent programs to start, grow, and survive, and they also become a mechanism for increasing service opportunities and enhancing coordination and family centeredness in the care of children. Partnerships can be informally based on a person's word or a handshake. Formal partnerships based on Memorandums of Understanding, Declarations of Unity, or merger pacts should not be entered into without legal consultation. Communicating, collaborating, negotiating, and communicating assertively are all skills that can be learned and improved. Taking time to invest in developing these skills will be worthwhile for you and your program.

REFERENCES

Cegelka, P., & Mendoza, J. (1986). *Parents and professionals advocating for collaborative training: Component I.* San Diego: San Diego State University.

Fisher, R., & Ury, W. (1981). *Getting to yes: Negotiating agreement without giving in.* New York: Houghton/Mifflin.

Individuals with Disabilities Education Act (IDEA) Amendments of 1997, PL 105-17, 20 U.S.C. §§ 1400 *et seq.*

RESOURCES

Burnett, K. (1996). *Relationship fundraising: A donor based approach to the business of raising money.* Chicago: Precept Press.

DiVenere, N. (1992). *Families and professionals pulling together.* Paper presented at the Family Network Meeting of the Association of the Care of Children's Health, Parent to Parent of Vermont ([802] 655-5290).

Dunst, C.J. (1990). Family support principles: Checklist for program builders and practitioners. *Family Systems Intervention Monograph*(2, Serial No. 5).

Edelman, L. (Ed.). (1991). *Getting on board: Training activities to promote the practice of family-centered care.* Bethesda, MD: Association for the Care of Children's Health.

Jardins, C.D. (1980). *How to get services by being assertive.* Chicago: Family Resource Center on Disabilities.

Kelker, K.A. (1987). *Working together: The parent/professional partnership.* Portland, OR: Families as Allies Project.

Lynch, E.W., & Hanson, M.J. (Eds.). (1998). *Developing cross-cultural competence: A guide for working with children and their families* (2nd ed.). Baltimore: Paul H. Brookes Publishing Co.

National Center for Clinical Infant Programs. (1984). *Equals in this partnership: Parents of disabled and at risk infants and toddlers speak to professionals.* Arlington, VA: Author.

Poyadue, F.S. (1998). *Assertiveness—In a nut shell.* Santa Clara, CA: Parents Helping Parents.

13

Evaluating Your Program

What Difference Are You Making?

"If you don't know where you're going, you probably won't get there . . . if you don't know where you are, it is hard to know how far you are from where you want to be, and if you don't know where you have come from, you may end up walking in circles."

—Alan S. Gurman and David P. Kniskern

You have read in the last several chapters about the activities that go into developing and directing a Parent to Parent program—pulling together a program development team, finding funding, preparing supporting parents, establishing the referral system, making parent matches, adding program components, promoting the program, and building collaborative partnerships with others. After putting all of their energy, fiscal resources, and staff time into these program development and operation activities, some program directors find that the last thing they want to think about is evaluating their program. And yet, documenting the outcomes of program services is an essential part of demonstrating program accountability to referral sources and to parents as consumers of the program. Moreover, most funding sources require evidence that the program activities they have funded have been accomplished and have made a difference to those who have participated in the program.

As Parent to Parent programs grow in their national visibility and availability, many newcomers to Parent to Parent (e.g., parents, service providers, funders, policy makers) are interested in learning more: "What services are provided by Parent to Parent, to whom, how, and with what results?" Similarly, Parent to Parent program directors also may have questions about their programs. "Is the program meeting its objectives?" "How many people are being served?" "How could the program be improved to meet the needs of families?" "How can the impact of Parent to Parent be documented?" Family stories and testimonials about parent to parent support are a compelling way to collect information and tell others about Parent to Parent and its importance, but those who provide funds and serve as referral sources to Parent to Parent are reluctant to support programs based solely on anecdotal evidence. Program evaluation offers a way to answer questions about and document the importance of Parent to Parent.

In this chapter you will learn about 1) what program evaluation is and why it is important, 2) different types of program evaluation used by Parent to Parent programs, and 3) steps you can use to evaluate your own program.

WHAT IS PROGRAM EVALUATION?

Program evaluation is the process through which questions about Parent to Parent can be asked in systematic ways and answered with data. Program evaluation involves answering questions about the types of services provided, how they are provided, who provides them, who receives them, how much they cost, and how well they work and includes a range of approaches for analyzing program operations. Program evaluation methods range from simple systems for documenting the number of parent matches that are made to sophisticated quantitative studies of the impact of one-to-one parent to parent support on the referred parent. Whatever the type of program evaluation and its level of sophistication, program evaluation can, and should, be built into every Parent to Parent program.

WHY CONDUCT A PROGRAM EVALUATION?

There are several reasons why program evaluation is important and Parent to Parent programs should consider it as a component. When you conduct a program evaluation, the results allow you to demonstrate what your program does and its effect on families. Program evaluation activities will give you descriptive and evaluative information about your program that you can share with others and use in your future program planning to better serve families.

Documenting the Need for Parent to Parent

If your program is in development or if you are considering bringing parent to parent support to a new segment of your community, you may want to begin by conducting a needs assessment to document the need for parent to parent support in your community. The results of this assessment can justify the need for parent to parent support and help you clarify your program goals and objectives so that they are responsive to the community needs.

Documenting the Implementation of Program Activities

As your program grows and you want others to understand what parent to parent support is all about and what your program does for and with families, you may want to document and describe the services you are providing. It is important to be able to cite concrete facts; for example, "Our Parent to Parent program trained 56 supporting parents in the past 6 months," or, "We matched 92 referred parents." These data can be obtained from record-keeping systems. You also will find that by documenting program activities you can learn more about who is participating and can monitor progress in achieving your program goals and objectives.

Documenting Satisfaction with Program Activities

To strengthen existing program activities and to plan for new ones, you may want to document user satisfaction. This information will help you to adapt or expand your program activities so that the users of your program's services report a greater level of satisfaction.

Documenting the Impact of Your Program

You may choose to document your program's impact by collecting data about the differences that the services offered by your program are making in the lives of children with special needs and their families. You can use the data to encourage fund-raising and referral sources to support your program.

DIFFERENT TYPES OF PROGRAM EVALUATION

Although the purposes of program evaluation vary from program to program and from time to time, there are several steps that all programs can follow in developing and conducting program evaluation. In this section you will read about four Parent to Parent programs and how they used the same program evaluation steps to collect data to answer questions that were important to their program development and expansion.

The Family Connection of South Carolina

The Family Connection of South Carolina, founded in 1989 by parents and professionals, is the statewide Parent to Parent program that matches parents across the state. The Children's Hospital of the Greenville Hospital System contacted The Family Connection for help in addressing the concerns of parents who have infants in the neonatal intensive care unit (NICU) and those who participate in or perhaps should be participating in the neonatal follow-up clinic. Was there an opportunity for these parents to be a part of a parent to parent match? Was there a need for parent support groups and parent matching for families within this particular hospital setting? To answer these questions, The Family Connection and staff at the hospital conducted their own program evaluation to document the need for Parent to Parent. *The resulting data enabled The Family Connection to offer a parent support group and matching program at the hospital.*

Family Support Network of North Carolina

Family Support Network (FSN) of North Carolina, a statewide program founded in 1985, developed a comprehensive system for tracking the number of referrals and matches and the progress of matches. The network has procedures and forms for documenting the number and types of incoming calls, the information about referred and supporting parent families that will be used to make matches, the number of matches made, which referred parents are matched with which supporting parents, and the number and timing of contacts between matched parents. This continual program evaluation looks at the implementation of the matched experience and allows FSN to make refinements on an ongoing basis. Many of the local programs in North Carolina use or adapt the program evaluation procedures and forms developed by FSN. One program, FSN of the High Country in Boone, wanted to evaluate its procedures for implementing matches. They adapted the FSN program evaluation methods to document the implementation of program activities. *The resulting data meant that FSN of the High Country could confidently report about their matching activities.*

Families Together

*Families Together, the parent training and information center (PTI) in Kansas, launched Kansas Parent to Parent, the statewide Parent to Parent program, in 1992. After a year or two of growth during which the number of local Parent to Parent programs in Kansas grew from 5 to 15, staff at Families Together wanted to learn more about how satisfied the local program coordinators and the supporting parents were with the training and technical assistance they received from Families Together. They decided to develop two questionnaires—one for local program coordinators and one for supporting parents—*to document satisfaction with program activities. *The resulting data collected through the surveys helped Families Together justify the supports provided to local coordinators and parents and helped the group make modifications to enhance training and technical assistance.*

Parent to Parent of Vermont

Parent to Parent of Vermont has been providing support and information to parents in Vermont since 1985, and the parents providing these services frequently heard from families about the benefits of parent to parent support. And yet, other than these testimonials from parents, there were no data on the effectiveness of parent to parent support. In 1993, Parent to Parent of Vermont joined a consortium of parents and researchers to conduct a national study to document the impact of parent to parent support. *The resulting data have been useful in convincing fund-raising and referral sources that Parent to Parent makes a difference for referred parents.*

STEPS TO DEVELOPING AND CONDUCTING PROGRAM EVALUATION

Each of these Parent to Parent programs followed the same seven steps in developing and conducting its program evaluation.

Step 1: Specifying Program Goals and Objectives

Parent to Parent programs have multiple goals because they are responsive to the differing needs of families. Clarifying your program's goals and objectives is the first step in the program evaluation process. Begin by reviewing your mission statement, goals, and objectives to identify any aspects of them that may seem ambiguous. Define key words and find ways to make them measurable. For example, if you want to determine the effectiveness of the parent match, you will need to define what *parent match* means. How many and what type of contacts over what length of time constitute a parent match?

Each of the four Parent to Parent programs, while having its own collection of program activities, shares the same comprehensive program goals:

- Increasing the emotional support that is available to parents who have a child with special needs
- Increasing the informational support that is available to parents who have a child with special needs
- Providing the emotional and informational support by offering parents the one-to-one matched experience with a veteran parent

To be specific about what is meant by *emotional support, informational support,* and the *one-to-one matched experience,* parent leaders defined these terms as follows:

- *Emotional support* has five components: 1) a sense of having a reliable ally, 2) a sense of empowerment, 3) a sense of social support, 4) a sense of being able to cope, and 5) a sense of acceptance about disability issues.
- *Informational support* is knowledge about services for the child with special needs.
- The *one-to-one matched experience* comprises at least four contacts from a veteran parent during an 8-week period.

The Family Connection of South Carolina was hoping to accomplish its program goal of providing emotional and informational support to parents by expanding its services to the NICU hospital setting, and they wanted to use program evaluation to justify the need for this expansion.

FSN of the High Country intended to document the implementation of its parent matching to ensure that its program goals were being accomplished. Specifically, FSN of the High Country wanted to ensure that 1) matches between supporting parents and referred parents began as soon as possible after the local coordinator connected the two parents, 2) an adequate number of contacts (based on the needs of the referred parent) were occurring, and 3) supporting parents and referred parents were comfortable with the progress of their matches.

As specified in the grant application submitted by Families Together to the Kansas Developmental Disabilities Council to establish Kansas Parent to Parent, the primary goal of Kansas Parent to Parent was that parents of children and youth with disabilities would receive emotional and informational support. Families Together believed that by providing training and technical assistance to local program coordinators and parents wishing to be supporting parents, the coordinators and supporting parents would be in a better position to ensure that parents received the emotional and informational support that were part of Families Together's program goals for Kansas Parent to Parent.

Parent to Parent of Vermont wished to collect efficacy data to determine whether the goals of Parent to Parent were effective in meeting parents' emotional and informational needs.

Step 2: Identifying the Purposes and Audiences for Program Evaluation

Before you develop your evaluation strategy, you will need to figure out your purposes for the evaluation and who will use this information. As you consider your reasons for conducting a program evaluation, think about who is or might be interested in particular aspects of your program.

- *Program developers* who are considering launching a Parent to Parent program may want to find out whether people want one-to-one parent to parent support in their community. Documentation of the need for parent to parent support answers their questions.
- *Those who provide funds* may want to know how a Parent to Parent program helps children and families before they agree to commit financial support to the program. Documentation of the impact of Parent to Parent answers their questions.
- *Referral sources* may want to know about the supports and services that the Parent to Parent program provides to parents they refer to the program. Documentation of the implementation of program activities answers their questions.
- The *board of directors* of a Parent to Parent program may want to know whether program staff carried out the program activities that were proposed and funded to meet the program's goals and objectives. Documentation of the implementation of program activities answers their questions.
- *State legislators* may want to know about the impact of one-to-one matching when considering whether to include support for Parent to Parent programs in state budgets and policy regulations. Documenting the impact of parent to parent support answers their questions.
- *Parents* may want to know more about the benefits of being matched with a supporting parent who has *been there* and understands. Documenting the effectiveness and impact of Parent to Parent would answer their questions.

The purpose of The Family Connection of South Carolina's program evaluation effort was to determine the support preferences of parents involved with the NICU at Children's Hospital of Greenville. If the parents expressed a need for emotional and informational support, then perhaps The Family Connection could help to meet those needs. The audience for the program evaluation consisted of officials at the hospital who were to decide whether to fund an effort to establish a Parent to Parent program for NICU families. The board of directors at The Family Connection needed to make decisions about expanding the one-to-one match opportunity to the NICU.

FSN of the High Country's purpose in evaluating their matching process was to learn how this process was happening. They wanted to be sure that the referred parent began receiving support from the supporting parent within a short time, ideally within 24 to 48 hours. The audience for the program evaluation was staff of FSN of the High Country—they could consider ways to improve their system for matching parents.

Families Together's purpose in its program evaluation was to learn how satisfied local program coordinators and supporting parents were with the technical assistance and the supporting parent orientation. Parent leaders at Families Together partnered with researchers at the Beach Center on Families and Disability at The University of Kansas to conduct a satisfaction survey of local program coordinators and supporting parents. Satisfaction data would help the staff at Families Together know how effectively they were carrying out their goals and objectives as specified in the grant and would assist them in designing future training and program development. These data would also be of interest to the Kansas Developmental Disabilities Council as a way of confirming the effective use of council funds. The audiences for the program evaluation consisted of staff at Families Together and the Kansas Developmental Disabilities Council.

Parent to Parent of Vermont joined a national research consortium to conduct an efficacy study for the purpose of generating quantitative data on the effectiveness of parent to parent support—data, combined with family stories, that would provide a comprehensive picture of the impact of parent to parent support. Parent to Parent of Vermont believed that quantitative data would strengthen the credibility of Parent to Parent programs. The intended audiences for this program evaluation thus were referral sources, parents, and possible funding sources.

Step 3: Defining Evaluation Roles and Responsibilities

Program evaluation can be a team effort, and the prospect of carrying out program evaluation may seem less intimidating if more than one person has this responsibility. Many people within a Parent to Parent program can carry out program evaluation activities, and you also may be able to collaborate with specialists and outside consultants. After you have decided what type of program evaluation you are going to do and have considered the types of skills and expertise you need to carry it out, you need to build your evaluation team. If you decide to work with an outside person, you will want to find someone who has evaluation skills and previous experience working with family service programs. Ask service providers in your area or other Parent to Parent programs for a referral to an evaluator who was helpful to them. You might also look for an outside evaluator at nearby universities and conferences.

As you talk with possible collaborators for your program evaluation, you may want to find out if they have had any previous experience with participatory action research (PAR). PAR has emerged from the work of researchers and families that believe that those who are affected by research should be involved in the full range of research activities. Several principles of PAR family research reflect the theme of participation:

- Research is a means, not an end. Its goals are to develop information and to test strategies and interventions that are designed to be useful to individuals with special needs and their families.
- Research should be a collaborative endeavor based on mutual respect, trust, and acceptance of each party's responsibilities and strengths.
- Research should be sensitive to cultural, socioeconomic, ethnic, lifestyle, and life-span diversities.
- Research should allow for a combination of methods, based on the expertise and preferences of the members of the research team.

Working to build a PAR team can ensure that more relevant research questions are asked, better intervention and dissemination strategies are developed, and more interest and commitment to the use of the research results occur. Let's look at how each of the four Parent to Parent programs defined evaluation roles and responsibilities.

The Family Connection of South Carolina benefited from the work of a researcher from the Medical University of South Carolina who had already conducted an evaluation with parents in the waiting room of the NICU at the hospital. In essence, the roles and responsibilities of the evaluation team had been previously decided as a part of this earlier research project. This evaluation team had decided who would 1) provide information about research design and research methods,

2) suggest or lead the development of evaluative instruments that might be used in the study, 3) recruit parents to participate in the program evaluation, 4) run the statistical analyses and summarize the data, and 5) write about the findings in a way that they would be meaningful to the intended audience. The Family Connection took advantage of the research activity that had been carried out. Initial meetings with the research team confirmed for the parent leaders at The Family Connection that the evaluation could provide The Family Connection with the data it needed.

As the program staff at FSN of the High Country considered their evaluation of parent matching, they decided that the roles and responsibilities of program staff included 1) developing the step-by-step procedures for the matching process, 2) developing the forms and questionnaires used to document the matched experience, and 3) recruiting parents by requesting that referred and supporting parents complete the documentation forms at certain times during their matched experience.

The evaluation teams for Families Together and Parent to Parent of Vermont (a member of the national consortium that researched the efficacy of parent to parent support) consisted of parents and researchers. The parents had firsthand knowledge of Parent to Parent, both as program directors and as parents of children with special needs. The researchers brought years of professional training and experience in conducting quantitative research. Although the roles and responsibilities varied depending on the tasks at hand, the researchers took on the following roles and responsibilities: 1) providing information about research design and research methods, 2) suggesting or leading the development of evaluative instruments that might be used in the study, 3) running the statistical analyses and summarizing the data, and 4) writing about the findings so that they are clearly understood by parents and respected by researchers. The parents took on the following roles and responsibilities: 1) providing information about Parent to Parent—showing how it works and what it does for local program coordinators and supporting parents, 2) suggesting modifications to the research design and research methods so that the evaluation was comfortable for parents, and 3) recruiting parents to participate in the program evaluation.

Step 4: Identifying Evaluation Questions to be Answered

Once you have determined the reasons for the program evaluation and for whom you are collecting the information, you will need to decide what specific questions you want to have answered. Start with key questions, and be precise as you work to break your key questions into a series of smaller, specific items. You will need to develop questions whose answers can be observed and measured. For example, finding out how many supporting parents were trained by your Parent to Parent program in the last 6 months is easy to measure by having parents sign in at each training session and counting the signatures. You also will need to word your questions carefully. For example, if you want to know the number of participants who have contacted your Parent to Parent program, you will need to define *participants* clearly. Is a participant a parent, a sibling, a service provider, or a child with special needs? Your definitions affect the answers to your questions, and the more precise you are, the more meaningful your data will be. As you form your questions, remember to select only a few related questions as the focus for any one evaluation effort. Not all evaluation questions can be answered with the same evaluation methods. If your evaluation effort involves many different questions, chances are it also will require many different evaluation methods and will become overwhelming. Save your other questions to be answered in a later evaluation activity. Be sure that you choose questions that 1) can be answered by data that you have or can get and 2) will give you useful answers for your audience.

The evaluation questions had already been determined for The Family Connection of South Carolina by the researcher from the Medical University of South Carolina:

- How do parents feel about the NICU experience and their child care demands?
- How interested are NICU parents in a parent support group, and what format and times would be best for them?
- What topics would be of most interest to NICU parents?

FSN of the High Country identified several questions to be answered in its evaluation of the implementation of the parent match:

- Are supporting parents contacting the referred parent within 24–48 hours of being matched?
- Do contacts occur between the supporting parent and the referred parent during the match, and are referred parents satisfied with the number of contacts they received?
- How satisfied are referred parents and supporting parents with the progress of their match?

Families Together took the lead in identifying several questions to be answered in its evaluation of program coordinators' and supporting parents' satisfaction with the training and technical assistance offered:

- How satisfied were local coordinators with the training they received from Families Together?
- How satisfied were local coordinators with the ongoing support they received from Families Together?
- How important was the training and ongoing support offered by Families Together to the local coordinators?
- How satisfied were supporting parents with the orientation that they received from Families Together before they were matched?
- How satisfied were supporting parents with the information and support they received from Families Together after they began serving as supporting parents?
- How important was the orientation, information, and support from Families Together to the supporting parents?

Parent to Parent of Vermont and the consortium identified several evaluation questions to be answered in their effort to evaluate the impact of the parent match:

- What is the impact of the one-to-one matched experience on referred parents' 1) sense of having a reliable ally, 2) acceptance of the disability and related issues, 3) sense of family empowerment, 4) sense of being able to cope, and 5) sense of social support?
- What is the impact of the one-to-one matched experience on referred parents' perceived stress levels?
- What is the impact of the one-to-one matched experience on referred parents' satisfaction with parent to parent support?
- What is the impact of the one-to-one matched experience on referred parents' sense that their needs have been met?
- How does the number of contacts with the supporting parent affect the referred parents' satisfaction with parent to parent support?

Step 5: Choosing Your Evaluation Methods

The next step in program evaluation is to design an evaluation plan that details the methods you will use in your evaluation.

- Who can provide the information you need to answer your questions *(sampling methods)?*
- What information will be collected *(measurement methods)?*
- How and when will you collect the information *(data collection methods)?*
- How will you analyze all of the information you collect *(data analysis issues)?*

The decisions and plans you make for sampling methods, measurement and data collection methods, and data analysis issues will be your blueprint for your overall evaluation.

Who Will Participate? You will need to decide whom to include in your evaluation effort. Who will have the information to answer your evaluation questions? If you are interested in how satisfied supporting parents are with the training that your program offers to them, then you will want to include supporting parents in your sample. But will you want to collect information from all supporting parents or just a few? Your answer to this question may be influenced by your own program budget and time issues—you may not have the resources to conduct a large-scale evaluation that involves all supporting parents. You need to consider which supporting parents should be a part of your evaluation. Perhaps you will decide to collect data from supporting parents who have been trained in the last 6 months *(purposive sample);* or perhaps you will decide to collect data from every fifth supporting parent on an alphabetical listing of all supporting parents *(random sample).* Do you need to be sure that fathers are represented in your sample? If only a few fathers are supporting parents, then you may want to include all of them *(oversampling)* so that fathers will be represented.

Your decisions about sampling also will be affected by the kind of evaluation you are doing. If you are evaluating the impact of the one-to-one match on referred parents to see whether parents who are matched do better because of the match, then you will need to have a standard of comparison. The comparison group may be parents before they were matched or other parents who were not matched. Without some basis for comparison, it would be difficult to determine whether the one-to-one match had any effect or to ascertain what might have happened to the parents if they had not been matched.

Information to Collect Your decisions about what information to collect should flow from your evaluation questions and definitions, which focus on certain characteristics or variables that are of interest to your audience. For example, state legislators might be interested in the cost benefits of parent to parent matching; referral sources to your program may want to know about the impact of parent to parent matching on children with disabilities; or a program coordinator may want to know about the number and timing of contacts in a match. For each of these examples, you need to collect different types of information. If you find that your questions and definitions do not provide clear guidelines about what information to collect, then you may need to go back and refine them. Be specific about what it is that you want to know. If your evaluation questions concern complex concepts (e.g., social support), finding ways to measure them may be difficult.

Another measurement decision you will need to make is whether to collect qualitative data or quantitative data. *Qualitative data* are collected through open-ended questions (e.g., How has Parent to Parent been helpful?) and can be summarized in a narrative form. *Quantitative data* are collected through closed questions (e.g., How many contacts did you have with your supporting parent in the last 6 months?) and require a single numerical response. Your decisions about whether to collect quantitative data or qualitative data may be based on your own program resources and your evaluation questions. Quantitative data are generally easier and faster to collect and are of great use when your evaluation questions can be answered numerically (e.g., How many hours of supporting parent training did you receive?). Qualitative data may take longer to gather but provide a depth of understanding that cannot be obtained from quantitative data. Collecting both qualitative and quantitative data offers a balance between precise measurement and the power of the descriptive word.

Collecting the Information There are different ways to collect information, and your data collection methods will depend on the kind of data you wish to collect and the time and resources you have for your program evaluation. If you are interested in collecting qualitative data from parents about their experiences in Parent to Parent, then you may want to use in-person or telephone interviews. Because interviews provide an opportunity for dialogue, you may find that you gain a better understanding of parents' views with this method than you would from responses to a multiple-choice questionnaire. However, interviews require more staff time and are not as anonymous as a written form.

Written questionnaires are used to collect quantitative data and ask participants to rank various items in terms of their importance or level of satisfaction. Most questionnaires are read and completed by the respondent and mailed back to the program evaluator, although information can be collected over the telephone or in person if there are literacy challenges. Data gathered from a questionnaire are often easier to score than interview data, although they offer less detail.

Some guidelines for formulating the questions and creating the data collection instrument are as follows:

- Find and review several instruments that have been useful to others in gathering similar information. Look at the types of questions they asked and the format and phrasing used.
- Keep your questionnaires brief. The more questions you ask, the longer it will take you to interpret the answers. It is better to get good answers to a few questions than to have too much information that will take time to evaluate.

- State each question simply, and be sure you are asking only for one piece of information per question so that there is little room for differing interpretations. Use neutral phrases and clear, objective language.
- Keep in mind that closed-ended (yes–no) questions are easier to answer and that the data are easier to enter and analyze than open-ended questions. As you develop your closed-ended questions, anticipate all possible answers to each question and include these choices on the questionnaire. A choice of *Other* will give you additional information as well.
- Open-ended questions are useful in understanding opinions, suggestions, and impressions about your program, but they take longer for people to answer and for you to interpret. After the responses have been entered, you will need to code the answers into meaningful, broad categories.
- When offering respondents an opportunity to rate services and supports, consider how many choices to give them. A scale with an odd number of choice options (e.g., 1 = Very unsatisfied, 2 = Somewhat unsatisfied, 3 = Neither unsatisfied nor satisfied, 4 = Somewhat satisfied, 5 = Very satisfied) allows people to give a neutral response. A scale with an even number of choice options (e.g., 1 = Very unsatisfied, 2 = Somewhat unsatisfied, 3 = Somewhat satisfied, 4 = Very satisfied) forces respondents to give you either a positive or a negative response. The decision you make about the number of choices you use on your questionnaires depends on the purpose of your evaluation.
- Make sure that your instruments are relevant for your target audience and for your evaluation questions. Once you have drafted your questionnaire or interview questions, it is a good idea to test them with a group that matches the individuals with whom you will be using it.

Interpreting the Information Two types of data analysis are used in program evaluation. *Quantitative analysis* uses basic mathematical calculations 1) to get a sum total of bits of information that can be counted (e.g., How many matches did the program make in the last 12 months?), 2) to get a percentage figure (e.g., What percentage of parents matched in the last 12 months were culturally diverse?), 3) to obtain a frequency distribution (e.g., How many supporting parents rated their training with a 5 for *excellent,* a 3 for *so-so,* or a 1 for *poor?*), and 4) to find an average (e.g., What was the average rating that supporting parents gave to their training?). *Qualitative analysis* looks systematically at written comments, interview responses, and other narrative information to identify major themes, trends, and relationships within the data. You will be able to determine the kind of analyses that are best for your program evaluation by referring back to your list of evaluation questions and thinking about how you would like to state the answers to each question.

The sample for a survey for The Family Connection of South Carolina needs assessment included parents who were in the NICU waiting room and who were willing to respond to the survey. Because the survey had already been developed, there was no need to develop a new instrument. The survey had 12 closed-ended questions that yielded quantitative data about parents' preferences for parent support. The data collection methods used in the study included having the written survey available in the NICU waiting room and requesting that parents complete it while they waited. The data analysis methods consisted of a quantitative analysis to summarize and interpret the data collected through the questionnaires. By using different types of mathematical calculations, a researcher was able to provide different numerical answers to the evaluation questions. The data provided a picture of how NICU parents felt about the need for and the different types of parent support (e.g., 73% of the parents either agreed or strongly agreed that it would be comforting to discuss their concerns with other parents of infants with similar problems).

FSN of the High Country decided that their sample would include all parents (either supporting parents or referred parents) who were matched by the program. Obtaining the sample was straightforward—all parents who are matched, either as a supporting parent or as a referred parent, were asked to participate by completing the necessary forms. FSN of the High Country decided to address measurement issues by collecting quantitative data so that they could objectively document the timing and the number of contacts within each match. Some of the forms that referred parents were asked to complete also contained open-ended questions so that the program staff could learn about referred parents' satisfaction with the number and timing of the contacts in their match. The data collection methods that FSN of the High Country used in the program evaluation included a number of forms for documentation of the progress of the match once it has been made:

- A letter from the network's coordinator to the supporting parent reminding him or her of the name of the referred parent and of the importance of early and frequent contacts
- A reporting form for the supporting parent to let the coordinator know the dates of each contact that is made with the referred parent

- A form to be completed by the supporting parent to let the coordinator know how the first contact went
- A follow-up form to be completed by the coordinator after the referred parent is called 2 weeks after the match to see how it is going
- A postcard to be sent to the supporting parent by the local coordinator to encourage contacts between the supporting parent and the referred parent
- A feedback form and a follow-up form for referred parents to complete after they have been matched for 3 and 6 months, respectively, that inform the coordinator about the progress of and their satisfaction with the matched experience

FSN of the High Country uses quantitative data analysis to summarize and interpret the data collected through the various documentation forms. Some qualitative data are gathered through the follow-up calls made by the match coordinator to the referred parents. By using different types of mathematical calculations, FSN of the High Country is able to provide numerical answers to the evaluation questions (e.g., What percentage of the matches have a first contact within 24 to 48 hours? How many matches are made during any given time period? How many and how frequent are the contacts in a match?). These findings help FSN of the High Country staff to be precise about what is happening in the matching process.

As Families Together considered its evaluation methods, they decided that because Parent to Parent of Kansas is a statewide resource, the sample would involve as many local coordinators and supporting parents in Kansas as possible. All local coordinators and supporting parents were invited to participate in the program evaluation effort. The team decided to collect quantitative and qualitative data for this study. Having both types of data would provide a comprehensive picture of the effectiveness of the supports being provided by Families Together. The data collection methods that the team used in the study included two written questionnaires—one for local coordinators and one for supporting parents. Each of these questionnaires was developed by the team and contained questions about the orientation and support that parents received before and after taking on the roles of either local coordinator or supporting parent. The questionnaires also had some questions about the characteristics of the local coordinator's or the supporting parent's family (e.g., size and structure of family, ages of family members, marital status, racial and ethnic background, education, income, disability of the child) so that Families Together could learn more about people who participate in Parent to Parent of Kansas. Each questionnaire also had an open-ended question at the end so that respondents could add any information that they felt had not been addressed in the questionnaire.

The researchers on the team primarily used quantitative data analysis to summarize and interpret the data collected through the questionnaires. Several mathematical calculations yielded data about parents' satisfaction with information provided to them by Families Together and its importance.

The team also used qualitative analyses to look at the responses to the open-ended question at the end of each questionnaire. Families Together found this qualitative information to be useful in expanding their understanding of how local coordinators and supporting parents felt about the supports provided to them by Families Together.

As a member of the consortium evaluating the effectiveness of Parent to Parent programs, Parent to Parent of Vermont worked to design evaluation methods that would produce relevant data. Because Parent to Parent is a national resource, the team wanted the sample to include referred parents from several states with regional and ethnic diversity. The team also wanted to recruit parents in states that had existing Parent to Parent programs. Parents and researchers from New Hampshire, Vermont, North Carolina, South Carolina, and Kansas agreed to work together to recruit parents in these five states. They decided that all parents who would participate in the study would be natural, adoptive, or stepparents of children and youth (ages birth to 21) who experience a developmental disability that qualifies them for special education services under the Individuals with Disabilities Education Act (IDEA) Amendments of 1997. The team also wanted the sample to include parents who had not been a part of a one-to-one parent to parent match. Because recruitment of people to participate in research is challenging, the team decided to enroll any parent who met all of these criteria and who understood and was comfortable with the design of the study.

The team decided to collect quantitative data for this study. Parent to Parent programs already had a lot of qualitative data (e.g., family stories, testimonials) about the impact of Parent to Parent. Quantitative data from the evaluation questions would be useful to Parent to Parent to support the qualitative data that had already been collected. The team did, however, decide to collect some qualitative data from a small sample of parents to expand its understanding of Parent to Parent.

The data collection methods used in the study included written questionnaires for all participating parents, to be completed at specific intervals before and during their one-to-one matched experience. The team used five different instruments—three that were well established and accepted in the research world and two that were developed by the consortium team. The team also conducted telephone interviews to selected parents to enhance its understanding of the quantitative data and of Parent to Parent.

The consortium primarily used quantitative data analysis to summarize and interpret all of the quantitative data that were collected through the questionnaires. The numerical scores on each of the questionnaires helped the team to be precise about what was happening in Parent to Parent and the impact of parent to parent support.

The team also used qualitative analyses to look at the written transcripts of telephone conversations with parents to identify major themes and issues that were not visible in the quantitative data. They discovered, for example, that for a few parents the one-to-one matched experience began later than the program coordinator thought it did. In another case a parent mentioned that the timing of the contacts affected their value (more frequent contacts led to greater satisfaction). This information suggests some recommended practices that Parent to Parent programs can implement to help matches be more effective—a follow-up call to both parents shortly after the match is made to be sure that an initial contact has occurred—including more information in the training of supporting parents about being sensitive to the referred parents' preferences about when contacts occur. This combination of quantitative and qualitative analyses gave the team a comprehensive snapshot of the one-to-one matched experience and its impact on referred parents.

Step 6: Preparing a Summary of Your Evaluation Results

After the information you collect through your evaluation has been analyzed, you need to consider how to present your findings. The type of summary you prepare depends on the audience with whom you will be sharing it. Some audiences (e.g., an agency that is funding a grant to your program) may expect a comprehensive written report and may provide you with a format for the report. Other audiences (e.g., the board of directors for your program) may only need a set of charts and tables verbally explained to them. You may find it useful to prepare several versions of the summary of your evaluation to use with different audiences.

A comprehensive evaluation report should contain most, if not all, of the items on the sample outline in Figure 13.1. Following this outline allows you to provide your audience with a description of your program and the results of your evaluation. Tables and charts can be used to present your data efficiently, but be sure to include interpretations and explanations in your text, as well as a discussion of the implications of your findings and suggested next steps.

Each of the four Parent to Parent programs prepared an evaluation report similar in content to the sample in Figure 13.1. A summary report of the results of the survey of NICU parents was prepared and presented to hospital staff and to the board of directors at The Family Connection of South Carolina. Because the program evaluation of the implementation of the match is ongoing at FSN of the High Country, staff are constantly using the results and making changes and refinements to the matching process. However, they know that at any moment they can prepare a summary of the evaluation results that reports and interprets the results and discusses the implications of the findings for the program.

Families Together prepared a summary report of Parent to Parent of Kansas for the Kansas Developmental Disabilities Council that included results of the satisfaction questionnaires and results of other types of program evaluation documenting the need and impact for Parent to Parent. In addition, a summary report of the satisfaction questionnaires was prepared for the parents who completed the questionnaires.

Parent to Parent of Vermont and the consortium developed different summaries of the evaluation results—three articles about the findings and implications were published by professional journals, and an abridged summary of the results was prepared for parents and service providers. A listing of articles about parent to parent support appears in the resources at the end of this chapter.

Step 7: Incorporating Your Findings in Program Planning

Although program evaluation answers many questions about your program and its effectiveness, it leaves some questions unanswered and even raises new ones. Use of your evaluation findings may be a gradual, cumulative process in which you change some questions and add others as you build your knowledge base. For example, in the national study to determine the effectiveness of Parent to Parent, the consortium asked, "What is the impact of the one-to-one match on the referred parent?" As the research progressed, the team discovered that in a few cases a referred parent was matched with a supporting parent who had not been trained. A new question arose: "What is the impact of a match between an untrained supporting parent and a referred parent?" The research answered some questions while presenting new ones.

Look at your program mission, goals, objectives, and activities to decide how your findings can be used. Do your findings suggest that changes need to happen or that new questions need to be asked? Perhaps you will discover the format for your supporting parent training needs to be revised because parents can no longer commit to a full day

Outline for an Evaluation Report

Description of the program

Target population and community characteristics

Program mission, goals, and objectives

Program structure, content, and service delivery model

Description of evaluation

Evaluation questions

Design, including sampling procedures and time frames

Data collection procedures

Measurement instruments (include copies in an appendix)

Reliability and validity of measures

Limitations in the design, data collection, or measurement procedures

Results

Description of participants

Documentation of program resources and activities

Interpretation of results

Recommendations for dissemination and utilization of the findings

Figure 13.1. Outline for an evaluation report. (From Littell, J.H. [1986]. *Building strong foundations: Evaluation strategies for family resource programs* [p. 54]. Chicago: Family Resource Coalition; reprinted by permission.)

of training on Saturday. Maybe you will find that your new follow-up system for tracking the progress of matches is one that supporting parents are satisfied with and you know that you are moving in the right direction. An important piece of the evaluation is that you use the results to shape the focus and direction of your program.

The data from its survey enabled The Family Connection of South Carolina to expand talks with hospital officials about the need for parent to parent matching for NICU families. With this information, and supported by a grant from the hospital foundation, The Family Connection of South Carolina expanded the Parent to Parent program and its own visibility in the hospital and clinic. Support activities and visibility in the hospital have made an impact on families. In the first 5 months of the new NICU program, nearly 40 parents completed the 12-hour support parent training program and more than 70 referrals and 50 parent matches were made. The success of the program has garnered additional support from the hospital and the community.

As the program evaluation of the implementation of the matched experience continues, FSN of the High Country keeps refining their procedures for making and documenting the matches based on what they learn from referred parents and from supporting parents.

Families Together needed to provide the Kansas Developmental Disabilities Council with evidence that their funds had been put to good use. The satisfaction data confirmed the usefulness of the supports provided to local coordinators and supporting parents by Families Together. Families Together also has been able to use the data to strengthen the orientation and ongoing support provided to local coordinators and to supporting parents. Training for local coordinators had originally been held over 2 days, beginning on Friday evening and ending Saturday afternoon. The results of the satisfaction survey indicated that local coordinators preferred to have the training only on Saturday. Families Together is considering how to modify the training to be responsive to local coordinators' preferences.

The research and the precision that research demands have documented what is happening in parent to parent matches, and Parent to Parent of Vermont and the other program coordinators on the consortium team have described this learning experience as being like going to "Parent to Parent school." On the basis of the results of this study, new procedures have been initiated by program coordinators to ensure that matches begin as quickly as possible after the initial referral and that at least four contacts occur during the first 8 weeks of the match. The data also suggest ways in which the training for supporting parents might be modified to add to the overall quality of the matched experience. New questions for research also have been identified (e.g.,

What is the impact of the one-to-one matched experience on the supporting parent?). The consortium shared the findings of this study and discussed the implications of the results for Parent to Parent programs nationwide.

SUMMARY

Coordinating a Parent to Parent program is a busy job with many responsibilities to the parents served by the program, to professionals who refer and learn from parents, to the board of directors who govern the program, and to funding agencies that support the program. And although program evaluation may seem like one more responsibility that may not have an obvious or immediate benefit, the four Parent to Parent programs featured in this chapter used program evaluation to enhance their services. The Family Connection of South Carolina expanded its services into the NICU of a large hospital. FSN of the High Country uses ongoing program evaluation activities to continually refine its matching procedures. Families Together used its program evaluation to satisfy its funding source and strengthen its training and technical assistance for local program coordinators and supporting parents. Parent to Parent of Vermont and the consortium demonstrated that Parent to Parent works, and the efficacy data are being used to enhance the credibility of Parent to Parent programs.

REFERENCES

Gurman, A.S., & Kniskern, D.P. (1981). Family therapy outcome research: Knowns and unknowns. In A.S. Gurman & D.P. Kniskern (Eds.), *Handbook of family therapy* (p. 744). New York: Brunner/Mazel.

Individuals with Disabilities Education Act (IDEA) Amendments of 1997, PL 105-17, 20 U.S.C. §§ 1400 *et seq.*

RESOURCES

Following are several articles about Parent to Parent that provide descriptive and evaluative data. Parent to Parent programs are citing these articles in their promotional and program evaluation activities:

Ainbinder, J., Blanchard, L., Singer, G.H.S., Sullivan, M., Powers, L., Marquis, J., & Santelli, B. (1998). How parents help one another: A qualitative study of Parent to Parent self-help. *Journal of Pediatric Psychology, 23,* 99–109.

Parent to Parent Program Evaluation Manual, developed by the team of parents and researchers that conducted the national study to determine the effectiveness of Parent to Parent, is available through the Beach Center on Families and Disability at The University of Kansas (see Appendix C).

Santelli, B., Singer, G.H.S., DiVenere, N., Ginsberg, C., & Powers, L. (1998). Participatory action research: Reflections on critical incidents in a PAR project. *Journal of The Association for Persons with Severe Handicaps, 23*(3), 211–222.

Santelli, B., Turnbull, A.P., & Higgins, C. (1996). Parent to Parent support and health care. *Pediatric Nursing, 23*(3), 303–306.

Santelli, B., Turnbull, A.P., Lerner, E., & Marquis, J. (1993). Parent to Parent programs: A unique form of mutual support for families of persons with disabilities. In G.H.S. Singer & L.E. Powers (Eds.), *Families, disability, and empowerment: Active coping skills and strategies for family interventions* (pp. 27–57). Baltimore: Paul H. Brookes Publishing Co.

Santelli, B., Turnbull, A.P., Marquis, J., & Lerner, E. (1993). Parent to Parent programs: Ongoing support for parents of young adults with special needs. *Journal of Vocational Rehabilitation, 3*(2), 25–37.

Santelli, B., Turnbull, A.P., Marquis, J., & Lerner, E. (1995). Parent to Parent programs: A unique form of mutual support. *Infants and Young Children, 8*(2), 48–57.

Santelli, B., Turnbull, A.P., Marquis, J., & Lerner, E. (1997). Parent to Parent programs: A resource for parents and professionals. *Journal of Early Intervention, 21*(1), 73–83.

Santelli, B., Turnbull, A.P., Marquis, J., & Lerner, E. (2000). Statewide Parent to Parent programs: Partners in early intervention. *Infants and Young Children, 13*(1), 74–88.

Santelli, B., Turnbull, A.P., Sergeant, J., Lerner, E., & Marquis, J. (1996). Parent to Parent programs: Parent preferences for support. *Infants and Young Children, 9*(1), 53–62.

Singer, G.H.S., Marquis, J., Powers, L., Blanchard, L., DiVenere, N., Santelli, B., & Sharp, M. (1999). A multi-site evaluation of Parent to Parent programs for parents of children with disabilities. *Journal of Early Intervention, 22*(3), 217–229.

IV

Growing to the Future

14

Developing Statewide Programs

Expanded Opportunities for Support

"Nationwide thinking, nationwide planning, and nationwide action are the three great essentials to prevent nationwide crises for future generations to struggle through."

—Franklin D. Roosevelt

As you have learned in previous chapters, local Parent to Parent programs exist in every state in the United States. These community-based programs provide support to families in the local area. In 30 states, a statewide Parent to Parent program exists to ensure that families across the state have access to information and emotional support through parent to parent matching. In many of these states, the statewide Parent to Parent program also maintains a database of families that are willing to be matched around specific disability issues so that if a local parent match cannot be found, the parent may be able to find a match with another parent living in the same state. Statewide programs often provide training and technical assistance to the local efforts to support the development of new local programs and to nurture the growth of existing programs.

In a few states, the statewide Parent to Parent program also serves as the federally funded parent training and information center (PTI). When a statewide Parent to Parent program also is the PTI, then the program offers the one-to-one parent matching that Parent to Parent programs provide and the information and training to parents about the educational needs and rights of children with disabilities that PTIs provide. In other states, the statewide Parent to Parent program has a close tie with the state's early intervention agency or with a university. Statewide Parent to Parent programs sometimes evolve from existing local programs that are seeking statewide coordination and technical assistance; in other cases the statewide Parent to Parent program comes first, with local efforts following later. No two state Parent to Parent programs are exactly alike, and the program in your state will be unique to your state.

In this chapter, you learn about guidelines for developing a statewide Parent to Parent program and creative strategies that are utilized by statewide Parent to Parent programs to enhance services for people with disabilities and their families.

DEVELOPING A STATEWIDE PARENT TO PARENT PROGRAM

If you are thinking about starting a Parent to Parent program in your state, most of the local program development strategies presented in Chapters 5–10 can be applied to statewide program development as well. Some aspects of statewide Parent to Parent programs, however, are unique, and this chapter introduces you to these elements.

As you begin to plan a statewide Parent to Parent program, remember that there are resources to help you get started—you don't have to do it all from scratch. There are many excellent information and training materials on Parent to Parent program development and implementation available from established statewide Parent to Parent programs (see the resources in Chapters 5 and 6). You also may want to find out whether any Parent to Parent programs exist in your state. Talk with other parents and providers about parent support programs that they may know of in your own region or in other regions of your state. The PTI in your state may maintain lists of resources and may know of Parent to Parent programs in the state. Similarly, representatives of state agencies (either programs with a specific disability focus such as an attention-deficit/hyperactivity disorder group or noncategorical programs such as The Arc) may know of local programs offering parent to parent support. If you are able to attend statewide conferences for parents and professionals who are involved in the families and disability field, you may learn about Parent to Parent programs in other parts of your state. The Beach Center on Families and Disability at The University of Kansas maintains and updates a list of Parent to Parent programs in each state (see Appendix C for contact information).

If there are already local Parent to Parent programs in your state, you may find it helpful to bring them into the early planning for the state program. Local program coordinators are wonderful resources to an emerging statewide program, and their participation in the initial planning should minimize any turf issues later. Even if the local program coordinators do not want to take an active role in the development of the statewide program but want to keep serving families locally, they will appreciate being asked and being informed about developments at the state level.

ORGANIZATIONAL MODELS OF STATEWIDE PARENT TO PARENT PROGRAMS

The 30 statewide Parent to Parent programs are unique in how they are organized and how they meet the needs of local efforts, and they vary considerably in terms of how they implement their program activities and how they interact with parents and/or local programs. The statewide programs, however, have some common organizational styles and themes.

Centralized Statewide Parent to Parent Programs

Some statewide programs are *centralized,* with all major program activities happening at the state level. In a centralized program, there are no local Parent to Parent programs, but rather there are trained supporting parents residing in communities across the state. The statewide program trains these local supporting parents and matches them with parents who are referred to the program. With a centralized statewide program, a community may have only one supporting parent or it may have many, but there is no local autonomous Parent to Parent program in the community.

Parent to Parent of Vermont

Parent to Parent of Vermont began in 1984 as a peer support program of the Champlain Arc providing one-to-one parent support to parents in Chittenden County. In 1988, in response to the need for parent matching across the state, Parent to Parent of Vermont incorporated as a public nonprofit statewide support and information network for families whose children have a chronic illness, disability, or were born prematurely.

Because Vermont is a small state, Chittenden County is only a few hours away from all of the state's rural communities. Therefore, coordinating Parent to Parent activities out of the statewide office is quite manageable. All referrals come to the Parent to Parent of Vermont central office staff through a single access telephone number. The staff at the central office maintain the roster of trained supporting parents and make all of the matches. Once a match is made, the statewide program staff document the progress of the match and provide follow-up support to the match as needed.

Parent to Parent of Vermont develops all of the training and promotional materials that are needed and used throughout the state. Brochures, public service announcements, and fliers are all produced in the central office and all have the same look and access number for families all across the state. Local supporting parents help to distribute these promotional materials in their communities on behalf of the statewide effort.

Because many of the local communities in Vermont are small and rural, there may be only a few parents of children with special needs who live close by. In these communities there may not be enough parents to develop and sustain a local Parent to Parent program. Given the geography and demographics of the state of Vermont, it makes perfect sense for the statewide Parent to Parent program to be centralized.

Decentralized Statewide Parent to Parent Programs

Other statewide programs are *decentralized,* with the statewide program providing training and technical assistance to autonomous local Parent to Parent programs. The local programs carry out Parent to Parent activities in their communities, with the statewide program assisting as requested.

Family Support Network of North Carolina

In 1985, with a grant from the North Carolina Council on Developmental Disabilities, a physician and a social worker developed two local Parent to Parent programs and an initiative to involve families in the education of medical students. From this beginning, Family Support Network (FSN) of North Carolina has evolved to include a statewide network of 25 local Parent to Parent programs for which FSN's central office serves as the coordinating arm.

Local programs develop at their own pace in their home communities, and each local program may look very different. Each local program within FSN has its own name and identity. The local programs in North Carolina either have their own 501(c)3 nonprofit status or are sponsored by another nonprofit organization in the community. Some local programs have paid coordinators, some do not, and most local program coordinators are part time and have the full responsibility for carrying out program activities. Local programs have their own local governing or advisory boards that work with them to raise funds and plan programs.

Each local program handles its own promotional efforts by producing its own brochures and fliers, and each has its own telephone number for taking referrals. The coordinator makes the matches and also may provide training to the supporting parents. Some of the local programs only offer parent matching and others have a wide variety of other program activities.

FSN, as the statewide program, provides technical assistance in all aspects of program operation to these autonomous local programs or chapters across the state. FSN trains local coordinators and supports the local efforts but does not control the programs' development. As a resource to the local programs, they also offer training for parents wishing to be supporting parents if a local program requests it. When a local coordinator cannot find a match, FSN can search its database of parents to make a statewide match.

Given the size of North Carolina, the distance between communities, the diversity of its communities (some large and urban, others small and rural), and the interest of parents in several communities to develop local Parent to Parent programs, it makes perfect sense for North Carolina to adopt a decentralized model for its statewide Parent to Parent program.

Somewhere in the Middle

Most programs fall somewhere in the middle on the continuum of centralization, and some programs are more centralized in some activities and more decentralized in others. For example, promotional activities may occur at the statewide level, although the training and matching of supporting parents may be implemented regionally or locally. These statewide programs often employ several regional coordinators to assist and personalize the statewide services in their respective regions. Over time, perhaps in an effort to enhance its services statewide or to respond to funding realities, a statewide program may adapt its organizational structure, becoming more or less centralized or decentralized. Parent to Parent of Georgia started as a decentralized program, moved toward a more centralized structure, and is now somewhere in the middle.

Parent to Parent of Georgia

Parent to Parent of Georgia started in 1980 as a 3-year project of the Governor's Council on Developmental Disabilities. A group of parents trained and supported other parents in communities across Georgia to develop their own local Parent to Parent programs. For several years, these local programs handled their own referrals and matches, with technical assistance from the central office in Atlanta. Over time, however, some of these programs lost their coordinators, and when replacement coordinators could not be found, the local programs ceased to exist. To ensure that parent matching services continued for parents across the state, even in communities without a local program, Parent to Parent of Georgia moved toward a more centralized model.

Parent to Parent of Georgia has a toll-free telephone number that connects all families to the statewide office, with all parent referrals coming directly to the statewide office. Four paid regional coordinators make matches for parents living within their regions. The statewide office maintains a database of parents and assists with matches when a local or regional match cannot be found. Regional coordinators provide training to parents who wish to be supporting parents in their region and assist with promotional activities on behalf of Parent to Parent of Georgia. Parent to Parent of Georgia has trained more than 2,000 parents representing 140 of Georgia's 159 counties. The shift from a decentralized to a more centralized model with regional activities means that Parent to Parent of Georgia has been able to continue to meet the needs of parents throughout the state.

The organizational structure that seems most appropriate for you depends on the "lay of the land" in your state. You may want to consider the following:

- *Size and geography of your state:* In smaller states it is possible for all of the Parent to Parent activities to be provided statewide from the state office—shorter distances from one end of the state to the other make it feasible for statewide program staff to get to local communities to train supporting parents. Statewide programs in larger states need to consider the distance factor in delivering training and support to local communities. In smaller and/or more rural states, the local communities may be small and may not have enough parents to support the development of a local program, whereas in larger, more populated states many communities will have more than enough parents to support a local program.
- *Presence of existing Parent to Parent programs:* An important fact to consider is whether Parent to Parent programs exist in your state and whether there is statewide support for these programs. Sometimes an existing Parent to Parent program in a state that is developing a statewide program may wish to retain its full autonomy—in which case a centralized model most likely would not work.

- *Presence of other statewide organizations providing support to families and how these services are organized across the state:* It may make sense to organize the statewide Parent to Parent program to fit in with existing statewide systems. For example, Parent to Parent of New Hampshire took advantage of existing (and funded) regional family support councils and was able to add the Parent to Parent component in each region.

DETERMINING LEADERSHIP

Once you have identified existing local Parent to Parent programs, you also may want to consider who else in your state is interested in being a part of the development of the statewide program. Building a broad participatory action team for the development of a statewide program will bring a range of perspectives and resources to your effort. Consider the following questions as you build your team of partners:

1. *Who might use the services of a statewide Parent to Parent program by referring families?* As you learned in Chapter 5, most referrals to Parent to Parent programs come from the medical and educational communities. Many statewide Parent to Parent programs are launched simply by bringing representatives from key referral sources together for an informational meeting and a chance to brainstorm about the role that a statewide Parent to Parent program can play in the state.
2. *Who might be able to help you secure funding for the program?* Chapter 9 provides information about possible funding sources for a Parent to Parent program (e.g., state agencies, private foundations), and you may want to invite representatives from these entities to participate in the early conceptualization of the program. They may be sufficiently enlightened during these early discussions that they offer financial support later.
3. *Who is a part of the existing statewide service system for families who have a family member with a disability?* Every state has different agencies that offer particular services to children with special needs and their families (e.g., Department of Health, Department of Education, Department of Human Services). Because a statewide Parent to Parent program also will be offering services to families across the state, representatives from these other state resources may be interested in how best to integrate complementary services.

You also will need to be sure that parents are well represented at this meeting so that the family perspective informs the discussion. At the meeting you may want to include the following items on your agenda:

- Overview of parent to parent support and how it is different from other types of support to parents; invite parents to share their personal experiences
- Statewide Parent to Parent programs—how they are structured in other states and what they do for families and for local Parent to Parent efforts
- Current resources for families in your state and how Parent to Parent might collaborate with and enhance these efforts
- State funding options for Parent to Parent in your state—both public and private
- Your vision for statewide Parent to Parent in your state
- Plans for next steps

Parents in New Jersey started this way, and at the end of their initial meeting with key stakeholders, the representative from the Department of Public Health promised significant funding support for the statewide program. Another important reason for beginning this way is that it is participatory—when other key players in the realm of family support in your state have the opportunity to be involved (even if they choose not to), they will feel less threatened by the developing statewide Parent to Parent program and more invested in its success.

As you read in Chapter 7, one key to the success of any Parent to Parent program is parent leadership in the development and implementation of the program. A visible parent commitment to the program from the outset will enhance the program's credibility in the eyes of other parents. When professionals have the opportunity to learn from parents in leadership positions about the unique support provided by Parent to Parent programs, they often are able to support the development of the statewide program in ways that enhance the program's credibility in the eyes of other professionals. Most statewide Parent to Parent programs were started by a team of parents and professionals in partnership. As you pull together your leadership team, think about other parents who might work with you and consider which professionals might be your reliable allies as well.

DECIDING SPONSORSHIP AND AGENCY SUPPORT

A statewide Parent to Parent program may be established as an entirely volunteer organization with its own nonprofit status, or it may be sponsored by a service provider agency, disability organization, or existing parent group. A majority of statewide Parent to Parent programs prefer the autonomy that a nonsponsored status permits. Chapter 7 provides you with detailed information about sponsorship issues for local programs, and these same issues apply to statewide programs as well.

The most common sponsoring agency for a statewide Parent to Parent program is the federally funded PTI. In Florida, Kansas, Arizona, and New Mexico, the statewide Parent to Parent program is a component of the PTI. In some cases, as in Kansas, the PTI came first and then the Parent to Parent component was added. In most cases, the statewide Parent to Parent program evolved first and competed for the federal grant for the PTI. The statewide Parent to Parent program in New Jersey is an autonomous program with its own line of funding, but it has chosen to have the PTI serve as its fiscal agent.

FUNDING CONSIDERATIONS

Statewide Parent to Parent programs sometimes start on a volunteer basis with little or no funding, and the dedication and commitment of a core group of parents is the force behind a program's success. But for Parent to Parent activities to occur across the state in a timely and coordinated fashion, a minimal funding base needs to be established in the first 12 months, with a more substantial funding base needed later to hire staff and to support the breadth and depth of activities of a mature program. At the end of their first 12 months, more than 75% of statewide programs reported an annual budget of less than $100,000, whereas in the year 1997, more than 75% of the programs reported an annual budget of more than $100,000. Clearly, statewide programs have been successful in expanding the size of their initial annual budgets (see Table 14.1 in Appendix A).

Where to find funding to support a newly developing statewide Parent to Parent program and to support the program for the long term is a critical question, and the funding experiences of existing statewide Parent to Parent programs may provide you with some ideas. (See Table 14.2 in Appendix A). Statewide programs often are supported financially by funds from several different public and private sources at the state and national levels.

State Funding Opportunities

Almost one third of statewide Parent to Parent programs receive early funding support from their state developmental disabilities councils. These councils often provide 2–3 years of seed money to support the initial development of statewide resources for individuals with disabilities and their families. Sometimes applying for developmental disabilities council funds requires a grant application in response to a request for proposals (RFP). In other cases, the council may elect to award discretionary funds to support the development of the program. Developmental disabilities councils traditionally have been wonderful supporters of newly developing statewide Parent to Parent efforts; however, they typically fund only one initial cycle of funding (usually 2–3 years) and expect a fledgling program to secure alternative funding to support its ongoing and long-term existence.

Sometimes a newly developing statewide program receives funding from more than one state agency, and often a single state agency is more willing to fund a new state resource if other state agencies have also agreed to support it. When you begin to search for funding, you may find it helpful to convene a meeting of representatives from the state agencies that you believe would support the mission of a statewide Parent to Parent program. Possible representatives include state agencies that oversee education, health, mental health, and social services. The names of these agencies may differ in each state, but most states have state-level agencies that oversee services in these respective areas.

Universities also may be willing to support a statewide Parent to Parent program. Most major universities have a university affiliated program (UAP) that helps to translate research into practice. UAPs often fund and conduct research and model programs to develop state-of-the-art procedures for meeting the needs of children and adults with disabilities and their families. They also train future service providers. Since the 1990s, universities, and UAPs in particular, have shown a greater interest in Parent to Parent as a unique form of support for parents who have a family member with a disability. UAPs have come to recognize the power of involving parents and offering one-to-one parent to parent support in their model programs. A number of UAPs also are involving parents as community faculty in the preparation of future service providers. Be sure to check with your state's universities about possible partnerships and funding opportunities.

Federal Funding Opportunities

A few statewide Parent to Parent programs have been able to get federal funding for their program development activities, but statewide efforts have been more successful at securing state funding than federal funding. The Division of Services for Children with Special Health Care Needs at the Maternal and Child Health Bureau (MCHB) in the U.S. Department of Health and Human Services often offers competitive grant opportunities in family support, and their funding priorities sometimes fit with the proposed activities of statewide Parent to Parent programs.

Federal funding for early intervention services (Part C of the Individuals with Disabilities Education Act [IDEA] Amendments of 1997) has supported the start-up of some statewide Parent to Parent programs and supported the existence of 39% of statewide programs in 1997. Although developing and existing statewide programs do not apply directly to the federal government for Part C funds, they have been able to take advantage of the fact that each state has received Part C federal funds to support their early intervention services. Because family-centered early intervention services are mandated by Part C of IDEA and because Parent to Parent programs provide family-centered services, there has been an increase in the number of partnerships (with funding) between local and state early intervention efforts and Parent to Parent efforts.

A few statewide programs receive funding from their PTI. Statewide Parent to Parent programs and PTIs are recognizing that parents need the information and advocacy support that are provided by PTIs and the one-to-one emotional support and personalized information that are provided through a parent to parent match. This enhanced awareness and understanding explains, at least in part, why more statewide Parent to Parent programs received funding in 1997 from their PTI than during their first 12 months of existence. The Office of Special Education Programs, within the Office of Special Education and Rehabilitative Services in the U.S. Department of Education, funds the PTIs. Regardless of whether your statewide program ever receives funding from the PTI in your state, hopefully you will be able to develop a positive, noncompetitive relationship with your PTI. Families are the ultimate beneficiaries when services are delivered collaboratively.

Statewide Parent to Parent programs rely on a variety of other funding sources to support their activities. Many of these funding sources are local (e.g., civic clubs, churches, hospitals, school districts), private, or rely on the generosity of others (e.g., donations, in-kind services). Chapter 9 includes comprehensive information about funding sources for Parent to Parent programs and a detailed description of fund-raising strategies.

Organizational and Funding Stories

Two parents and a professional started RAISING Special Kids in Phoenix in 1979 as a Parent to Parent program for matching parents of young children with disabilities. The Arc of Arizona served as the fiscal agent and the sponsor for the developing program. In 1985, because the Parent to Parent program had grown considerably and wanted to expand to offer support to families with school-age children, the founders of the program applied for and were awarded a federal grant to serve as the PTI for Arizona. Additional state funding from the developmental disabilities council supported the continued expansion of the parent matching component. The program formally incorporated as a not-for-profit corporation, with a board of directors composed of a majority of parents of children with various disabilities along with other interested community people.

Parent to Parent of Connecticut was initiated in 1987 by the collaborative efforts of parents and staff members from the University of Connecticut Health Center. In its first year, the program, which received in-kind support from the University of Connecticut, provided training and start-up assistance to two local Parent to Parent programs. In its second year, Parent to Parent of Connecticut received a small grant from the Connecticut Department of Mental Retardation and launched two more local programs. In 1989, the developmental disabilities council in Connecticut awarded Parent to Parent of Connecticut with a 3-year grant, allowing the program to hire a parent to coordinate the development of a statewide network of local Parent to Parent programs. In 1991, Parent to Parent Network of Connecticut, along with other parent programs from the university, collaborated to open the Family Center, a statewide resource that is located in the Connecticut Children's Medical Center and offers support, information, and training to families who have a child with special needs. Presently, the Parent to Parent network is housed within the Family Center, with funding to the Family Center (and to Parent to Parent) coming from private grants, training contracts, and an ongoing financial commitment from the Connecticut Children's Medical Center. Parent to Parent of Connecticut is unique in its affiliation with the Connecticut Children's Medical Center. Although the hospital has made a significant financial contribution to Parent to Parent of Connecticut, the statewide program has been able to maintain complete parent ownership and autonomy with no constraints on its ability to serve families through this affiliation. Thus, Parent to Parent of Connecticut has been able to maintain a broad-based grass roots component while centralizing the funding and administration pieces.

Parent to Parent of New Hampshire started in 1989 as the local Parent to Parent program (Upper Valley Support Group) and expanded to meet the needs of parents statewide. With a grant from the MCHB, the Upper Valley Support Group launched a statewide networking project in collaboration with the Institute on Disability (a UAP) and the Bureau of Special Medical Services (Title V). In 1991, the MCHB project funded four regions to begin or expand their own local Parent to Parent programs, and in 1994 additional funding from the New Hampshire Bureau of Developmental Services supported the development of local programs in 12 regions. Funds for the local programs have been reallocated within the existing New Hampshire Family

Support Legislation, and funding to the local programs is renewed on a yearly basis. Parent to Parent of New Hampshire provides leadership, training, and technical assistance to this network of local Parent to Parent programs.

In 1995, the Northwest New Jersey Regional Early Intervention Collaborative, funded under federal early intervention Part C money, initiated a demonstration Parent to Parent program. In 1996, at the initiative of the parents, representatives from disability organizations, several state agencies, parents, community members, and professionals working in related fields met together to explore ways to bring the vision to reality. One year later, New Jersey Statewide Parent to Parent, with funding from the New Jersey Department of Health and Senior Services under Special Child and Health Services, launched its activities statewide. The program also has collaborative relationships with the PTI in New Jersey (Statewide Parent Advocacy Network [SPAN]) and the Family Support Center of New Jersey. SPAN serves as the fiscal agent for New Jersey Statewide Parent to Parent, and the Family Support Center shares their toll-free telephone number and their resource library with New Jersey Statewide Parent to Parent. New Jersey Statewide Parent to Parent is divided into four regions, and each one has a part-time regional associate who conducts outreach, provides training for support parents, coordinates parent matches, and offers technical assistance to local Parent to Parent programs. An advisory board, comprising mostly parents, meets quarterly.

A small group of parents and professionals started Parent to Parent of New York State in 1984 to offer one-to-one emotional and informational support to parents of children with disabilities. They developed their own by-laws, launched a publicity campaign, and began making parent matches—all on a volunteer basis. During the next 2 years, the program grew quickly and soon needed a permanent office and telephone line. The program founders approached the New York Easter Seals Society and received donated office space and the use of the Easter Seals toll-free telephone number. From 1986 until 1994, the program remained at the New York Easter Seals and grew to a statewide network of more than 500 trained support parents. In 1994, with funding from a family support grant awarded by the New York State Office of Mental Retardation and Developmental Disabilities, Parent to Parent of New York State established its own statewide office. The PTI in upstate New York served as the fiscal agent for Parent to Parent of New York State. Currently, Parent to Parent of New York State oversees program activities in seven regional offices, with each office employing one full-time paid coordinator and receiving in-kind support from a related agency.

Several parents in Pennsylvania were so united in their determination to create a statewide Parent to Parent program that after some unsuccessful initial grant writing efforts, they approached administrators from three state agencies—the Office of Mental Retardation, the Office of Mental Health, and the Office of Children and Youth—to discuss funding possibilities. In 1996, with funding from these three departments, the parents launched Parent to Parent of Pennsylvania. The program takes advantage of many in-kind services (e.g., the toll-free telephone number is shared with and funded by Special Kids Network, a Department of Health initiative; several computers have been donated by the Department of Education; printing needs are being met by a vocational-technical school). Part-time regional coordinators work to recruit and train support parents, match parents and support the matches, and provide technical assistance to those wishing to start a local program.

Parents and supportive professionals founded The Family Connection of South Carolina, and in 1989 The Family Connection incorporated as a non-profit organization. In 1990, with funding from the developmental disabilities council, the South Carolina Department of Disabilities and Special Needs, and private donations, a full-time program coordinator and a part-time executive director were hired to work in donated space at the Easter Seals Society. In 1992, The Family Connection was awarded a contract by the state of South Carolina to provide parent to parent support through its Family Partners Program to parents of infants and toddlers who are eligible for the state's early intervention program. The Family Partners Program provided the springboard for statewide parent to parent support for families that have children with special needs of all ages. Although most of the services of The Family Connection are centralized, a local Parent to Parent program in partnership with Children's Hospital of Greenville also is supported by the The Family Connection staff.

Washington State Parent to Parent began in 1982 as a local program sponsored by The Arc of King County. As the program grew to meet the needs of parents in the Seattle area, parents in other parts of the state expressed interest in replicating the model. In 1988, replication efforts began across the state, and in 2000, 25 community-based Parent to Parent programs and a Washington State Parent to Parent Coordinating Office served families in all 39 counties. Each local program is either autonomous or has a sponsoring agency, and each program has its own advisory board, paid parent coordinator, and core of trained helping parents. The Washington State Parent to Parent Coordinating Office serves as the umbrella organization and provides training and technical assistance to the local programs. Local programs are responsible for training helping parents and matching and providing information to referred parents in their area of the state.

Initial funding for the statewide initiative in Washington came from the Office of the Superintendent of Public Instruction that continues to use IDEA-619 Part B (Early Childhood Discretionary) funds to support the programs. The program also receives a state-level contract from the Washington State Department of Health, Office of Children with Special Health Care

Needs (Title V funds). But most of the program operating costs come from local sources—school districts, educational service districts, county and regional developmental disability programs, the United Way, service clubs, and fundraisers.

IMPLEMENTING AND COORDINATING PROGRAM ACTIVITIES FOR FAMILIES

How centralized or decentralized a statewide Parent to Parent program is determines how the major program activities of a statewide Parent to Parent program (e.g., recruiting and training supporting parents, making parent matches, adding other program activities for families) are implemented and coordinated. In a centralized program, these program activities are accomplished by the statewide program itself, whereas in a decentralized program, each local program carries out its own program activities with support from the statewide program as needed. Many statewide programs rely on both the statewide staff and the regional staff to coordinate program activities. Regardless of whether program activities are carried out at the local, regional, or state level, there are different strategies to consider when implementing the program activities for families (see Chapters 5–9 and Table 14.3 in Appendix A).

PROGRAM ACTIVITIES FOR PROFESSIONALS

In addition to offering program activities for families, many statewide programs are involved in the preservice and in-service training of professionals who will be or are already working with families who have children with disabilities. Parents as trainers and community faculty bring an important perspective to service delivery that cannot be fully captured in a textbook or classroom setting.

Training Professionals

RAISING Special Kids in Arizona collaborated with Southwest Human Development Inc. to form the Southwest Institute for Family-Centered Practice, an innovative professional development entity. The Southwest Institute for Family-Centered Practice offers a variety of in-service training opportunities for professionals to help them learn about, adopt, and incorporate into their work the principles of family-centered care. At the Southwest Institute for Family-Centered Practice, family members are equal partners in the develop-

ment of the training content and the training methods and in the delivery of the training sessions as co-trainers.

The Family TIES program in Massachusetts collaborated with the Institute for Community Inclusion at Children's Hospital on a pilot project titled Learning Together. Through the project, family members co-develop and co-present in-service training sessions on family-centered care for health professionals. An offshoot of the Learning Together project has been the Family Grand Rounds series—a project in collaboration with the American Academy of Pediatrics. Through this project, Family TIES hosts discussion forums with local health care providers that enhance their understanding of the family perspective.

Parent to Parent of Vermont coordinates a number of different preservice training opportunities for medical, education, and health professionals. In partnership with the Department of Pediatrics at the University of Vermont Medical School, the Medical Education Project provides third-year medical students with a four-part seminar titled "The Practice of Family Centered Care." Parent to Parent of Vermont staff serve as co-faculty teaching the first two sessions of the seminar along with physician faculty members at the University of Vermont Medical School. For the third part of the seminar, each medical student is matched with and visits a family who has a child with special needs. The family experience is the learning experience. A final session consists of a facilitated discussion to help the medical students reflect on their home visit with the family and consider this experience within the context of the entire seminar. In 12 years, 687 medical students had the privilege of learning from families who have opened their homes and shared their wisdom and experiences.

The success of the Medical Education Project has prompted Parent to Parent of Vermont to work in partnership with other faculty at the University of Vermont to broaden the education of those preparing to work with children and families. Between 1996 and 2000 all first-year graduate students in the Communication Sciences Department had been matched with families. In addition, Parent to Parent of Vermont staff and parents have been involved as adjunct faculty for the Early Childhood Specialist Certification program at the University of Vermont. Parent to Parent of Vermont teaches seven 3-hour sessions in family-centered care over the course of an academic year. A third teaching opportunity that Parent to Parent of Vermont has is with the Vermont Interdisciplinary Leadership Education for Health Professionals Program. The goal of this program is to ensure appropriate family-centered community-based training for advanced students working with children with or at risk for developmental disabilities.

PROVIDING TECHNICAL ASSISTANCE TO LOCAL PROGRAMS

Statewide Parent to Parent programs, particularly those that are more decentralized and have a network of local programs, provide a variety of technical assistance and other supports to local Parent to Parent programs in their state. These supports range from training and technical assistance in program development to financial and administrative support for the maintenance of the local program (see Table 14.4 in Appendix A).

Most statewide programs support the promotional efforts of local programs by producing a statewide program brochure that can be used by local/regional programs as well. The brochure often provides contact information for the statewide program itself but then also may list local programs and their contact information. Or in some cases, the brochure developed by the statewide program leaves a space within the brochure for the local/regional program to affix its own relevant contact information. Local/regional programs often find that their own credibility and visibility efforts are enhanced when they are seen as being a part of a statewide entity.

In a similar way, most statewide programs offer technical assistance in the development of a local Parent to Parent program. The format for this technical assistance varies—some statewide programs bring all new local program coordinators together for a group training session; others provide technical assistance on an as-needed basis as new programs emerge. Many statewide programs have a program development manual that is a resource to those wishing to start a local program. Once a new local program is on its way, the statewide program often provides opportunities for local program coordinators to meet with other local program coordinators to share information, recommended practices, and mutual support.

FSN has a unique system for supporting the coordinators of new local programs in North Carolina—a system that is modeled on the parent to parent match. As new local efforts identify themselves to the statewide office, the statewide office collects descriptive information about their newly developing program (e.g., setting, fiscal realities, program development team, priorities) and then, based on these factors, makes a program to program match with a veteran local program coordinator in North Carolina whose program has had program development experiences similar to those being addressed by the developing program. The veteran local program coordinator provides individualized information and support to the new local program coordinator in a flexible and responsive way just as supporting parents do for the parents with whom they are matched.

SUMMARY

Statewide Parent to Parent programs are important resources in their home states—to parents; local and regional Parent to Parent program coordinators; and other statewide efforts on behalf of families, professionals, and policy makers. Although each statewide Parent to Parent program is unique in its organizational style and how it provides its services, the programs share a common commitment to the importance of the carefully made one-to-one parent match as the foundation of its support to families. As the number of statewide programs continues to grow, perhaps Parent to Parent support will become an integral part of every state's comprehensive system of support services for families who have children with special needs.

Many statewide Parent to Parent programs across the country have developed manuals, printed information, videotapes, newsletters, training curricula for parents and practitioners, and guides for program development. When contacting statewide directors to learn more about their resources, you may want to request a mutually convenient telephone appointment time to talk in more detail about your specific request. In the spirit of generosity that is so much a part of Parent to Parent, the directors of the statewide programs are committed to responding to inquiries as the needs of their own families and programs will allow. In the same way that parent matches are always made based on the time availability of the parents, so, too, *matches* around program issues and the need for technical assistance will happen as time permits. The grids of *Gifts and Talents* identify which statewide programs have resources or information to share in each of the various components of program development (see Figures 14.1, 14.2, 14.3, and 14.4). For example, Arizona, California, New Hampshire, New Mexico, New York, North Carolina, South Carolina, and Vermont have Parent to Parent programs that train professionals on how to work with families who have children with disabilities. In addition, New Hampshire, New Mexico, North Carolina, South Carolina, and Vermont have gifts that they can share about evaluating Parent to Parent program efforts. Use these figures, plus the contact information for statewide programs that appears in the resources section at the end of Chapter 3, to get in touch with the statewide program that has expertise that interests you. Or you may contact the Parent to Parent Project at the Beach Center on Families and Disability for additional information (see Appendix C for contact information).

REFERENCES

Individuals with Disabilities Education Act (IDEA) Amendments of 1997, PL 105-17, 20 U.S.C. §§ 1400 *et seq.*

RESOURCES

Maternal and Child Health Bureau, 5600 Fishers Lane, Rockville, MD 20857; telephone: (301) 443-2370; http://www.mchb.hrsa.gov

Office of Special Education Programs, Office of Special Education and Rehabilitative Services, U.S. Department of Education, Room 3006, Switzer Building, 330 C Street, SW, Washington, DC 20202-2500; telephone: (202) 205-9161; http://www.ed.gov/offices/OSERS/OSEP/index.html

Organizational characteristics																														
State	AR	AZ	CA	CO	CT	FL	GA	ID	IN	KS	KY	LA	MA	MI	NC	ND	NH	NJ	NM	NV	NY	OH	PA	SC	TN	UT	VA	VT	WA	WV
Decentralized statewide Parent to Parent			X		X	X																	X				X		X	
Centralized statewide Parent to Parent				X				X		X						X			X	X								X		
Decentralized/centralized mix		X					X						X		X		X	X	X		X		X	X	X	X				
Parent to Parent and PTI partnering efforts		X	X	X		X			X	X		X	X					X	X		X							X		
Parent to Parent and PDFRC			X						X			X						X	X											
Parent to Parent and university partnership			X	X											X	X			X	X										
Board of directors		X	X	X			X	X	X										X		X		X	X						
Strategic planning		X	X	X			X								X								X	X						
Newer statewide programs				X				X			X					X		X					X							
Veteran statewide programs		X	X			X	X		X					X	X		X		X	X	X	X		X	X		X	X	X	

Figure 14.1. Statewide Parent to Parent gifts and talents: organizational characteristics. (PTI, parent training and information center; PDFRC, parent-directed family resource center)

Funding characteristics

State	AR	AZ	CA	CO	CT	FL	GA	ID	IN	KS	KY	LA	MA	MI	NC	ND	NH	NJ	NM	NV	NY	OH	PA	SC	TN	UT	VA	VT	WA	WV
Parent to Parent as a line item in state budgets							X								X				X									X		
Parent to Parent as a part of state or federal grants		X	X	X		X	X			X			X		X	X	X		X		X		X		X		X	X	X	
Funded in part through early intervention			X	X			X			X		X	X		X				X					X			X	X		
Funded in part through private foundations		X	X				X										X		X					X				X		
Hired a fundraising expert			X				X												X					X				X		

Figure 14.2. Statewide Parent to Parent gifts and talents: funding characteristics.

Referral and matching characteristics

State	AR	AZ	CA	CO	CT	FL	GA	ID	IN	KS	KY	LA	MA	MI	NC	ND	NH	NJ	NM	NV	NY	OH	PA	SC	TN	UT	VA	VT	WA	WV
Research-based recommended practices in matching															X	X	X						X	X				X		
Payment for supporting parents																								X	X					
Programs for new populations (e.g., children/adults with mental health issues, adults with disabilities)		X				X						X			X		X		X		X			X	X		X	X		
Recommended practices for matching culturally diverse populations		X	X			X	X	X											X					X	X		X		X	
Computerized database of disabilities		X	X	X		X	X					X			X	X	X		X	X	X		X	X	X		X	X		

Figure 14.3. Statewide Parent to Parent gifts and talents: referral and matching characteristics.

Training supporting parents characteristics																														
State	AR	AZ	CA	CO	CT	FL	GA	ID	IN	KS	KY	LA	MA	MI	NC	ND	NH	NJ	NM	NV	NY	OH	PA	SC	TN	UT	VA	VT	WA	WV
Training program available for supporting parents		X	X	X	X	X	X	X	X	X	X	X	X		X	X	X	X	X	X	X		X	X	X	X	X	X	X	
Manual developed for training			X	X	X	X	X	X	X	X	X	X	X		X	X	X	X	X	X	X		X	X	X	X	X	X	X	
Videotapes used/developed for training			X												X				X	X					X		X			
Training materials available for independent use						X	X																							
Program for nurturing supporting parents		X	X				X								X			X						X			X	X		

Figure 14.4. Statewide Parent to Parent gifts and talents: training supporting parents characteristics.

15

Looking Ahead

Parent to Parent

"The future stands not there like a statue to be uncovered, but lies like clay in our hands to be shaped."

—Florene Stewart Poyadue

Because Parent to Parent programs are now available in communities across the country, each with many different service components in addition to the one-to-one parent match, capturing the future for Parent to Parent will no doubt prove as elusive as defining its scope in the present. Although looking into the future for Parent to Parent is an awesome task, it is as exciting and heartwarming as reviewing its heroic past. As you anticipate the future of Parent to Parent, you may find it helpful to revisit the past, reflect on the present, and ask yourself some questions about the future.

This chapter encourages you to start thinking and planning for the future with your mind wide open to possibilities for Parent to Parent—as a resource for systems change, for the professionals within the systems, and most importantly for parents themselves. Beginning the dialogue, the discussions, and the conversations about what Parent to Parent's future role will be and where it will fit in the scheme of caring for children and families is the first priority. As parent leaders have discovered in the past, the simplest way to develop the solutions is just to begin. Begin with the vision, and know that the future for Parent to Parent will be nurtured by your visions.

PARENT TO PARENT: A RESOURCE FOR SYSTEMS CHANGE

The role of parents as caregivers and advocates for their children with special needs has changed dramatically over time, and these changes have resulted largely from the persistent efforts of parent leaders and supportive professionals. In the early 1900s, parents were seen as the cause of their child's disability, and parents often were shunned and their children were put into institutions. Yet, parents believed that these societal responses to their children's needs were inaccurate and inadequate, and in the 1940s they began to organize at the local, state, and national levels to advocate for alternative solutions for their children. As parents connected with other parents in these early advocacy activities, they realized that they also were important resources to each other. And they realized that together they could change systems.

Parents have been very successful in bringing about significant changes in the educational system for children with special needs. The Individuals with Disabilities Education Act (IDEA) of 1990 mandates a free and appropriate public education for all children and is in place largely because parent leaders would accept nothing less. Parents also have been influential in bringing the principles of family-centered care to all service systems and in educating professionals about the family perspective and the importance of partnerships between those caring for children at home and those providing professional services. Parents have invited professionals to work in partnership on behalf of children with disabilities, and parents have implemented community faculty programs in which parents teach present and future service providers about how to work with families in compassionate and respectful ways. Early parent organizations, including Parent to Parent programs, helped to energize parent leaders and to bring them together around their own visions for the future. These parent visions have become the realities of today, and children with special needs and their families have many more opportunities.

For too long advocacy has been considered a four-letter word. Actually its true meaning is very nonthreatening—*pleading the cause of another; speaking or writing in favor of something or someone.* And, in its most simple form, *to advocate is to provide a voice for another.* We invite you to take a closer look at how the advocacy efforts of parents in the past might continue to influence the role of Parent to Parent in systems change and serve as a resource for families and professionals in the future. From what platform will Parent to Parent find the most effective voice on behalf of children with special needs in the new millennium? Consider the following as you begin to find your own answers and create your own vision:

- Will the current legislation mandating a free, appropriate public education in the least restrictive environment for children with disabilities in elementary and high schools extend to the college campus? Will the same legal guarantees that children with disabilities have through age 21 be available to adults with disabilities who choose higher education? Will legislation be drafted to guarantee children with special needs and their families the same kinds of safeguards in health care?
- How will future policy and regulation changes in welfare reform; supplemental security income, Medicaid, Medicare, the Family Support Act of 1998, and managed care affect Parent to Parent programs? Might the opportunity for Parent to Parent support be included as a mandated component of federal legislation in these areas?
- Will there be a parent leader who is hired as a parent liaison on the White House staff or in the U.S. Department of Health and Human Services, as there is now in the U.S. Department of Education? Will there be paid parent liaisons to work with care teams of professionals in all settings in all communities—schools, hospitals, clinics, and social services agencies? Because there may be some who will have a hard time accepting parent members on their teams, will there be policies that reflect how parents and professionals can be supportive to each other and enhance their respective efforts? Policy must support the concept that each participant in the care of children has his or her job to do and neither replaces the other. If someone is replaced, policy has been ignored, prudent management has not prevailed, and an opportunity has been missed. Perhaps in the future, parents will be even more respected and valued than they are today for their unique contributions to service providers in the community.
- Will there will be more programs that facilitate the involvement of parents in the preservice and in-service training of professionals in the field of families and disabilities? Will parents work alongside medical school faculty to design medical education curricula? Family as Faculty programs exist today that might be replicated routinely by colleges and universities across the country.

These are some possible new directions for Parent to Parent programs. A few programs and parents are already beginning work in these areas, and others most likely will explore these opportunities more fully or in diverse ways in the future.

PARENT TO PARENT: A RESOURCE FOR PARENTS

Parent to Parent programs provide relationship-based emotional and informational support by carefully matching parents of children with special needs who want support and information with other parents who have *been there.* Because Parent to Parent is as broad as its name suggests, one parent will always reach out to another, whether the connection is made on the Internet, through the television, on the telephone, in the home, in the classroom, or via satellite. And because the concept of parents helping other parents is so simple, in the future perhaps parent to parent support will be available for caregivers in a variety of settings. Perhaps parent matching will happen for all parents who want a reliable ally, and not just for those who have children with special needs. Consider a future in which parent to parent support opportunities are available to all who are involved in any aspect of caring for others:

- Because the majority of people in the United States are Caucasian, sometimes Americans forget that the majority of people in the world are culturally diverse. As the demographic make-up of families in America changes and becomes more like the rest of the world, how will parent to parent matching be affected? Many culturally diverse families manage the challenges of a child's or an adult family member's disability as well as the challenges of language and poverty. Connecting with another family who shares their cultural background and speaks the same language is especially important. Some local and statewide Parent to Parent programs are discovering ways in which the original Parent to Parent model works and can be adapted to meet the needs of culturally and linguistically diverse families. Parent to Parent manuals and training materials for culturally diverse communities are becoming more widely available. In the future, perhaps Parent to Parent programs will exist in all communities with support provided in culturally responsive ways to all families.
- Although parent to parent support is generally available for parents of children with special needs who are young, in the future, parent to parent support might be available to families across their

life span. Families with adult children with special needs often have new and different issues to address—independent living, supported employment, and recreation and leisure activities. Will the road toward supported employment and independent living in the community that adult children with special needs choose be easier because Parent to Parent programs add new components to support adult children and their families? What if young adults with disabilities preparing for their transition to the adult world of supported living and employment could be matched with other young adults who have successfully managed this transition? What if their families were matched with other families who have already responded to the challenges that come with letting go but continuing to be a resource to their adult child with a disability? A supporting parent or a supporting adult with a disability who has dealt with some of these same issues can be just as helpful in this phase of life as at the beginning. Perhaps in the future, Parent to Parent programs will develop collaborative relationships with adult advocacy organizations, such as independent living centers, and will bring the one-to-one matched opportunity into this arena as well.

- Perhaps, too, as adults with disabilities move out of their family home and into a different community, "nearby parent" programs might match the young adult with a parent or family nearby. As "nearby parents," they would help to support the young adult's integration into the community and would be able to respond quickly in emergencies. And as "nearby parents," they would also stay in touch with the young adult's parents about how their adult with a disability is doing.
- Perhaps parent to parent support will be available to the caregivers of aging parents with Alzheimer's disease and other debilitating diseases—for example, matching an adult daughter who is caring for her parent(s) with another adult daughter with a bit more experience in doing the same thing. The supporting caregiver knows all about systems for the care of older adults and can share this information with the newcomer in compassionate ways.
- Will the broader community begin to see Parent to Parent as a model for solving other family issues and not just those related to disability? Wouldn't it be wonderful if parent matches were available for parents who are experiencing any family life challenge? For example, single parents might be matched with other single parents for support about parenting alone; parents who are challenged by substance abuse could be matched with other parents who have

successfully managed their own substance abuse issues; parents who have found their way out of the welfare system may be matched with other parents who are still seeking their own way; or likewise, parents who have experienced homelessness might be matched with parents for whom homelessness is still a part of their reality. Foster parents with foster parents; adoptive parents with adoptive parents; teen parents with other parents who started parenting as teens. The concept remains the same—support and information from another person who has *been there.*

- Maybe one day parent to parent support will be routinely made available to all families beginning at birth—even those without a specific challenge. Parenting is one of life's most important responsibilities, and yet too often new parents know very little about how to be parents. Hospitals might routinely inform parents about the parent to parent match with a supporting parent who lives nearby and whose child is a bit older. The two sets of parents connect even before the new parents leave the hospital, and support and information is shared about caring for a newborn almost before the new parent has time to ask questions.
- Will the future find Parent to Parent programs aligned with all family and community support systems—not just educational and medical but also the recreational, occupational, legal, and social services systems? Will Parent to Parent programs be a catalyst for more community programs, especially for children—perhaps helping to develop neighborhood integrated play groups for children with and without disabilities? Perhaps in the future, Parent to Parent programs will work more closely with legal and judicial systems to create programs to serve children and young adults with disabilities who have become entangled with the law. Although much training already has been done for health and education professionals, wouldn't it be useful if these same training opportunities were extended to legal professionals and others who now have contact with people who have disabilities? Wouldn't it be wonderful if Parent to Parent programs were a part of collaborative satellite sites at schools, hospitals, the workplace, community programs, and at houses of worship? Being on site and in sight would not only make parent to parent support more readily available to all families but also would increase their own visibility and capacity.

It is exciting to think about the possibilities for extending the basic principle of matching parents and families around similar issues for emotional and informational support from someone who has *been there.* Parent to Parent programs today can be models for replication tomorrow in these and other new settings, and the possibilities for Parent to Parent are as endless as the arenas of family support. And these possibilities will continue to become realities because there will always be parent leaders who are like eagles—willing to fly alone, above the crowd, and with a clear vision for what's up ahead.

PARENT TO PARENT IN THE NEW MILLENNIUM

Family Visions

Visions can be the road map to innovative programs and services, suggesting new directions and new possibilities, and this chapter would not be complete without the visions of some other families. Their visions, plus your own, will determine the future for Parent to Parent.

Two Fathers from the Silicon Valley

Parent to Parent programs will become places where parents can have easy access to modern technology—giving every family a fair chance at using technology to get information, services, and resources for their children.

Because it is impossible for a family to be concerned about a child's individualized education program when they are trying to locate food, shelter, medicine, and clothing for their children, Parent to Parent programs will offer its support and information to families who are seeking financial help for meeting the needs of their entire family. Parent to Parent programs will be aware of local, state, and federal assistance programs to help these families.

Parent to Parent programs will go from being government driven to being government supported; from being dependent to being self-sufficient; from being just community based to being community embraced; from being culturally isolated to being culturally appreciated; and from being parent represented to being parent directed.

A Parent from New Jersey

It is my hope that Parent to Parent will one day be a name commonly referred to by all families, not just a hidden support that only the "world of disability" knows. Everyone—parents, grandparents, siblings, neighbors, school teachers, and community members—would have the opportunity to be connected with another person who has a relationship with a child with a developmental delay or disability.

Imagine if Parent to Parent were known and accessible to all people in their communities. A toll-free telephone number posted not only in doctors' offices and hospitals but also in community centers and schools would allow all people to be connected with others who have similar life experiences. Suppose a new family with a child with multiple disabilities has just moved into your neighborhood. You have never met anyone with a disability, you want to reach out to welcome this family, but your lack of knowledge about and experience with people with disabilities keeps you away. You call the toll-free telephone number and get a match for yourself—with someone who has had a lot of experience connecting with people with disabilities. This person shares with you how they included new neighbors into their community, offers informational resources to you about disabilities, and helps ease your fears so that you and your family can reach out. You then help that child and his or her family become truly significant members of your community.

Or suppose you are the coach of a soccer team. As you are reading through the registration forms, you see that one child is deaf and uses sign language to communicate. You could take a sign language class so that you can talk with him or her, but soccer practice starts next week and there is not enough time for that. You remember seeing information about how a Parent to Parent program can help you connect with a family member of someone who has a disability. After making a simple telephone call, you are matched with a family member or friend of a deaf person, or a deaf person him- or herself. Now you can ask questions about the best way to include this child and how to be the best coach for all of the children on your team.

The one-to-one match of parents is the key to empowering families and getting them in touch with the rich and often abundant resources available for their child. To go the next step and make Parent to Parent a resource for all members of the community is my vision.

A Parent from Arizona

Parent to Parent programs first started in the 1970s, when the right-to-education legislation was passed. Since then, a whole generation of children has been raised in a different world and has had new and far better opportunities than the generation born before. To be fully responsive to these new and more visionary families, Parent to Parent programs must rely on them to be a catalyst for our own visions for the future.

As inclusive educational settings become more commonplace, our country is becoming more accepting of and comfortable with diversity. In Arizona, we are finding that more and more families want to know how to negotiate and better manage their child's involvement in integrated settings in the community—ways to foster friendships, dignity, and respect. As individual families navigate these inclusive communities, their needs and dreams vary greatly. Parent to Parent programs will grow to appreciate and respect the diversity of these families and the dreams that they have for their children, and Parent to Parent programs can be natural resources for families as they create new ways of being involved in more inclusive communities. In the future, perhaps Parent to Parent programs will be able to count on these same communities to help fund support for these same families.

For too long, families have been part of the "disability world" that existed parallel to the "real world." With a more inclusive society, families do not have the same need to "join" the disability world, but they do have a need to "connect" to it. My vision is that Parent to Parent will always be the one connecting point for families as they journey through all phases of their lives.

A Parent from California

My vision unfolds as a challenging, exciting, and rewarding future for Parent to Parent programs—one in which parent-directed family resource centers (PDFRCs) offer not only the one-to-one parent match but also a host of other family support services and are the conduit through which major national efforts on behalf of children and families are implemented. For example, America's Promise—The Alliance For Youth (http://www.americaspromise.org) was created out of a 1997 Presidential Summit for America's Future. This national program to save our children might find PDFRCs to be the missing link between the national headquarters' ideas, funding, and resources, and the local implementation of the program. Parent to Parent programs in communities across the country could provide important local feedback to the national leaders of America's Promise that they would then incorporate into their plans and future budgets. In the same way, the federal government has put a priority on family-centered, community-based, culturally competent, coordinated care as a recommended practice in the care of children. Parent to Parent programs naturally provide family-centered, community-based, culturally competent, coordinated care, and their involvement in this movement could be a large part of the answer to getting the theory implemented at the local level.

A WORD OF CAUTION

As you read and think about all of these possibilities for Parent to Parent programs, it is important to remember that there are two sides to every coin. In order for visions to become realities, the dreams must be shared. But the possible obstacles and challenges need to be addressed as well so that you can plan to prevent, negate, and steer clear of them.

Although there are many who envision a future in which a Parent to Parent program will be strategically located in each neighborhood and will serve all families in a variety of ways, it will be important that the one-to-one parent matching component is not lost. This threat is very real because a quality matching program takes more energy and time than some of the other possible program components envisioned in this chapter. And because sometimes people will follow the path of least resistance when their hours are limited, there is the risk that the parent matching component will be diminished. Then, as fewer parents experience the benefits of a one-to-one parent match, fewer will be interested in volunteering as support parents. The parent matching component then becomes jeopardized or even lost. However, nature and human behavior are cyclical—what goes around comes around. So, *if* in the future parent matching is diminished, parents in time *will* notice its absence, and their needs will be the catalyst for reinstating this core component.

Another possible challenge in the future is that because of the efforts of a whole generation of parents who fought for services for people with disabilities, parents in the future will be experiencing a system that is much improved. Parents in the future may not have the same "fire in the belly" to maintain quality programs, create new programs, and especially to serve in leadership positions alongside other parents. Unless new parent leadership is nurtured and supported in its efforts to follow in the footsteps of today's leaders and carry on the work of the future, there is a risk that the important gains that have been made will not be maintained.

These are simply possible barriers to be aware of as you hold on to and work toward your visions. Don't let them discourage you, but do let them remind you that the visions of the future will require the same strong parent commitment that brought us to where we are in the new millennium.

REACHING THE VISION THROUGH A NATIONAL PRESENCE FOR PARENT TO PARENT

You have learned that Parent to Parent programs are local, community-based resources that provide emotional and informational support to parents of children who have special needs. To provide this support, trained and experienced veteran parents are carefully matched in one-to-one relationships with parents who are newly referred to the program. The support is provided by a parent who lives in the same community as the parent seeking support, so the two parents are dealing with similar contexts and service systems. The geographic proximity of the available support means that the parent providing support is close by and can respond in a timely manner. Because the support is community based, parents are encouraged to get involved at the grass roots level, and their own growth as tomorrow's community leaders is nurtured.

Since 1980, Parent to Parent has benefited from a strong, solid, informal national network that is itself relationship based, with a generous sharing of resources, recommended practices, and mutual support. A lot of activities have happened nationally for Parent to Parent even though there never has been a formal national organization to coordinate these national opportunities.

And yet as Parent to Parent continues to grow as a national resource for families seeking individualized support through a parent match, the national opportunities for Parent to Parent are increasing. Parent to Parent programs are beginning to do national consulting about the implementation of the Parent to Parent model and to represent the voices of families in communities in conversations about federal policy. Yet without a national organization, it is difficult for Parent to Parent to participate in these national opportunities.

Consequently, and with some trepidation that a national organization for Parent to Parent might have a negative effect on the local autonomy that contributes to the strength of Parent to Parent, Parent to Parent leaders are beginning to think about the benefits of a national hub and what it might look like and do. An early decision was made to explore a possible collaboration between Parent to Parent and Grassroots Consortium on Disabilities in this effort.

Grassroots Consortium on Disabilities is a national coalition of community-based, parent-directed, family support and information programs serving culturally and linguistically diverse families who have children with disabilities and other special needs and who are living in traditionally underserved communities (see Chapter 3). The services provided are individualized, flexible, and comprehensive (just as they are in Parent to Parent) and often include assistance with meeting basic life needs related to poverty along with the disability-related needs. Fostering leadership development is a key component of Grassroots Consortium on Disabilities, just as it is in Parent to Parent. Parent to Parent and Grassroots Consortium on Disabilities both exist to ensure that children and adults with disabilities, chronic illnesses, and special health care needs and their families receive individualized, culturally responsive, and community-based family support and information services.

The decision has been made to explore partnership opportunities that would help to establish a strong and well-funded national infrastructure for Parent to Parent and Grassroots Consortium on Disabilities. This infrastructure would support the work of community-based family support and information programs, facilitate the mutual sharing of recommended practices and resources, and forge new partnerships with other national efforts. Parent to Parent and Grassroots Consortium on Disabilities leaders are moving ahead united by the following common values:

- Mutual respect and trust between parents who have *been there*
- Individualized, one-to-one support from one parent to another
- Information based on family needs and preferences
- Community-based supports that support the child within the context of the family within the community
- Family-centered and culturally responsive care
- Parent-directed programs
- Meaningful solutions found through collaboration among families and between families and professionals
- Choices—parents know best about the kind of support and resources that are most helpful to them
- Leadership development to build the capacity of parents in communities
- Equal opportunities for a full and meaningful life for all people, including those with disabilities

With a strong and well-funded infrastructure for the community-based family support and information programs of Parent to Parent and Grassroots Consortium on Disabilities, parent leaders representing these two networks would then be able to participate in national conversations about how best to coordinate all of the national resources that exist for families who have family members with special needs. Parent to Parent and Grassroots Consortium on Disabilities would be at the national table to consider how their strengths can be shared nationally and how Parent to Parent and Grassroots Consortium on Disabilities can benefit from the strengths and resources of other national parent-directed efforts. Perhaps the efforts of Parent to Parent will contribute to an eventual collaborative parent network of many different national resources that are each working to support families in their own way. Some of these other possible partners you read about in Chapter 3:

- Family Voices provides families with meaningful and relevant information about health care issues and advocates for federal policies that will benefit families who have children with special health care needs. As a part of a national collaborative parent network, the health care information from Family Voices might reach more families at the community level and might be shared from one parent to another.

- Parent training and information centers (PTI) train parents to be their own successful advocates on behalf of the educational needs of their children with disabilities. Over the years, PTIs have developed wonderful training resources for parents about the educational and legal rights of children with special needs and their families. PTIs share information through workshops and conferences nationwide. As a part of a national collaborative parent network, PTIs' excellent training materials also could be shared through the individualized and ongoing support that Parent to Parent and Grassroots Consortium on Disabilities as community-based family support and information programs provide.
- The National Center for Parent-Directed Family Resource Centers at PHP, Inc. has developed a comprehensive set of training materials for developing and directing a community-based PDFRC. These materials, and an annual training institute for those who are interested in starting or expanding their own program, mean that newly developing programs don't have to start from scratch. As a part of a collaborative national parent network, the National Center for Parent-Directed Family Resource Centers would be a wonderful resource for supporting the technical assistance needs of emerging parent programs.
- Research in the family and disability field is occurring in universities across the country, and the partnership that the Beach Center on Families and Disability at The University of Kansas has forged with parent leaders can be used as a model for other parent–researcher partnerships. Such partnerships, perhaps facilitated by a national collaborative parent network in partnership with universities, might mean that more parents are involved in all phases of research as members of participatory action research teams and that research would lead to results that are relevant and beneficial to families sooner rather than later.
- National and international parent matches are still sometimes difficult to find for parents whose children have very rare disabilities. A national collaborative parent network might ensure that parents know about the few national/international databases (e.g., Mothers United for Moral Support, National Organization for Rare Disorders) that exist for parents and that there is some coordination be-

tween and among these matching services and the matching efforts that occur locally and statewide.

- National Coalition for Family Leadership is an informal coalition of parent leaders that has been meeting annually to 1) identify emerging trends and needs for families who have children with disabilities, 2) create innovations in service delivery, 3) nurture and prepare a new cadre of parent leaders to carry on, and 4) be mutually supportive of each other. These parent leaders have been instrumental in building the Parent to Parent movement, and they carry with them a wealth of historical knowledge. As part of a national collaborative parent network, National Coalition for Family Leadership offers a way for the accomplishments of the past to be carried forward by emerging parent leaders as lessons for the future.
- Specific disability support groups exist nationally and are important resources for parents who wish to participate in support group meetings with other parents whose children have the same disability. Group support opportunities complement one-to-one parent support activities. As part of a national collaborative parent network, there might be a greater coordination of services for families and a mutual sharing of recommended practices and resources.
- National information and support programs for siblings and fathers: The National Fathers Network and the Sibling Support Project have benefited from some federal funding, but regrettably this funding has not been long term. As part of a national collaborative parent network, these two national resources might benefit from a concerted national mobilization on behalf of siblings and fathers in families that have a child with special needs.
- National Parent Network on Disabilities (NPND) is a parent organization that keeps families informed about legislation, regulations, what laws mean to the lives and well-being of children and families, and how to be effectively involved with the legislative process. NPND works to ensure that while parents are supported in communities, their voices are heard at the federal level, and parents are informed about legislation that will affect their families' quality of life. As part of a national collaborative parent network, those representing families in Washington, D.C., would have easy access to the experiences and voices of families in communities across the country. Through the nationwide network of community-based programs, information about legislation and opportunities for families to influence policy also could reach parents through their individual connections with other parents.
- Families as Faculty projects exist as partnerships between parents and university faculty teaching in preservice education programs.

> By reaching future service providers before they begin to work with children and families and by employing parents as community faculty members, Family as Faculty programs have an enormous potential to create a whole new wave of providers who are well trained in the family perspective and in the principles of family-centered care. As part of a collaborative national parent network, Family as Faculty programs would benefit from national connections with parents who might want to serve as community faculty. Replication of existing Family as Faculty programs also might occur more easily with technical assistance perhaps being coordinated by a partnership between the collaborative national parent network and universities.

A possibility for the future is that a national collaborative parent network might exist on behalf of all families with children who have special needs. A collaborative national parent network might serve as an anchor for each of these autonomous national resources—not controlling them at all but just facilitating a reciprocal sharing of resources between and among them all to ensure that families benefit from the best of what each has to offer. This is a different way of doing business—certainly *not business as usual,* but one in which the resources of the whole would be greater than the sum of each separate part.

Although families of children with disabilities may encounter challenges to providing the best care for their children, families are resilient and can successfully make their way, especially with a little help from another friendly, experienced parent. When one parent reaches out to help another, helplessness and hopelessness are cleared from their paths. Families not only survive, but they also thrive, and through Parent to Parent programs they return to help someone else.

The sharing of experiences and information that happens between parents through Parent to Parent programs is an important and unique resource for parents. Parent to parent support ensures that parents will have someone, somewhere, who can empathize with them in their good moments and more importantly in their worst moments. Often, just simply being there, ready to listen with ears and heart and soul is what is needed the most. Parent to Parent offers that friend who is just a telephone call away.

We hope that everyone who reads this book has learned something new. Perhaps you learned about some statistics demonstrating the efficacy of Parent to Parent that you can now use to promote your program. Or maybe you gathered enough how-to information that you now have the courage to start a Parent to Parent program. We hope that those of you who have been contemplating, but hesitating to start a program to serve children and families, now have the technical skills and resources you need to bring a Parent to Parent program to your community. Maybe you gained a new appreciation for your own capacity to use your personal experiences in partnership with professionals—to improve children's care and be a catalyst for systems change. Or perhaps you just came away with a new sense that you are not alone.

Each family you met in this book has a unique story but also shares countless common experiences with thousands of other families who have a child with special needs. If you are a parent, we hope that the perspectives and experiences of these families will have a familiar ring and provide comfort to you. If you are a service provider, we hope that the family stories shared in the book will become a guiding voice for you as you work with children and families—the lessons are theirs, the opportunity to learn from and with families is yours.

Regardless of your role in the lives of children with special needs, Parent to Parent programs are an important resource. Parent to Parent complements other supports and services for families. When Parent to Parent is an established part of a comprehensive set of services for children and families, everyone can be assured that emotional and informational support from Parent to Parent will follow families over the life span and that Parent to Parent programs will help to change attitudes, set trends, influence policy, and transform communities into the magnificent caring villages we all envision for our children.

SUMMARY

Because the needs that people have for both physical and emotional nourishment remain constant even as the world around them changes, the personal touch of Parent to Parent will be needed just as much in the future as it is now. And, a bright future for Parent to Parent is on an expanding horizon for those who will work together to successfully shape it. Good luck; the future *is in your hands.*

REFERENCES

Family Support Act of 1988, PL 100-485, 42 U.S.C. §§ 1305 *et seq.*

Individuals with Disabilities Education Act (IDEA) of 1990, PL 101-476, 20 U.S.C. §§ 1400 *et seq.*

Appendix A
Research About Parent to Parent

WHY IS RESEARCH IMPORTANT TO PARENT TO PARENT?

Research is useful to Parent to Parent programs because it can answer questions that people with an interest in Parent to Parent may have about the programs and the services they provide. Parent to Parent program developers (as well as those who have already developed a program) may be interested in learning about how other Parent to Parent programs are organized, funded, and staffed; what kind of training they offer to supporting parents; how matches are made; what other program activities exist in the program; and what materials other programs have to share. This kind of information will provide them with a description of Parent to Parent that may influence their own program development and expansion decisions. As their own programs get underway, program developers also may be interested in documenting their program activities to learn more about who is participating and in what ways, as well as how satisfied participants are with and the impact of the program services.

Parents who are considering whether to participate in a Parent to Parent program (as well as those parents who are already participating in the program) may want to learn more about what actually happens in parent to parent matches—how they are made, how long they usually last, and the nature of the support that is typically shared. Or, they may want to know about the training that Parent to Parent programs offer to supporting parents—what is covered, how long the training usually lasts, and what other training opportunities are available. Parent also may be interested in learning about the perspectives of other parents who have participated in the program as well. This kind of information may help parents to decide if and how they might like to be involved in a Parent to Parent program.

Potential referral and funding sources typically have a particular interest in learning about the effectiveness of parent to parent support so that they can be sure that the needs of parents they refer will be met and/or the program activities they decide to fund will make a difference in the lives of children with special needs and their families. Data that demonstrate the efficacy of parent to parent support help to enhance the visibility, credibility, and fundability of Parent to Parent. Efficacy data also may suggest new recommended practices that add to the value of parent to parent support.

HOW TO FIND AND USE PARENT TO PARENT RESEARCH

Prior to 1988, there was little research available about parent to parent support, and the few studies that did exist were published only in the professional journals and were not readily accessible to parents. Those with an interest in Parent to Parent had little research-based information about Parent to Parent. In 1988, the Beach Center on Families and Disability at The University of Kansas began a research partnership with Parent to Parent to generate research-based information about Parent to Parent. Parents identified research needs, and then three different research efforts with Parent to Parent program directors and parents were carried out:

1. National survey of local Parent to Parent programs
2. National study to determine the effectiveness of Parent to Parent
3. National survey of statewide Parent to Parent programs

Final data, products, and resources developed from the research data are available from the Beach Center.

The national survey of local Parent to Parent programs was conducted from 1989 to 1993, and three different surveys were completed: a survey of program directors of Parent to Parent programs nationally, a survey of supporting parents, and a survey of referred parents. More than 600 parents and 375 Parent to Parent program directors answered the survey questions, and their information provided a great deal of descriptive data about Parent to Parent.

The national study to determine the effectiveness of Parent to Parent was conducted from 1993 to 1996. This study came about because parents who were a part of Parent to Parent knew in their hearts that Parent to Parent made a difference for parents who were matched with a supporting parent. And yet there was no hard evidence that validated Parent to Parent as an effective support for parents of children with special needs. To have research results that documented the effectiveness of Parent to Parent might mean that Parent to Parent programs would be more credible in the eyes of referral sources and potential funders.

There were actually two studies within the efficacy research project—a quantitative study to determine whether Parent to Parent works and a qualitative study to understand more fully why Parent to Parent works and how it might work even better.

For the quantitative study, parents responded to several different questionnaires that measured the sense of having a reliable ally, how well parents felt they were coping, how much social support parents felt they were receiving, parents' level of acceptance, and how empowered the parents felt. Some parents were participating in a parent to parent match and some were not, and their responses to the questionnaires were compared.

For the qualitative study, 24 parents were interviewed about their matched experience. The results of these interviews indicated why Parent to Parent is helpful and how it can be even more helpful.

The third research study was the survey of statewide Parent to Parent programs that was conducted from 1996 to 1999. The purpose of this survey was to learn more about how statewide Parent to Parent programs are structured and funded and about the supports and services that they provide to parents and to local Parent to Parent program directors. Seventeen statewide Parent to Parent programs and 36 directors of local Parent to Parent programs in states that had a statewide Parent to Parent program participated in this study.

The results of these three research studies are referenced in many of the chapters in the book, and the tables that summarize much of the data from these research studies are included in this appendix. In addition, Chapter 13 includes a thorough discussion of different kinds of program evaluation research that can be helpful to Parent to Parent program directors and parents involved in Parent to Parent.

More information and details about Parent to Parent research can be found at http://www.brookespublishing.com/ptop/.

CHAPTER 4

Table 4.1. Age and size of Parent to Parent programs

Size	Percentage of programs reporting
Small (1–12 parents served)	31%
Small to medium (13–25 parents served)	40%
Medium to large (26–75 parents served)	12%
Large (more than 75 parents served)	18%
Age	**Percentage of programs reporting**
Young (0–4 years old)	24%
Middle (5–8 years old)	30%
Old (more than 8 years old)	46%

From Santelli, B., Turnbull, A., Marquis, J., & Lerner, E. (1993). Parent to Parent programs: Ongoing support for parents of young adults with special needs. *Journal of Vocational Rehabilitation, 3*(2), 30; reprinted by permission.

Table 4.2. Breakdown of children's disabilities

Child's disability	Percentage of parents reporting
Developmental delay	31%
Down syndrome	29%
Mental retardation	23%
Learning disability	20%
Physical disability	20%
Visual impairment	16%
Cerebral palsy	16%
Multiple disabilities	15%
Ongoing medical condition	15%
Prematurity	10%
Hearing impairment	10%
Epilepsy	8%
Autism	3%
Spina bifida	2%
Traumatic head injury	2%

From Santelli, B., Turnbull, A., Marquis, J., & Lerner, E. (1995). Parent to Parent programs: A unique form of mutual support. *Infants and Young Children, 8*(2), 50; reprinted by permission.

Table 4.3. Severity of the disability of the children of parents participating

Severity of disability	Percentage of parents reporting
Mild	33%
Moderate	39%
Severe	25%
Other	3%

Table 4.4. Ages of children with disabilities of parents participating

Age	Percentage of parents reporting
Birth–2 years old	40%
3–5 years old	25%
6–11 years old	20%
12–18 years old	9%
19–21 years old	3%
22–55 years old	2%

Table 4.5. Sponsorship status of Parent to Parent programs

Sponsorship status	Percentage of programs reporting
Nonsponsored	48%
Sponsored by an Arc	19%
Sponsored by a social services agency	11%
Sponsored by a disability organization	5%
Sponsored by the statewide Parent to Parent program	5%
Sponsored by a hospital	5%
Sponsored by a school district	3%

From Santelli, B., Turnbull, A., Marquis, J., & Lerner, E. (1993). Parent to Parent programs: Ongoing support for parents of young adults with special needs. *Journal of Vocational Rehabilitation, 3*(2), 30; reprinted by permission.

CHAPTER 5

Table 5.1. Supports provided through the match

Supports	Percentage of programs reporting
Someone to listen and understand	100%
Information about the disability	98%
Information about community resources	96%
Information about caring for a child with a disability	96%
Help with referrals to other agencies	95%
Help with problem solving	93%

From Santelli, B., Turnbull, A., Marquis, J., & Lerner, E. (1993). Parent to Parent programs: Ongoing support for parents of young adults with special needs. *Journal of Vocational Rehabilitation, 3*(2), 33; reprinted by permission.

Table 5.2. Factors considered when matching parents

Factors	Percentage of programs reporting use	Percentage of parents reporting most important
Similar disability	96%	56%
Similar issues	91%	21%
Supporting parent can respond in 24 hours	67%	7%
Members with disability are close in age	57%	7%
Families live close by	49%	1%
Similar family structure	47%	1%
Similar cultural or ethnic background	40%	0%
Parents are about the same age	36%	1%
Parents have similar education and income	32%	0%

Table 5.3. Timing of the first contact

Time between referral and first contact	Percentage of programs reporting
Within 24 hours	63%
Within 1 week	19%
Within 1 month	1%
No specified time, depends on the disability	17%

Table 5.4. Nature of the first contact

Type of first contact	Percentage of programs reporting
Telephone	96%
In person	23%
Other	12%

Table 5.5. Duration of parent matches

Length of match	Percentage of programs reporting
More than 1 year	17%
6–12 months	16%
1–6 months	41%
1–4 weeks	15%
Less than 1 week	5%

From Santelli, B., Turnbull, A., Marquis, J., & Lerner, E. (1993). Parent to Parent programs: Ongoing support for parents of young adults with special needs. *Journal of Vocational Rehabilitation, 3*(2), 32; reprinted by permission.

Table 5.6. Type of ongoing contact between parents

Type of contact	Percentage of programs reporting
Telephone	88%
In person	60%
Other	24%

CHAPTER 6

Table 6.1. Content of training for supporting parents

Content area	Percentage of programs reporting
Listening skills	94%
Communication skills	93%
Orientation to program	92%
Adjustment process	86%
Community resources	83%
Information about disabilities	81%
Positive philosophy	80%
Disability organizations	80%
Referral process	74%
Self-awareness	60%
Financial information	58%
Advocacy training	56%
Leadership training	39%
Cultural diversity training	37%

From Santelli, B., Turnbull, A., Marquis, J., & Lerner, E. (1995). Parent to Parent programs: A unique form of mutual support. *Infants and Young Children, 8*(2), 53; reprinted by permission.

Table 6.2. Format of training for supporting parents

Format	Percentage of programs reporting
Train parents in small groups	94%
Train parents individually in person	50%
Train parents individually by telephone	39%
Send written training materials	28%

Table 6.3. Amount of training provided to supporting parents

Number of hours of training	Percentage of programs reporting
More than 10 hours	44%
7–9 hours	15%
4–6 hours	19%
1–3 hours	15%

From Santelli, B., Turnbull, A., Marquis, J., & Lerner, E. (1995). Parent to Parent programs: A unique form of mutual support. *Infants and Young Children, 8*(2), 53; reprinted by permission.

Table 6.4. Other supports provided to supporting parents

Type of support	Percentage of statewide programs reporting
Supporting parent manual	83%
One-to-one consultation	78%
Reimbursement for long-distance telephone calls	78%
Ongoing training	67%
Reimbursement for postage expenses	61%
Retreat/conference	56%
Support group	44%
Reimbursement for travel expenses	44%

CHAPTER 9

Table 9.1. Size of annual program budgets of local Parent to Parent programs

Size of annual budget	Percentage of programs reporting
Less than $1,000	35%
$1,000–$4,999	20%
$5,000–$9,999	7%
$10,000–$24,999	21%
$25,000–$49,999	7%
$50,000–$99,999	4%
$100,000–$249,999	4%
$250,000–$499,999	2%
More than $500,000	0%

From Santelli, B., Turnbull, A., Marquis, J., & Lerner, E. (1993). Parent to Parent programs: Ongoing support for parents of young adults with special needs. *Journal of Vocational Rehabilitation, 3*(2), 31; reprinted by permission.

Table 9.2. Sources of funding for local Parent to Parent programs

Funding source	Percentage of local programs reporting
Sponsoring agency	44%
Private donations	41%
Fund-raising activities	33%
Local/state grants	30%
Membership fees	13%
Federal grants	7%
Statewide Parent to Parent program	5%

From Santelli, B., Turnbull, A., Marquis, J., & Lerner, E. (1993). Parent to Parent programs: Ongoing support for parents of young adults with special needs. *Journal of Vocational Rehabilitation, 3*(2), 31; reprinted by permission.

CHAPTER 10

Table 10.1. Program activities beyond the one-to-one match

Program activity	Percentage of local programs reporting
Parent informational group meetings	69%
Parent support group meetings	65%
Social events	63%
Group meetings for veteran parents	44%
Speakers' bureau	36%
Activities for other family members	31%
24-hour "warm line"	27%
Training of professionals	14%
Training for preservice students	13%

CHAPTER 12

Table 12.1. Collaborating partners with statewide Parent to Parent programs

State organization	Percentage of statewide programs in partnership
Lead agency—health	94%
Part C—early intervention	89%
Developmental disabilities council	82%
State disability organization	82%
Hospital	82%
Lead agency—education	77%
University affiliated program	77%
Lead agency—social services	70%
Parent training and information center	70%
Lead agency—rehabilitation	59%
School districts	50%
State Arc	47%

From Santelli, B., Turnbull, A., Marquis, J., & Lerner, E. (2000). Statewide Parent to Parent programs: Partners in early intervention. *Infants and Young Children, 13*(1), 81; reprinted by permission.

CHAPTER 14

Table 14.1. Annual budgets of statewide programs: End of the first year of the program and then in 1996–1997

Annual budget	At end of the first year of the program	1996–1997
Less than $1,000	6%	0%
$1,000–$4,999	6%	0%
$5,000–$9,999	0%	0%
$10,000–$24,999	33%	0%
$25,000–$49,999	11%	17%
$50,000–$99,999	22%	0%
$100,000–$249,999	17%	33%
$250,000–$499,999	6%	28%
More than $500,000	6%	22%

From Santelli, B., Turnbull, A., Marquis, J., & Lerner, E. (2000). Statewide Parent to Parent programs: Partners in early intervention. *Infants and Young Children, 13*(1), 80; reprinted by permission.

Table 14.2. Funding sources for statewide programs: At end of the first year of the program and 1996–1997

Funding source	End of the first year of the program	1996–1997
State funds		
Developmental Disabilities Council	33%	11%
State Title V/ Department of Health	28%	33%
State Department of Education	17%	17%
University	11%	28%
Line item on state budget	0%	11%
Federal funds		
Maternal and child health	11%	17%
Part C—early intervention funding	6%	39%
Parent Training and Information Center	0%	17%
Other funds		
Donations	22%	33%
In-kind services	17%	17%
Private foundation grants	17%	39%
Fund-raisers	11%	33%
Civic clubs	11%	17%
United Way	11%	11%
Hospitals	6%	17%
Churches	6%	17%
School districts	0%	6%

From Santelli, B., Turnbull, A., Marquis, J., & Lerner, E. (2000). Statewide Parent to Parent programs: Partners in early intervention. *Infants and Young Children, 13*(1), 80; reprinted by permission.

Table 14.3. Program activities for families

Program activity	Percentage of state programs offering
Conference	78%
Lending library	78%
Financial support	56%
Activities for siblings	39%
Activities for families	22%
Computer center	17%
Extended family member activities	17%
Toy library	0%
Equipment library	0%

Table 14.4. Technical assistance/supports offered by statewide programs for local program coordinators

Type of technical assistance or support	Percentage of statewide programs offering to local coordinators
A statewide program brochure or other promotional literature	56%
Technical assistance in program development/operation	56%
A program development manual for program coordinators	44%
Administrative office support to help with mailings	44%
Group meetings with other program coordinators	39%
Training to be a local/regional program coordinator	33%
A resource manual with information about disabilities and community resources	33%
Reimbursement for travel expenses	28%
Reimbursement for telephone expenses	28%
Reimbursement for postage expenses	28%
Printing services	17%

From Santelli, B., Turnbull, A., Marquis, J., & Lerner, E. (2000). Statewide Parent to Parent programs: Partners in early intervention. *Infants and Young Children, 13*(1), 83; reprinted by permission.

Appendix B
Suggested Readings

BOOKS FOR PARENTS AND PROVIDERS

Anderson, C., Richardson, V., & Binkard, B. (1996). *Choices: Opportunities for life.* Minneapolis: PACER Center.

Buck, P.S. (1992). *The child who never grew* (2nd ed.). Bethesda, MD: Woodbine House.

Cutler, B.C. (1993). *You, your child, and special education: A guide to making the system work.* Baltimore: Paul H. Brookes Publishing Co.

Duffy, S., Phillips, S., Davis, S., Maloney, T., Stromnes, J., Miller, B., Colling, K., & Larson, K. (1994). *We're all in this together, so let's talk: Effective communication between parents of children with disabilities and the professionals who work with them.* Missoula: Montana University Affiliated Rural Institute on Disabilities, Dynamic Communication Process Project.

Exceptional Parent Annual Resource Guide; Exceptional Parent magazine publishes an annual resource guide for families who have a child or adult with a disability and for professionals working with families and disability issues. The Parent to Parent list contains program names, addresses, telephone and fax numbers, and e-mail addresses of local and statewide programs in every state. Contact Exceptional Parent, 555 Kindercamack Road, Oradell, NJ 07649-1517; telephone: (201) 634-6550

Fialka, J., & Mikus, K. (1999). *Do you hear what I hear? Parents and professionals working together for children with special needs.* Ann Arbor, MI: Proctor Publications, LLC.

Greenstein, D. (1995). *Backyards and butterflies: Ways to include children with disabilities in outdoor activities.* Cambridge, MA: Brookline.

Haerle, T. (1992). *Children with Tourette syndrome: A parent's guide.* Bethesda, MD: Woodbine House.

Hartmann, T. (1995). *ADD success stories: A guide to fulfillment for families with attention deficit disorder.* Grass Valley, CA: Underwood Books.

Holbrook, M.C. (1996). *Children and visual impairments: A parent's guide.* Bethesda, MD: Woodbine House.

Kingsley, J., & Levitz, M. (1994). *Count us in: Growing up with Down syndrome.* San Diego: Harcourt, Brace & Company.

MacKenzie, L. (1996). *The complete directory for people with disabilities: Products, resources, books, and services.* Lakeville, CT: Grey House Publishing.

Malloy, J.M. (1995). *Benefits planning for children and youth with disabilities.* Durham: University of New Hampshire, Institute on Disability.

Mendelsohn, S.B. (1996). *Tax options and strategies for people with disabilities.* New York: Demos Publishing.

Moon, M.S. (1994). *Making school and community recreation fun for everyone: Places and ways to integrate.* Baltimore: Paul H. Brookes Publishing Co.

O'Brien, J., & Forest, M. (1989). *Action for inclusion: How to improve schools by welcoming children with special needs into regular classrooms.* Toronto: Inclusion Press.

Ogden, P.W. (1996). *The silent garden: Raising your deaf child.* Washington, DC: Gallaudet University Press.

Papazian, S. (1997). *Growing up with Joey: A mother's story of her son's disability and her family's triumph.* Santa Barbara, CA: Fithian Press.

Perske, R. (1988). *Circles of friends: People with disabilities and their friends enrich the lives of one another.* Nashville, TN: Abingdon Press.

Powers, M.D. (1989). *Children with autism: A parents' guide.* Bethesda, MD: Woodbine House.

Racino, J.A., Walker, P., O'Connor, S., & Taylor, S.J. (1993). *Housing, support, and community: Choices and strategies for adults with disabilities* (Vol. 2). Baltimore: Paul H. Brookes Publishing Co.

Rife, J.M. (1994). *Injured mind, shattered dreams: Brian's journey from severe head injury to a new dream.* Cambridge, MA: Brookline.

Schaffner, B.C., & Buswell, B.E. (1992). *Connecting students: A guide to thoughtful friendship facilitation for educators and families.* Colorado Springs: PEAK Parent Center.

Segal, M. (1988). *In time and with love: Caring for the special needs baby.* New York: New Market Press.

Siegel, B. (1996). *The world of the autistic child.* New York: Oxford University Press.

Smith, C., & Strick, L. (1997). *Learning disabilities: A to Z. A parent's complete guide to learning disabilities from preschool to adulthood.* New York: The Free Press/ Simon & Schuster.

Smith, R. (1993). *Children with mental retardation: A parent's guide.* Bethesda, MD: Woodbine House.

Smith, S.L. (1991). *Succeeding against the odds: How the learning disabled can realize their promise.* New York: Putnam.

Smith, S.L. (1995). *No easy answers.* New York: Bantam.

Staub, D. (1998). *Delicate threads: Friendships between children with and without special needs in inclusive settings.* Bethesda, MD: Woodbine House.

Stehli, A. (1996). *The sound of a miracle.* Westport, CT: The Georgiana Organization.

Stray-Gundersen, K. (1995). *Babies with Down syndrome: A new parents' guide.* Bethesda, MD: Woodbine House.

Sweeney, W. (1998). *The special needs reading list: An annotated guide to the best publications for parents and professionals.* Bethesda, MD: Woodbine House.

Van Dyke, D.C., Mattheis, P., Eberly, S., & Williams, J. (1995). *Medical & surgical care for children with Down syndrome: A guide for parents.* Bethesda, MD: Woodbine House.

Weber, J.D. (1994). *Transitioning "special" children into elementary school.* Boulder, CO: Books Beyond Borders, Inc.

Wehman, P., & Kregel, J. (1998). *More than a job: Securing satisfying careers for people with disabilities.* Baltimore: Paul H. Brookes Publishing Co.

Wehmeyer, M.L., & Palmer, S.B. (2000). Promoting the acquisition and development of self-determination in young children with disabilities. *Early Education and Development, 11,* 465–481.

White, B., & Madara, E. (Eds.). (1998). *The self-help sourcebook: Your guide to community on-line support groups* (6th ed.). Denville, NJ: American Self-Help Clearinghouse.

BOOKS FOR CHILDREN

Armenta, C.A. (1992). *Russell is extra special: A book about autism for children.* New York: Magination Press.

Buehrens, A. (1993). *Hi, I'm Adam: A child's story of Tourette syndrome.* Duarte, CA: Hope Press.

Gehret, J. (1991). *Eagle eyes: A child's guide to paying attention.* Fairport, NY: Verbal Images.

Gordon, M. (1992). *My brother's a world-class pain: Sibling's guide to ADHD/hyperactivity.* Dewitt, NY: GSI.

Janover, C. (1997). *Zipper, the kid with ADHD.* Bethesda, MD: Woodbine House.

Katz, I., & Ritvo, E. (1993). *Joey and Sam.* Northridge, CA: Real Life Story Books.

Kraus, R. (1971). *Leo the late bloomer.* New York: HarperCollins.

Lakin, P. (1994). *Dad and me in the morning.* Morton Grove, IL: Albert Whitman & Co.

O'Shaughnessy, E. (1992). *Somebody called me a retard today and my heart felt sad.* New York: Walker and Company.

Quinn, P.O., & Stern, J.M. (1991). *Putting on the brakes: Young people's guide to understanding attention deficit hyperactivity disorder.* New York: Magination Press.

Quinn, P.O., & Stern, J.M. (1993). *The "putting on the brakes" activity book for young people with ADHD.* New York: Magination Press.

Rheingrover, J.S. (1996). *Veronica's first year.* Morton Grove, IL: Albert Whitman & Co.

Schwier, K.M. (1988). *Edward's different day.* San Luis Obispo, CA: Impact Publishers.

Schwier, K.M. (1997). *Idea man.* Eastman, Quebec: Diverse City Press.

Thompson, M. (1992). *My brother, Matthew.* Bethesda, MD: Woodbine House.

Thompson, M. (1996). *Andy and his yellow frisbee.* Bethesda, MD: Woodbine House.

Wanous, S. (1995). *Sara's secret.* Minneapolis: Carolrhoda Books.

Yates, S. (1994). *Nobody knows!* Winnipeg, Manitoba: Gemma B. Publishing.

Young, R. (n.d.) *Mikey goes to our school.* Carbondale, CO: Hometown Press.

Appendix C
Contact Information/Resources

ORGANIZATIONS

Beach Center on Families and Disability
3111 Haworth Hall
University of Kansas
Lawrence, KS 66045
Telephone: (785) 864-7600
Fax: (785) 864-7605
beach@dole.lsi.ukans.edu
http://www.beachcenter.org

Family Voices
Post Office Box 769
Algodones, NM 87001
Telephone: (505) 867-2368
Fax: (505) 867-6517
http://www.familyvoices.org

Grassroots Consortium on Disabilities
Post Office Box 61628
Houston, TX 77208
Telephone: (713) 734-5355
Fax: (713) 643-6291
http://www.GCOD.org

Mothers United for Moral Support, National Parent to Parent Network
150 Custer Court
Green Bay, WI 54301-1243
Telephone: (920) 336-5333

National Center on Parent-Directed Family Resource Centers
PHP, Inc.
3041 Olcott Street
Santa Clara, CA 95054-3222
Telephone: (408) 727-5775
Fax: (408) 727-0182
http://www.php.com

National Coalition for Family Leadership
Indiana Parent Information Network (IPIN)
4755 Kingsway Drive
Suite 105
Indianapolis, IN 46205-1545
Telephone: (800) 964-4746

National Fathers Network
Kindering Center
16120 NE 8th Street
Bellevue, WA 98008-3937
Telephone: (425) 747-4004
http://www.fathersnetwork.org

National Information Center for Children and Youth with Disabilities
Post Office Box 1492
Washington, DC 20013
Telephone: (800) 695-0285
http://www.nichcy.org

National Organization for Rare Disorders
100 Route 37
Post Office Box 8923
Fairfield, CT 06812-8923
Telephone: (800) 999-6673,
(203) 746-6518
TTY: (203) 746-6927
Fax: (203) 746-6481
http://www.rarediseases.org

National Parent Network on Disabilities
1200 G Street, NW
Suite 800
Washington, DC 20005
Telephone: (202) 434-8686

The Sibling Support Project
Children's Hospital and Medical Center
Post Office Box 5371, CL-09
Seattle, WA 98105
Telephone: (206) 527-5712
Fax: (206) 527-5705
dmeyer@chmc.org

Technical Assistance Alliance for Parent Centers
PACER Center
8161 Normandale Boulevard
Minneapolis, MN 55437-1044
Telephone: (952) 838-9000
TTY: (952) 838-0190
Fax: (952) 838-0199
alliance@taalliance.org
http://www.taalliance.org

Grassroots Consortium on Disabilities Member Programs

COFFO, Inc.
305 South Flager Avenue
Homestead, FL 33030
Telephone: (305) 237-5093
Fax: (305) 237-5013

discapacitados abriendose caminos (d.a.c.)
608 Smith Avenue
St. Paul, MN 55107
Telephone: (651) 293-1748
Fax: (651) 293-1744
marlui@ix.netcom.com

Island Parents Educational Support and Training
202 Lake Street
Post Office Box 4081
Vineyard Haven, MA 02586
Telephone: (508) 693-8612
Fax: (508) 693-7111

Lakota Tiwahe Tokata Ho
Post Office Box 937
Pine Ridge, SD 57770
Telephone: (605) 867-1392
Fax: (605) 867-2761

Loving Your Disabled Child
4528 Crenshaw Boulevard
Los Angeles, CA 90043
Telephone: (323) 299-2925
Fax: (323) 299-4373
lydc@pacbell.net

Mentor Parent Program
Post Office Box 47
Pittsfield, PA 16340
Telephone: (814) 563-3470
Fax: (814) 563-3445

Parent to Parent Power
1118 South 142nd Street
Tacoma, WA 98444
Telephone: (253) 531-2022
Fax: (253) 538-1126

Parents of Watts
10828 Lou Dillon Avenue
Los Angeles, CA 90059
Telephone: (323) 566-7556
Fax: (323) 569-3982

Pyramid Parent Training
4120 Eve Street
New Orleans, LA 70125
Telephone: (504) 827-0610
Fax: (504) 827-2999

Special Kids Inc. (SKI)
Post Office Box 266958
Houston, TX 77207-6958
Telephone: (713) 643-9576
Fax: (713) 643-6291
speckids@pdq.net

United We Stand
312 South 3rd Street
Brooklyn, NY 11211
Telephone: (718) 302-4313
Fax: (718) 302-4315
uswofny@aol.com

Urban Pride
1472 Tremont
Roxbury, MA 02120
Telephone: (617) 445-3191
Fax: (617) 445-6309

Vietnamese Parents of Disabled Children
831 Park Vine Street
Orange, CA 92686
Telephone: (310) 370-6704
Fax: (310) 542-0522

VI-FIND
Post Office Box 11670
St. Thomas, VI 00801
Telephone: (340) 774-1662
Fax: (340) 775-3962

STATEWIDE PARENT TO PARENT PROGRAMS

Arizona
RAISING Special Kids
4750 Black Canyon Highway
Suite 101
Phoenix, AZ 85017-3621
Telephone: (602) 242-4366
Fax: (602) 242-4306

Arkansas
Parent to Parent
2000 Main
Little Rock, AR 72206
Telephone: (501) 375-7770
Fax: (501) 372-4558

California
Parents Helping Parents
3041 Olcott Street
Santa Clara, CA 95054-3222
Telephone: (408) 727-5775
Fax: (408) 727-0182
http://www.php.com

Colorado
Parent to Parent of Colorado
c/o UCPCO
2200 South Jasmine Street
Denver, CO 80222
Telephone: (877) 472-7201
Fax: (719) 336-2389
http://www.p2p-co.org

Connecticut
Parent to Parent Network of Connecticut
The Family Center
282 Washington
Hartford, CT 06106
Telephone: (860) 545-9021
Fax: (860) 545-9201

Florida
Family Network on Disabilities of Florida
2735 Whitney Road
Clearwater, FL 34520
Telephone: (727) 523-1130
Fax: (727) 523-8687
http://www.fndfl.org

Georgia
Parent to Parent of Georgia
3805 Presidential Parkway
Suite 207
Atlanta, GA 30340
Telephone: (770) 451-5484
Fax: (770) 458-4091
http://www.parenttoparentofga.org

Idaho
Idaho State Parent to Parent
129 West 3rd Street
Moscow, ID 83843
Telephone: (208) 885-3500
Fax: (208) 885-3628
http://www.parentsreachingout.org

Indiana
Indiana Parent Information Network
4755 Kingsway Drive
Suite 105
Indianapolis, IN 46205
Telephone: (317) 257-8683
Fax: (317) 251-7488

Kansas
Families Together, Inc.
501 SW Jackson
Suite 400
Topeka, KS 66603
Telephone: (785) 233-4777
Fax: (785) 233-4787
http://www.kansas.net/~family

Kentucky
Parent Information Network of Kentucky
3004 Taylorsville Road
Louisville, KY 40205
Telephone: (502) 479-7465
Fax: (502) 452-2145
http://www.kyp2p.org

Louisiana
Families Helping Families
4323 Division Street
Suite 110
Metairie, LA 70002-3179
Telephone: (504) 888-9111
Fax: (504) 888-0246

Massachusetts
Family Ties
Massachusetts Department of Public Health
SE Region
109 Rhode Island Road
Lakeville, MA 02347
Telephone: (617) 727-1440, (508) 947-1231
Fax: (617) 727-9296
http://www.massfamilyties.org

Michigan
Family Support Network of Michigan
1200 6th Street
3rd Floor
South Tower
#316
Detroit, MI 48226-2495
Telephone: (313) 256-2186, (800) 359-3722
Fax: (313) 256-2605

Nevada
Nevada Parent Network - UAP
College of Education/285
Reno, NV 89557-0082
Telephone: (775) 784-4921
Fax: (775) 784-4997
http://www.unr.edu/repc/npn

New Hampshire
Parent to Parent of New Hampshire
12 Flynn Street
Lebanon, NH 03766
Telephone: (603) 448-6393
Fax: (603) 448-6311
http://www.parenttoparentnh.org

New Jersey
New Jersey Statewide Parent to Parent
c/o SPAN
35 Halsey Street
4th Floor
Newark, NJ 07102
Telephone: (973) 642-8100
Fax: (973) 642-8080
http://www.taalliance.org/ptis/nj

New Mexico
Parents Reaching Out
1000A Main Street
Los Lunas, NM 87031
Telephone: (505) 865-3700
Fax: (505) 865-3737
http://www.parentsreachingout.org

New York
Parent to Parent of New York State
Balltown and Consaul Roads
Schenectady, NY 12304
Telephone: (800) 305-8817
Fax: (518) 382-1959
http://www.parenttoparentnys.org

North Carolina
Family Support Network of North Carolina
CB #7340
Chase Hall
University of North Carolina
Chapel Hill, NC 27699-7340
Telephone: (919) 966-2841
Fax: (919) 966-2916
http://www.med.unc.edu/commedu/familysu

North Dakota
Family to Family Project
UND School of Medicine and Health Science
Post Office Box 9037
Grand Forks, ND 58202
Telephone: (701) 777-2359
Fax: (701) 777-2353
http://www.medicine.nodalc.edu

Ohio
The Family Information Network
Ohio Department of Health
246 North High Street
5th Floor
Columbus, OH 43266-0118
Telephone: (614) 644-8389
Fax: (614) 728-9163

Pennsylvania
Parent to Parent of Pennsylvania
Gateway Corporate Center
6340 Flank Drive
#1200
Harrisburg, PA 17112
Telephone: (717) 540-4722
Fax: (717) 657-5983
http://www.parenttoparent.org

South Carolina
The Family Connection of South Carolina
2712 Middleburg Drive
Suite 103-B
Columbia, SC 29204
Telephone: (803) 252-0914
Fax: (803) 799-8017
http://www.familyconnectionsc.org

Tennessee
Parents Encouraging Parents
5th Floor
C. Hull Building
426 Fifth Avenue North
Nashville, TN 37247-4850
Telephone: (615) 741-0353
Fax: (615) 741-1063

Utah
HOPE-A Parent Network
2290 East 4500 South
Suite 110
Salt Lake City, UT 84117
Telephone: (801) 272-1051
Fax: (801) 272-8907

Vermont
Parent to Parent of Vermont
1 Main Street
69 Champlain Mill
Winooski, VT 05404
Telephone: (802) 655-5290
Fax: (802) 655-3507
http://www.partoparvt.org

Virginia
Parent to Parent of Virginia
c/o Arc of Virginia
6 North 6th Street
Suite 403
Richmond, VA 23219
Telephone: (804) 222-1945
Fax: (804) 222-3402

Washington
Parent to Parent Support Program
10550 Lake City Way, NE
Suite A
Seattle, WA 98125
Telephone: (206) 364-3814
Fax: (206) 364-8140
http://www.arcwa.com/parent2.htm

West Virginia
Common Bonds of West Virginia
1101 Hospital Drive
Hurricane, WV 25526
Telephone: (304) 757-8465
Fax: (304) 757-1003

Index

Page references followed by *f* or *t* indicate figures or tables, respectively.